AF334482

IX

Channelling in Intermediary Metabolism

IX

Other books in this series:

PORTLAND PRESS RESEARCH MONOGRAPH IX

Channelling in Intermediary Metabolism

Edited by

L. Agius

H. S. A. Sherratt

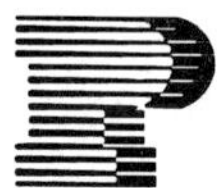

Portland Press
London and Miami

Published by Portland Press, 59 Portland Place, London W1N 3AJ, U.K.
In North America orders should be sent to Ashgate Publishing Co.,
Old Post Road, Brookfield, VT 05036-9704, U.S.A.

ISBN 1 85578 075 5   **ISSN 0964-5845**

British Library Cataloguing in Publication Data
A catalogue record for this book is available from the British Library

Although, at the time of going to press, the information contained in this publication is believed to be correct, neither the authors nor the editors nor the publisher assume any responsibility for any errors or omissions herein contained. Opinions expressed in this book are those of the authors and are not necessarily held by the editors or the publishers.

Typeset by Unicus Graphics Ltd, Horsham, Sussex and
Printed in Great Britain by Whitstable Litho Printers Ltd

Contents

Preface

The concept of metabolic channelling, whereby a pathway intermediate is transferred from the enzyme that catalyses its formation to the next enzyme in the pathway sequence, without the intermediate being released into free solution or without equilibrating with the pool of metabolites in free solution, has originated from many experimental observations. However, the evidence for direct transfer, or channelling of a metabolite between sequential enzymes, is not always unequivocal. Some metabolic pathways have been more extensively investigated in terms of channelling than others and, whereas there is clear evidence for channelling in the urea cycle, this is not the case for fatty acid oxidation. The idea for this book stemmed from a Biochemical Society colloquium on the Regulation of Fatty Acid Oxidation (December 1993, published in *Biochemical Society Transactions*, vol. 21: 4); this colloquium included contributions from Paul Srere and Athel Cornish-Bowden, who discussed channelling in mitochondrial fatty acid oxidation from different points of view.

The physiological implications of channelling are a topic of lively debate, as emerged from the colloquium on fatty acid oxidation and from a large number of theoretical and experimental papers on channelling over recent years. Some take the view that channelling has many metabolic advantages, whereas others argue that even if channelling occurs in metabolic pathways, it may not necessarily confer any advantages. In this book we have invited contributions from scientists with extensive experience in the study of metabolic channelling, as well as from theoretical scientists who discuss the kinetics and physiological implications of channelling.

The over-riding theme that emerges from the chapters which discuss experimental evidence in support of channelling is that metabolic fluxes in the intact cell cannot be explained by known kinetic and allosteric properties of the individual enzymes if these are assumed to function as isolated entities independently of their environment. The reader who is unfamiliar with the subject of channelling is advised first to read Chapters 9–12. Surprisingly, there is almost complete lack of mention of channelling in most textbooks of biochemistry or intermediary metabolism.

Recent advances in molecular biology techniques have enabled the elucidation of the structure of proteins and genes, and this tends to overshadow other important areas of biochemistry. However, to understand how flux through metabolic pathways is regulated in the intact cell, it is necessary to know the location of proteins within the cell; whether they are free in solution, or bound to cellular components, or in a microcompartment; what the associations are between sequential or non-sequential enzymes in metabolic pathways; whether metabolic intermediates equilibrate with the bulk phase or are transferred from the active site of one enzyme to that of the next; and what the implications are of enzyme–enzyme associations and intermediate transfer between enzymes.

We hope that the hypotheses and arguments presented in this book will stimulate studies on intermediary metabolism from the view of cellular organization and channelling. Further work in this field (and, accordingly, funding) is crucial for understanding the regulation of intermediary metabolism.

Loranne Agius
Stanley Sherratt
Newcastle, February 1996

Abbreviations

ACO	aconitase
ACP	acyl carrier protein
AICAR	5-aminoimidazole-4-carboxamide ribotide
AIR	5-aminoimidazole ribotide
AspAT	mitochondrial aspartate aminotransferase
AspAT-PLP	pyridoxal phosphate form of AspAT
AspAT-PMP	pyridoxamine phosphate form of AspAT
BCDHC	branched-chain 2-oxoacid dehydrogenase complex
CA-asp	N-carbamoyl-L-aspartate
CAIR	4-carboxy-5-aminoimidazole ribotide
CAP	carbamoyl phosphate
cMDH	cytosolic malate dehydrogenase
CPS	carbamoyl phosphate synthase
CS	citrate synthase
DHO	L-dihydro orotate
DHQ	dehydroquinate
DHS	dehydroshikimate
E3BP	E3-binding protein
ETF	electron transfer flavoprotein
FAICAR	5-formamidoimidazole-4-carboxamide ribotide
FAS	fatty acid synthase
FGAM	N-formylglycineamidine ribotide
FGAR	N-formylglycineamide ribotide
GAR	glycineamide ribotide
GDH	glutamate dehydrogenase
Glc 1-P	glucose 1-phosphate
Glc 6-P	glucose 6-phosphate
ICDH	isocitrate dehydrogenase
IMM	mitochondrial inner membrane
MAP	microtubule associated protein
(m)MDH	(mitochondrial) malate dehydrogenase
OAA	oxaloacetate
OCT	orientation conserved transfer
OGDHC	2-oxoglutarate (α-ketoglutarate) dehydrogenase complex
OMP	orotidine 5'-monophosphate
OTC	ornithine transcarbamylase
P-Rib-PP	5-phosphoribosyl-1-pyrophosphate
PALO	δ-N-phosphonacetyl L-ornithine
PC	pyruvate carboxylase
PCA	protocatechuic acid
PDG	phosphate-dependent glutaminase

PDHC	pyruvate dehydrogenase complex
PEG	poly(ethylene glycol)
PEPCK	phosphoenolpyruvate carboxykinase
PRA	5-phosphoribosylamine
SAICAR	*N*-succino-5-aminoimidazole-4-carboxamide ribotide
sAMP	*N*-succino-AMP
SPT	Scaled Particle Theory
TCA	tricarboxylic acid
THF	tetrahydrofolate
TPP	thiamin pyrophosphate

Introduction

Loranne Agius* and H. Stanley A. Sherratt†

Departments of *Medicine and †Neurology,
The Medical School, University of Newcastle, Framlington Place,
Newcastle upon Tyne NE2 4HH, U.K.

"When the guidance of theory is clear interest centres round the broad principles; when the theory is rudimentary, interest centres round technical details which are anxiously scrutinized as they appear to favour now one view now another."

Sir Arthur Eddington, Stars and Atoms (1927)

Background

Intermediary metabolism is now assumed to be well understood by many contemporary biochemists and its importance is often overlooked because of the recent progress in molecular biology. However, rates of metabolic flux in intact cells often cannot be described adequately from the kinetic and allosteric properties of enzymes as determined after purification. Many of these enzymes have been cloned and sequenced and are regarded as being very well characterized. The traditional view of intermediary metabolism is of free diffusion of intermediates between the enzymes involved. This is based on the assumption that most metabolic intermediates are present as a single homogeneous pool and that enzymes that are recovered in the high-speed supernatant fraction of tissue homogenates occur in the cell in free solution either in the cytoplasm or in subcellular organelles. However, studies using gentle techniques for cell disruption have shown that many enzymes that were assumed to be in solution in the intact cell, for example glucokinase (hexokinase IV) and enzymes of glycolysis and the citrate and urea cycles, have a much more complex organization and are partially associated with other enzymes, structural proteins and other cell components.

The idea of channelling of intermediates has often been invoked by several authors (see [1], and Chapter 11 of the current volume) to explain some features of metabolism, although it has been overlooked by most others. This idea is that in a biochemical pathway the product of an enzyme-catalysed reaction is transferred as substrate to the enzyme that catalyses the next reaction without complete equilibration with the pool of intermediates in the surrounding medium. The modern concept of channelling has arisen largely from experimental observations and was not apparently predicted theoretically. For example, the starting point for the elegant studies by L. Raijman and colleagues on channelling in the urea cycle was the observation that ornithine affects flux catalysed by carbamoyl phosphate synthase in intact hepatocytes and liver mitochondria, but not the activity of the isolated enzyme in solution (see below and Chapter 10). Similarly, an observation that stimulated the study of the organization of the enzymes of the citrate cycle was that the flux through the cycle is greater than predicted from the concentration of oxaloacetate and the kinetics of purified citrate synthase, as discussed by P.A. Srere and colleagues (Chapter 11). These and numerous other observations led to detailed analyses of enzyme organization and function *in situ*.

Although there is strong evidence for channelling in several metabolic pathways and that many enzymes conventionally thought to be in free solution are highly organized within cells, there is virtually no mention of this in most contemporary textbooks. One may suggest several reasons for this neglect: the importance of channelling may not be fully appreciated, or authors may find the subject too complex to deal with comprehensively. Alternatively they might feel that there is as yet insufficient information to assess its physiological significance. Most workers now accept the reality of channelling, although there is still some controversy about the evidence for its occurrence (see, for example, the contributions to a discussion on channelling in 1991 in *J. Theor. Biol.* [2]). Papers on channelling are generally of two types. On the one hand there are experimental papers concerned with whether or not it occurs in a given pathway. On the other hand there are theoretical papers concerned with the effects of channelling on the kinetics of metabolic pathways and on metabolite concentrations, and the physiological consequences of any proposed effects.

In this book we have invited reviews discussing the occurrence, mechanisms and possible roles of channelling. Theoretical papers deal with general principles of enzyme catalysis and kinetics that are relevant to the physical basis of channelling (Chapters 2–6). Some of the molecular processes which may be involved in channelling are described in detail by I.C. West and M.M. Garner in Chapters 2 and 3 respectively. The kinetic consequences of different channelling mechanisms are discussed by A. Cornish-Bowden, J.S. Easterby and B.N. Kholodenko et al. in Chapters 4–6. The experimental evidence for channelling in multifunctional enzymes is discussed by T.E. Roche and D.J. Cox, and by S. Smith (Chapters 7 and 8) and in several metabolic pathways by the other contributors (Chapters 10–16). Naturally some authors sometimes have different opinions, but we hope that these reviews may help readers to form their own conclusions, particularly since the literature on channelling is widely scattered. It has not been possible to deal with all aspects of metabolism where channelling may occur so as to keep this book within reasonable length, and we are aware that our choice of topics may sometimes appear arbitrary. The possible role of channelling in protein synthesis is not considered, and it is only briefly mentioned with regard to nucleic acid replication (Chapter 16).

Definition and mechanisms of channelling

> "Channelling will be used to mean that a reactant is transferred between soluble enzymes with little or no diffusion into the bulk aqueous medium. Soluble enzymes are defined as those which are released into solution when cells or subcellular structures are disrupted in the absence of detergents"
>
> N.S. Cohen et al., Chapter 10

> "Metabolic channelling of an intermediate can be defined as the passage of a common intermediate between two enzymes. The intermediate is localized and out of equilibrium with the bulk solution"
>
> P.A. Srere et al., Chapter 11

These two representative definitions of channelling are given in this book. It is usually thought that in most cases channelling is not complete and that there is *both* direct transfer of the intermediate between enzymes and diffusion of the intermediate between free enzymes. It is thought that the lifetime of an enzyme–substrate(s) complex is much longer (perhaps 100 times as long) than the average time taken for substrates to diffuse to an enzyme (Chapter 2). J.S. Easterby suggests that there may be a local pool of intermediates associated with an enzyme complex, which thus encounters a higher concentration of the intermediates than occurs in the bulk phase (Chapter 5); his analysis does not consider this to be a subcellular compartment. Indeed, the distinction between incomplete channelling and micro-compartmentation may not always be clearly defined in the literature. The above definitions of channelling do not necessarily specify *direct* transfer of a product from the active site of an enzyme (as a substrate) to the active site of the next enzyme in the pathway. The possibility may also be considered that the product is *indirectly* transferred within the complex. A transfer of intermediates directly between active sites without any release into the bulk phase is a limiting case. Examples include sequences of reactions in which the substrates remain covalently bound to a multienzyme complex, as in the mammalian fatty acid synthases and the 2-oxoacid dehydrogenases (T.F. Roche and D.J. Cox, Chapter 7; S. Smith, Chapter 8). There has been relatively little detailed consideration of the molecular mechanisms involved in channelling, with the exception of the mammalian multifunctional fatty acid synthases and 2-oxoacid dehydrogenases. In the reactions catalysed by these enzymes the intermediates are covalently bound throughout the reaction (although these reactions are not described as being channelled in textbooks).

Channelling may be dynamic or static, involving various types of enzyme associations, as discussed in several chapters. For the simplest cases, consider a pathway involving two enzymes:

$$A \xrightarrow{E_1} B \xrightarrow{E_2} C$$

Dynamic channelling of this pathway occurs if the first enzyme (E_1) first binds its substrate (A) and the E_1–A complex forms E_1–B. E_1–B then directly transfers B to the next enzyme (E_2) in the metabolic pathway and E_2–B forms E_2–C which dissociates releasing C.

$$A + E_1 \longrightarrow E_1\text{–}A \longrightarrow E_1\text{–}B$$

$$E_1\text{–}B + E_2 \longrightarrow E_1 + E_2\text{–}B$$

$$E_2\text{–}B \longrightarrow E_2\text{–}C \longrightarrow E_2 + C$$

E_1 is then able to bind another molecule of A for another catalytic cycle. Another mechanism for dynamic channelling is that E_1–B combines with E_2 without release of B to form E_1–B–E_2. This is followed by its conversion to E_1–C–E_2 which then dissociates releasing C.

$$E_1\text{–}B + E_2 \longrightarrow E_1\text{–}B\text{–}E_2 \longrightarrow E_1\text{–}C\text{–}E_2 \longrightarrow E_1 + E_2 + C$$

Alternatively, the E_1–A complex may combine with E_2 and the E_1–A–E_2 complex is then converted into E_1–B–E_2.

Static channelling occurs when two enzymes first form a complex ($E_1 \cdot E_2$) that accepts A, which is then converted into B and transformed directly to C while still bound to the $E_1 \cdot E_2$ complex. C is then released without dissociation of the $E_1 \cdot E_2$ complex, the lifetime of the $E_1 \cdot E_2$ complex being longer than the time required for the catalytic cycle.

$$E_1 + E_2 \rightleftharpoons E_1 \cdot E_2$$

$$E_1 \cdot E_2 + A \longrightarrow A\text{–}E_1 \cdot E_2 \longrightarrow E_1 \cdot E_2\text{–}B \longrightarrow E_1 \cdot E_2\text{–}C \longrightarrow E_1 \cdot E_2 + C$$

The enzymes may also function independently without channelling. A is converted by uncomplexed E_1 into B. B then diffuses to E_2 where it is converted into C. The looseness of channelling may be defined as the fraction of the total flux that goes through free B without any direct contact between the enzymes. The fraction of the flux which is channelled would be predicted to increase with increases in the concentrations of E_1 and E_2. It may be remarked, however, that theoretical discussions of channelling are often about enzymes assumed to have single substrates and products, although most enzymes catalyse reactions with two or more substrates and products. Indeed, for a multi-substrate reaction only one of the substrates may be channelled.

Fersht [3] argues convincingly that, contrary to what is often thought, *high* K_m values may facilitate enzyme catalysis (k_{cat}) more than lower values. Some of the binding energy of the formation of the enzyme–substrate complex is used to *lower* the activation energy of k_{cat} and many enzymes appear to have evolved to bind substrates weakly. It is easily shown that (if k_{cat}/K_m is kept constant) the rates of catalysis are maximized when the K_m is greater than the substrate concentration. High values of k_{cat}, therefore, more than compensate for high values of K_m (when a high V_{max} is required). If a high K_m means a high value of k_{off} for a substrate it might be thought that rapid dissociation of the E_1–S complexes would limit any dynamic channelling. However, when dynamic channelling occurs it must be assumed that the average life of the E_1–S complex is long enough for combination with E_2, even if E_1 has a high K_m and a high k_{cat} for its substrate.

Most attention has perhaps been devoted to dynamic channelling (for example, see Chapter 6). If a productive complex is formed between the E_1-substrate (or the E_1-intermediate) with E_2, the intermediate may be converted into product at the interface between the enzymes. If the product does not have direct access to the bulk phase, the enzymes must dissociate before the product is released and another catalytic cycle can occur. With a static channel the active sites of E_1 and E_2 must be juxtaposed so that the product can be released without dissociation of the complex. Static channelling may also involve a complex of three or more enzymes catalysing a longer sequence of reactions (see Chapter 12). The tryptophan synthase bi-enzyme complex has a tunnel in its centre where tryptophan is made from indole 3-glycerol phosphate and serine by two successive reactions without the release of free indole (which is an intermediate); this appears to be the only known example of this mechanism (Chapter 2).

Theoretically, some mechanisms might be more complex and combine both dynamic and static channelling (Chapter 6). In complexes between two oligomeric enzymes not all the active sites of the enzymes involved may be juxtaposed so as to enable channelling between them. The other sites might also catalyse unchannelled reactions. It cannot be assumed, however, that there is *necessarily* transfer of an intermediate between adjacent active sites in heterologous enzyme complexes. The product of the first reaction may have to be released into the bulk phase before it can diffuse to and bind to the second site on the same or a different molecule of the complex. There is evidence that static channelling is not complete in some enzyme complexes, for example the trifunctional mitochondrial long-chain acyl CoA dehydrogenase·enoyl-CoA hydratase:acyl-CoA thiolase complex (Chapter 15) and the pentafunctional AROM enzyme, since all their component activities can be assayed individually (at least *in vitro*). The AROM complex in fungi contains five enzyme activities in a single protein chain catalysing five reactions of the pre-chorismate pathway, and there is little evidence for channelling between the active sites, as discussed by H.K. Lamb et al. (Chapter 9). Further, there are some examples of two enzymes that catalyse unrelated reactions in *different* metabolic pathways forming complexes in which one enzyme may influence allosterically the activity of the other, and thus co-ordinate the activities of these pathways [4].

Experimental studies of channelling

Two techniques have been used to determine whether metabolic intermediates are channelled (Chapter 13): (1) measurement of the transient times for achieving a new steady-state reaction rate when the system is perturbed; and (2) the isotope dilution technique as discussed below. The transient time is determined and compared with that calculated from the kinetic constants of the enzymes in the sequence, assuming that the first enzyme has zero-order kinetics and that the following enzymes have *pseudo*-first-order kinetics (at low substrate concentrations). The results of such experiments may be extrapolated to cells, since most substrate concentrations *in vivo* are less than the K_ms of the enzymes involved. The total transient time of an enzyme-catalysed reaction, τ, is the sum of the diffusional transient time, τ_d, and the reaction transient time, $\tau_r = K_m/V_{max}$, while that of a reaction sequence catalysed by non-interacting enzymes is the sum of the individual τ values. A shorter transition time compared with that calculated from the kinetic parameters of the purified individual enzymes may suggest channelling. Alternatively, it might suggest allosteric effects on the kinetics of these enzymes due to complex-formation without necessarily any direct transfer of intermediates between the enzymes. However, channelling is indicated if the transient time is less than that calculated using the kinetic parameters of the individual enzyme reactions determined in the presence of the same concentrations of the other enzymes (see also Chapter 4). Enzyme–enzyme interactions leading to reversible complex-formation have been detected *in vitro* by changes in light scattering or by changes in anisotropy of fluorescently labelled enzymes when solutions of purified enzymes are mixed. Complex-formation occurs at much lower concentrations of enzymes than occur *in situ*. Enzymes in such complexes often have different kinetic properties from the uncomplexed enzymes (Chapter 12).

One of the most commonly used techniques to determine whether channelling occurs is to measure the flux through coupled enzyme reactions *in vitro* or through pathways in intact or permeabilized cells and organelles with a radiolabelled substrate. The extent to which the radioactivity of the end-product is diluted by the addition of various concentrations of unlabelled intermediates is determined (see also Chapters 11 and 16). This establishes by how much labelled intermediates derived from the substrate are diluted by unlabelled intermediates in the bulk phase and the proportion of the flux that is channelled (see also Chapter 16). (Alternatively the extent of incorporation of radioactivity into the end-product using an unlabelled substrate and exogenous labelled intermediates could be determined.) Other methods to detect channelling are to link two enzymes that form specific non-covalent complexes by gene fusion or to link both to an inert polymer, and then to determine any changes in their kinetic parameters (see Chapters 4, and 11–13). There is now much evidence indicating that substrate channelling occurs in several metabolic pathways, and that there is more than one mechanism of channelling (see Chapters 6, 10–13 and 16).

One may ask why enzymes are so large compared with the sizes of their catalytic sites, and why so many enzymes are oligomers. Large proteins are likely to have more stable three-dimensional structures, and the formation of oligomers may enable the evolution of co-operative allosteric behaviour [1,5]. It has been suggested that part of the surface of a large enzyme may serve as a 'funnel' trapping substrates in a two-dimensional walk around the catalytic site [6]. This idea might be extended to suggest that a funnel may be formed between juxtaposed catalytic sites on a complex of different enzymes which facilitates channelling. Some examples of proposed channelling involve interactions between oligomeric enzymes (Chapters 12 and 13), for example between glyceraldehyde-3-phosphate dehydrogenase and 3-phosphoglycerate kinase (see [2]). Oligomeric enzymes may facilitate the evolution of channelling if two different oligomers can associate more readily than two different monomers? L.A. Fahien and M.C. Chobanian suggest that a tri-enzyme complex may be formed if two different enzymes can associate with individual oligomers of a third enzyme (Chapter 12). Oligomer formation requires complementarity between some areas of the surfaces of the subunits. The specific associations between different enzymes for channelling also implies some complementarity between their surfaces (which may be allosterically modified by binding effectors), although such associations must not be too tight when dynamic channelling occurs. The amino acid sequences and the three-dimensional structures of several purified enzymes (at least in the crystalline state) which are thought be involved in channelling are known. Enzyme structures might be used to predict which pairs of enzymes may form complexes, and such studies might be very rewarding (as, for example, in characterizing actin–actomyosin interactions [7] and subunit interactions in the mitochondrial F_1-ATPase complex [8]).

If a reaction sequence is completely channelled there will clearly be no release of intermediates into the bulk phase. With partial channelling some of the intermediates will necessarily be present in the bulk phase and it is often thought that, for a given flux rate, their concentrations will be lower than if channelling does not occur. Of course, when fluxes change with different physiological conditions the concentrations of intermediates may change whether or not there is channelling (except, perhaps, in the rather unlikely situation where the activities of all the enzymes involved change by the same extent!). A. Cornish-Bowden argues strongly that partial channelling will have only small effects on concentrations of intermediates in the bulk phase (Chapter 4). Less of an intermediate, X, is released from E_1–X when there is significant channelling, but X is also taken up more slowly by E_2 (since the concentrations of E_1–X and E_2 are lower) and there may be an increase or decrease in the concentration of X [9]. He has also pointed out that changing the activity of an enzyme in a pathway by complex-formation with another enzyme will tend to have opposite effects on the concentrations of its substrate and product (crossover effects) which may not be due to channelling (Chapter 4). By contrast, both J.S. Easterby (Chapter 5) and B. Kholodenko et al. (Chapter 6) maintain that channelling will influence substrate concentrations and usually lower them. Kholodenko et al. base their arguments on a modification of classical Metabolic Control Analysis introduced by Kacser and Burns [10] using *elemental* flux control coefficients (C_i^J) and *elemental* concentration coefficients (C_i^X) for the forward and reverse reactions catalysed by enzyme i instead of the classical flux and concentration control coefficients, $C_{e_i}^J$ and $C_{e_i}^X$. The effects of channelling on [X] are discussed in terms of all the reactions catalysed by the various free and complexed forms of each enzyme. For non-ideal pathways these are defined for the catalytic activity of enzymes rather than for their concentrations. Both dynamic and static channelling are analysed, and it is concluded that channelling can increase or decrease, or have little effect on intermediate concentrations, but that concentrations are usually lowered.

These discussions are theoretical and depend on the models and assumptions used (Chapters 4–6). It may appear surprising to many readers that there should be such disagreement. However, the effects of channelling on the concentrations of intermediates are perhaps more complex than might at first appear (Chapters 4–6). We do not know of any attempts to investigate the effects of partial channelling between pairs of purified enzymes by *measuring the concentrations* of intermediates and comparing these with those predicted from kinetic constants assuming no channelling although, as mentioned above, transient times have been measured in similar experiments.

The biological role of channelling

The diffusion of macromolecules is slow compared with that of most metabolites, and it might seem improbable kinetically that a pathway would proceed by collisions between macromolecules. Such interactions would be facilitated by the very high protein concentrations in cells, as discussed in Chapters 2, 3 and 10. A. Cornish-Bowden asks whether channelling of metabolites, when this occurs, necessarily has biological advantages, and could these have explained its evolution (Chapter 4)? J. Ovádi and F. Orosz discuss several advantages for channelling (Chapter 13). These include conserving the solute capacity of cells when (apparently) high concentrations of metabolites only occur locally and not in the bulk phase, and overcoming problems of diffusion between enzymes by decreasing the transit time, separating intermediates from possible competing reactions and protecting chemically unstable intermediates. Channelling has also been suggested to facilitate rapid changes in metabolic rates in response to physiological need by minimizing buffering by lowering concentrations of intermediates (Chapter 5). These suggested advantages are discussed in several chapters in this book.

Dynamic channelling may allow an enzyme to partition between complexes with different enzymes. This may be important in determining the distribution of flux in branched (non-processive) metabolic pathways. Aldolase forms a complex with glyceraldehyde-3-phosphate dehydrogenase which catalyses the subsequent reaction in glycolysis. Glycerol-3-phosphate dehydrogenase can also bind to aldolase. Glyceraldehyde phosphate can therefore be an intermediate of glycolysis or form glycerol 3-phosphate required for triacylglycerol synthesis. Both dehydrogenases also transfer NADH directly to lactate dehydrogenase, enabling coupling between the formation of NADH and its oxidation by lactate dehydrogenase [11]. The evidence for channelling involving some combinations of enzymes including citrate synthase, malate dehydrogenase, aspartate aminotransferases, 2-oxoglutarate dehydrogenase, pyruvate carboxylase and carbamoyl phosphate synthase in the regulation of oxaloacetate metabolism in the citrate cycle is discussed by P.A. Srere et al. and by L. Fahien and M.C. Chobanian (Chapters 11 and 12 respectively).

The urea cycle spans both the cytoplasmic compartment and the mitochondrial matrix in hepatocytes. It was found by L. Raijman and colleagues (Chapter 10) that ornithine stimulates the synthesis of carbamoyl phosphate (from CO_2, NH_4^+ and 2ATP) by carbamoyl phosphate synthase. Ornithine only stimulates the activity of carbamoyl phosphate synthase in the matrix of intact liver mitochondria, but not that of the purified enzyme in solution. The carbamoyl phosphate formed then reacts with ornithine to form citrulline and P_i, catalysed by ornithine transcarbamylase. This observation raised the question whether the association of two enzymes which act sequentially can affect the kinetics of the first enzyme? The formation of argininosuccinate, and then arginine and its conversion into ornithine and urea, occurs in the cytoplasm. Recent immunocytochemical evidence also indicates that the cytoplasmic enzymes are closely associated with the mitochondrial outer membrane. There is an exchange carrier for ornithine/citrulline in the mitochondrial inner membrane. In the matrix, some of the enzymes involved also bind to specific proteins in the mitochondrial inner membrane. This suggests that the cytoplasmic and matrix enzymes are located at regions of contact between the inner and outer membranes.

E. Meléndez-Hevia et al. present an hypothesis which invokes channelling in gluconeogenesis for thermodynamic reasons (Chapter 14). They suggest that, in gluconeogenesis, glucose 6-phosphate formed from lactate is not directly dephosphorylated to glucose but is converted into glycogen and then back again to glucose 6-phosphate, which is finally dephosphorylated to glucose. This extended pathway requires seven molecules of ATP:

$$2\text{Lactate} + 7\text{ATP} + 7H_2O \longrightarrow \text{glucose} + 7\text{ADP} + 7P_i$$

instead of six for the classical pathway, and would therefore increase the $\Delta G^{o'}$ for gluconeogenesis by $-34\,kJ\cdot mol^{-1}$ (or the physiological $\Delta G'$ by approx. $-50\,kJ\cdot mol^{-1}$). This mechanism requires two pools of metabolites, each containing glucose 6-phosphate and glucose 1-phosphate, separated by channelling. We think that this is a novel view which should be considered. Further, a similar argument could be extended to other metabolic pathways such as the indirect pathway for glycogen synthesis. However, it must be recognized that it has not been established whether the greater exergonism of an extended pathway would have physiological advantages, or whether an extended pathway would have (or also have) advantages for non-thermodynamic reasons. J. Ovádi and F. Orosz also discuss the interactions between glycolytic/gluconeogenic enzymes and the cytoskeletal components, and the effects of these interactions on the kinetics of these enzymes and on the organization of the cytoskeleton (Chapter 13). Channelling of metabolic intermediates may result from the proximity of sequential enzymes that bind to specific epitopes of cytoskeletal filaments. There is evidence for the separate compartmentation of the glycolytic and gluconeogenic fluxes in vascular smooth muscle. It would clearly be of interest to establish whether any compartmentation occurs in other tissues, particularly in liver where it might be relevant for the indirect pathway of gluconeogenesis via glycogen suggested by Meléndez-Hevia et al. (Chapter 14).

The *de novo* synthesis of fatty acids from acetyl-CoA is catalysed in higher animals by seven enzymes that are different domains of a single peptide chain, while the growing fatty-acyl chain remains covalently attached to the complex. By contrast, the dodecameric fatty acid synthase complex ($\alpha_6\beta_6$) in lower organisms consists of six trifunctional α-chains containing three of the enzymes of fatty acid synthesis, and six tetrafunctional β-chains containing the other four activities. This indicates that a completely *covalently channelled* mechanism is not necessary for fatty acid synthesis (Chapter 8, Fig. 4). Mitochondrial β-oxidation of long-chain fatty acids involves several recurring cycles of four steps, including the reactions catalysed by the trifunctional long-chain acyl-CoA dehydrogenase:enoyl-CoA hydratase:acyl-CoA thiolase enzyme. It is not yet established whether there is any channelling of intermediates in β-oxidation even though they occur at extremely low concentrations, as discussed by H. Osmundsen et al. (Chapter 15).

The biosynthesis of pyrimidine and purine nucleotides in mammals is discussed by R.I. Christopherson and E. Szabados (Chapter 16). A bifunctional and a trifunctional enzyme are involved in pyrimidine synthesis. The trifunctional L-dihydro-orotate synthase in the cytoplasm has carbamoyl phosphate synthase activity (which is distinct from the carbamoyl synthase in the matrix), and there is evidence that the two intermediates of this enzyme complex are partly channelled. Two trifunctional enzymes and two bifunctional enzymes are involved in the biosynthesis of purine nucleotides. The reactions catalysed by one bifunctional and one trifunctional enzyme may be partly channelled; no information is apparently available about the others. It has been proposed that there is a metabolon for the *de novo* synthesis of purine nucleotides, but this is speculative. The evidence is also discussed for channelling in a complex which synthesizes pyrimidine deoxyribonucleotide triphosphates in the cytoplasm and which is associated with the outer face of the nuclear membrane. This complex provides deoxyribonucleotides for a replitase involved in DNA replication in the nucleus (Chapter 16).

Conclusions

The chapters of this book present a range of opinions about channelling in intermediary metabolism. Overall they present evidence that channelling occurs in many metabolic pathways but that it does not occur in all. Thus there is little doubt that channelling occurs in the urea cycle and in tryptophan synthesis. However, the evidence in some other systems is indirect and circumstantial. There are several different mechanisms of channelling, and the reason why these different forms have evolved is unknown. As illustrated by fatty acid synthase, a pathway may be completely channelled in some organisms but not necessarily in others. Channelling has not been demonstrated in mitochondrial β-oxidation and does not appear to be important for the pentafunctional AROM enzyme of the pre-chorismate pathway. We hope that there will be a continuing interest in the roles of channelling in biology and that there will be more integration between experimental and theoretical studies. We anticipate the development of new non-invasive physical methods to investigate channelling in both single cells and higher organisms.

References

1. Srere, P.A. (1987) Annu. Rev. Biochem. **56**, 81–124
2. Ovádi, J. (1991) J. Theor. Biol. **152**, 1–22 and following papers
3. Fersht, A. (1985) Enzyme Structure and Function, pp. 311–346, W.H. Freeman and Co., New York
4. Kellershohn, N. and Ricard, J. (1994) Eur. J. Biochem. **220**, 955–961
5. Goodsell, D.S. and Olson, A.J. (1993) Trends Biochem. Sci. **18**, 65–68
6. Paycn, T.A.J. (1983) Trends Biochem. Sci. **8**, 46
7. dos Remedios, C.G. and Moens, P.D.J. (1995) Biochim. Biophys. Acta **1228**, 99–124
8. Abrahams, J.P., Leslie, A.G.W., Lutter, R. and Walker, J.E. (1994) Nature (London) **370**, 621–628
9. Cornish-Bowden, A. (1995) Fundamentals of Enzyme Kinetics, 2nd edn., pp. 264–265, Portland Press, London
10. Kacser, H. and Burns, J.A. (1979) Biochem. Soc. Trans. **7**, 1149–1160
11. Srivastava, D.K. and Bernhard, S.A. (1987) Biochemistry **26**, 1240–1246

Molecular and physicochemical aspects

2

Ian C. West

Department of Biochemistry and Genetics, The Medical School, University of Newcastle, Newcastle upon Tyne NE2 4HH, U.K.

Introduction: two types of channelling concept and the fundamental issues they raise

It has been widely suggested that some enzymes that operate on sequentially related substrates lie closely juxtaposed in the cell, and that this arrangement has evolved because of some advantage it confers on metabolism. It is usually assumed that this advantage is kinetic, that the close juxtaposition of two enzymic active sites cuts down on diffusion time between sites, or raises local concentrations of substrate while lowering local product concentrations. Other conceivable advantages are in minimizing side reactions or lag times. This whole concept, or bundle of concepts, has been called channelling.

The concept of channelling has arisen in a quite separate way from a second type of observation. There are a number of cases where a presumed intermediate in the enzymic transformation of a substrate is not found in the cytoplasm at the expected concentrations. In some cases, the intermediate reacts poorly, if at all, when added to the purified enzyme that releases the final product. It looks as though intermediates may be trapped, either by being bound (i.e. thermodynamically) or by barriers to free diffusion (i.e. kinetically). Rather obvious cases of this sort are where intermediates are bound covalently to the enzyme or enzyme complex, as in the 2-oxoacid dehydrogenases (see Chapter 7), or mammalian fatty acid synthase (see Chapter 8), but more interesting, and perhaps debatable, cases exist where the nature of the trapping has not been adequately investigated, nor its metabolic advantage established. A fascinating and well studied example is tryptophan synthase, a bienzyme in which the product of the α subunit (indole) appears to dart down a protein tube to reach the β subunit more quickly than it can reach it from free solution (see Fig. 8). The metabolic advantages of this type of channelling might include the raising of the thermodynamic potential of the trapped intermediate, as advocated by Peter Mitchell [1], though not, of course, if the intermediates are trapped thermodynamically, for then their thermodynamic potential must be lowered by the binding energy.

This whole channelling concept is contentious and has been both widely disputed and widely ignored. The literature resembles that on the Loch Ness monster, with some authors seeing, and some not seeing, channelling effects (see, for example, the commentary papers that follow ref. [2]). It has been argued (e.g. [3], and see below) that, after making very reasonable assumptions about catalytic-centre activities, diffusion coefficients, diffusion paths, enzyme and substrate concentrations, etc., the transit time between successive enzymes in a metabolic pathway would seem to be very small compared with the time taken on the enzyme; or, to look at it from another point of view, concentration gradients in the cytoplasm will be very shallow, and negligible kinetic benefit would be expected to accrue from juxtaposition.

In order to assess these arguments it will be necessary to test rather carefully some of the assumptions made. For example, the following questions should be answered: what are realistic diffusion constants in cytoplasm? Does cytoplasm present a structured medium? Does the high protein concentration affect the viscosity of the medium or the availability or activity of water in some other way? If, after careful appraisal, the concept of channelling for kinetic advantage remains absurd, one presumably looks for non-kinetic advantages, or scrutinizes the reality of juxtaposition.

Enzymic channelling of the second sort, by a trapped intermediate, raises its own questions, in particular the role of concentration and activity in the kinetics and thermodynamics of reaction pathways.

It is the objective of the present chapter to delve a little into the fundamental biophysical principles that underlie these questions. Some consideration will be given to questions of distance scales, time scales, protein hydration, diffusion, viscosity, unstirred layers, cell water, molecular crowding, activity coefficients, and the role of concentration and activity in the kinetics and thermodynamics of reaction pathways.

Cytoplasm as an aqueous solution

Physical dimensions, intermolecular distances and cell size

Diffusion times are obviously sensitive functions of distance from source to sink (see calculation of metabolite diffusion rates, below). The longest path we can naively visualize will run from the cell exterior to the centre of the cell. The shortest diffusion path will be the average intermolecular distance between molecules uniformly dispersed in the cytoplasm, and that will depend only on concentration. For example, molecules of a solute will be 11.84 nm apart (on average) at 1 mM concentration (Fig. 1), and ten times that at 1 μM (Table 1).

If substrate and enzyme are each uniformly dispersed at a concentration of 1 μM, the mean distance between them that a substrate molecule would have to travel (assuming that the smaller molecule does all the diffusing) would be 94 nm.

Fig. 1   Hydration shell on a spherical soluble protein

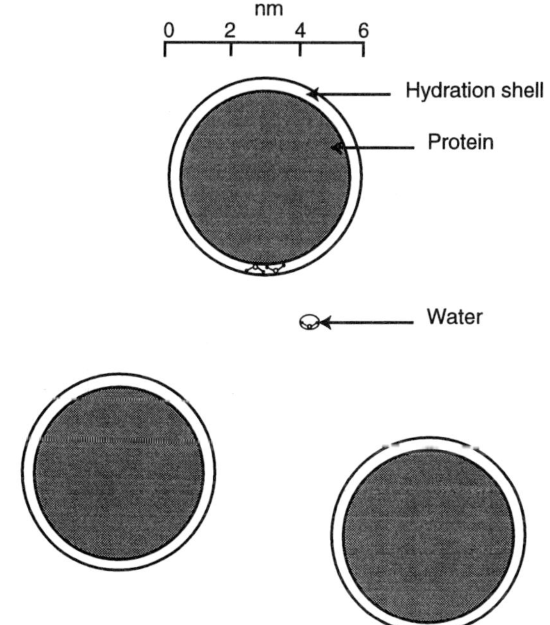

From its size and dispersion, this could be haemoglobin at 1 mM (67 g·l⁻¹). See the text for details.

Table 1   **Relationship between mean intermolecular distance and concentration**

c (mol/litre)	d (nm)
1	1.184
1×10^{-1}	2.55
1×10^{-2}	5.50
1×10^{-3}	11.84
1×10^{-4}	25.51
1×10^{-5}	55.0
1×10^{-6}	118.4

The mean intermolecular distance (d) is given (in nm) by the relationship: $d = 1.184c^{-1/3}$, where c is the molar concentration.

Fig. 2   **Approximate sizes of different cell types**

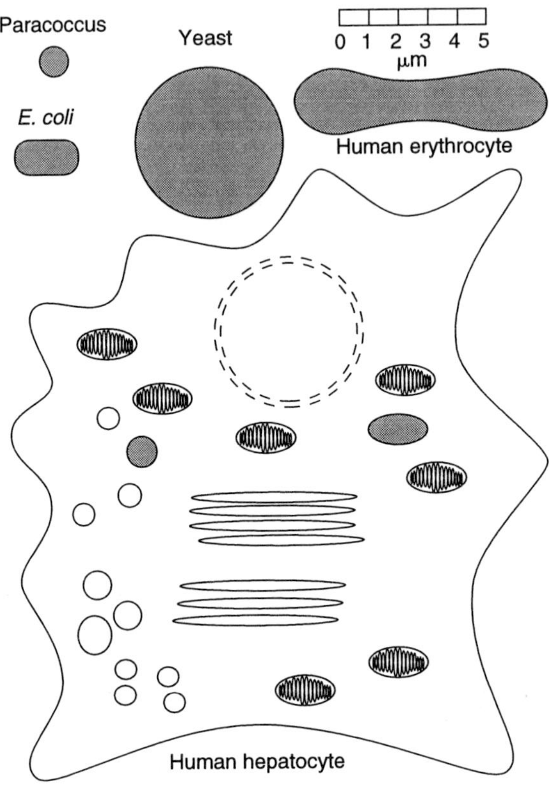

Cells come in different sizes (Fig. 2). For example, *Escherichia coli* is 2–4 μm in length, *Saccharomyces cerevisiae* 5 μm, a human erythrocyte 8.5 μm in diameter, while an hepatocyte may be 40–50 μm across. Thus the maximum distance from the cell exterior is 0.50 μm in *E. coli*, 1.20 μm in the erythrocyte, but 20 μm in the hepatocyte. It could turn out (see the Conclusions section) that what works in a bacterium is too slow for an hepatocyte.

If we consider the structures inside a eukaryotic cell, as visualized by the electron microscope (Fig. 3), we realize that diffusion paths may be considerably longer than those calculated naively above. Endoplasmic reticulum clearly consists of double sheets of phospholipid membrane, and presents an impenetrable barrier to the diffusion of most solutes, as do mitochondria, lysosomes, droplets, granules, etc. This is not easily allowed for. If the organelles are regarded as uniform, rigid, close-packed spheres the diffusion path would be lengthened surprisingly little (a trivial 4%). On the other hand, the cross-sectional area available for diffusion would be decreased 4-fold. However, that is an inadequate model of the cytoplasm, and even more inadequate for the mitochondrial matrix. The obstacles are not spherical, but neither are they close-packed, and the gaps between them are themselves obstructed by impenetrable globular proteins which, if close-packed, would lead to another 4-fold decrease in transmission area. In a later section the problem of diffusion in the cytoplasm will be raised again in terms of viscosity and diffusion coefficients. These three effects (viscosity, diffusion coefficients and transmission area) are probable *not* additive; they may in part be different ways of looking at the same problem

Protein hydration

Most proteins retain a certain amount of water, which will be referred to as the water of hydration. This has been the subject of considerable study and indeed debate, but the topic has been well elaborated [4,5]. It is important to understand the nature of this water; to know if the water is bound, or how tightly it is bound; to know if it is available for dissolving other solutes; to know the diffusional mobility of that water and of any solutes that may be dissolved in it.

A wide range of soluble proteins examined by a variety of techniques are found to have water of hydration of around 0.2–0.3 g/g of

---

Fig. 3   **The texture of eukaryotic cytoplasm**

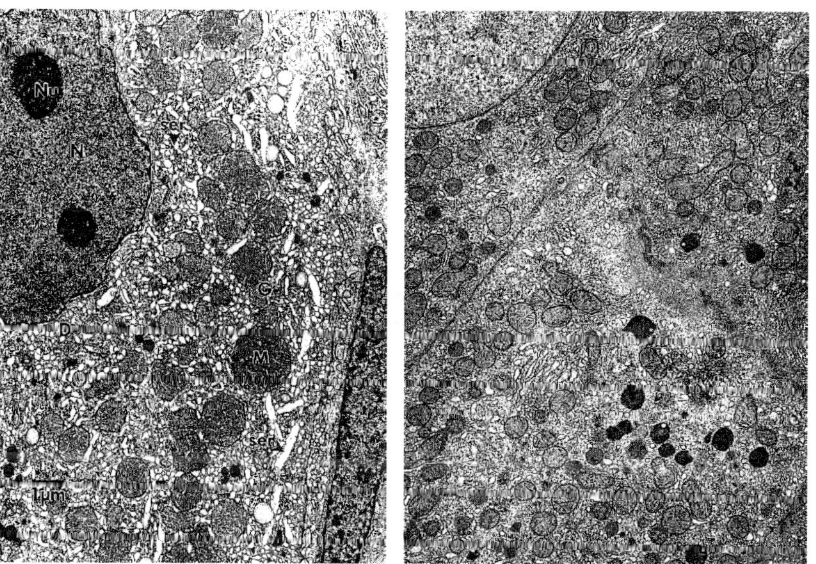

Left: electron micrograph of primate corpus luteum showing nucleus (N), smooth endoplasmic reticulum (ser), dictyosomes (D), nucleolus (Nu), mitochondria (M) and glycogen granule (G). Reprinted from [65], with permission. Right: electron micrograph of rat liver at similar magnification showing nucleus, mitochondria, cell membrane, endoplasmic reticulum and other membrane-bound cytoplasmic granules. (Photograph by courtesy of Professor F. Van Hoof.)

protein. This amounts to 750–1100 molecules of water for a protein of M_r 67000 (such as haemoglobin). For the most widely studied proteins (lysozyme, myoglobin, serum albumin) a consensus picture does emerge. There appears to be a single layer of water molecules covering essentially all the surface of these soluble proteins. In the case of a protein of M_r 67000, this would be a 3 Å (0.3 nm) layer of water on a sphere of radius 27 Å; equivalent to 20 Å^2 per molecule of water (see Fig. 1). However, the water probably does not stick to the protein evenly; charged groups on the surface are likely to be more heavily hydrated than areas that are merely polar.

This water does not freeze at the same temperature as bulk water (whatever that temperature is; see section on ideal and non-ideal solutions, below), but seems rather to melt with the protein itself. The molecules in this first layer have slowed rotational and translational mobilities (compared with bulk water), but only by a factor of 10–100 [mean residence time (τ) 10^{-9}–10^{8} s instead of 10^{-10} s for bulk water]. The heat capacity and partial molar volume of water in this hydration shell are only 10–15% different from bulk-water values, and the molar free energy of transfer of water into this shell is only -2.1 kJ·mol^{-1} (-0.5 kcal·mol^{-1}). So this water is slowed but not immobilized, and it is only weakly bound. {In addition to the thousand-odd molecules of this loose hydration shell, haemoglobin carries a mere five molecules of more tightly bound water ($\tau > 10^{-8}$ s) [5].}

Time scales

Different physical methods observe motions on different time scales. Thus neutron scattering detects motions in the ps range, NMR operates in the ns range, Mössbauer spectroscopy in the 100 ns range and EPR in the μs range. It is possible for one technique to find a molecule static or bound whereas another finds it mobile or essentially not there. This can generate apparent conflict and real confusion. One example of this is the long-running controversy between NMR people and EPR people over the existence of a phospholipid annulus round intrinsic membrane proteins; what looked like immobilized phospholipid to the former was to the latter as mobile as bulk phospholipid, and therefore indistinguishable from it. In the present context it is relevant to note that molecules of the hydration shell (see above) are only immobilized in relation to very rapid processes, with τ of the order of 10^{-9} s. Although on a time-average the hydration shell is always there, water itself can diffuse into and out of this zone, albeit some 10-fold more slowly than through bulk water. In some contexts it is relevant to ask how much free water there is in cytoplasm; careful thinking may be required to decide whether to include the water of hydration (see section on water activity, below).

Classical calculation of metabolite diffusion rates

How fast are the processes in which we are interested from the point of view of channelling: the processes of rotation, lateral diffusion, substrate binding, reaction and release? The classical or orthodox answer [3,6] is that the time taken for substrate to diffuse from one enzyme to the next is very short compared with the processes of binding, reaction and release. We shall take this orthodox view as our starting point, and I shall therefore reproduce here the arguments of Webb [3].

Molecules in solution 'jig' around, each possessing kT joules of kinetic energy (where k is the Boltzmann constant and T is absolute temperature). The mean speed of each molecule between collisions (û) will depend on its mass (M):

$$\hat{u} = (8RT/\pi M)^{1/2} \tag{1}$$

where R is the gas constant. For a molecule of M_r 100 at 310 K, this comes to $260\ \mathrm{m \cdot s^{-1}}$ or 580 miles per h. Of course, in condensed media such as water, frequent collisions interrupt this very rapid motion, and macroscopic diffusion laws have to be used. Of these there are two: (a) Fick's law, and (b) the Einstein–Smoluchowski relation. Fick's law, like Ohm's law, specifies a *linear* relationship between rate of flow (J_i) and the distance (x) between source and sink (Fig. 4A):

$$\mathrm{d}n_i/\mathrm{d}t = J_i = A\,\mathrm{D}\,(c_1 - c_2)/x \tag{2}$$

where A is the cross-sectional or transmission area of the relevant diffusion path, D is the macroscopic diffusion coefficient, c_1 is the source and c_2 the sink concentration. On the other hand, the Einstein–Smoluchowski equation relates mean *square* displacement (d^2) to transit time (τ):

$$\tau = d^2/2\mathrm{D} \tag{3}$$

The value 2 may be approximate only [7], and should be 6 if three dimensions are considered [8].

These two equations may appear mutually contradictory, and indeed it is not immediately obvious which is the more appropriate. However, they are not really in conflict. If the concentrations of source and sink are maintained, there will be a linear concentration gradient between them, and flux will halve if the path is doubled, according to Fick's law (Fig. 4A). On the other hand, if a source is created instantly at a point, molecules will spread out in each direction entirely at random (Fig. 4B). Part of the population will move away from the source, but the *mean displacement* (the sum of the displacements of each particle divided by the number of particles) will be zero. Only the mean of the squares of the displacements (always positive) will give us a quantity that increases with time. It is this *mean square displacement* (d^2) of the population that is described by the Einstein–Smoluchowski relation [7]. Progress will slow as the gradient flattens, which is why transit time goes up as the square of the distance travelled. At any time, 68% of the particles lie within $\pm d$ of the origin.

Most authors use the Einstein–Smoluchowski equation to calculate the transit time expected for given displacements. Webb, for example, tabulates [3] the following values (Table 2) using a diffusion coefficient of $5 \times 10^{-6}\,\mathrm{cm^2 \cdot s^{-1}}$, as might be appropriate for a molecule of M_r 500 diffusing in water (*not* cytoplasm). As mentioned above, with two enzymes each uniformly dispersed at 1 μM concentration, the diffusing metabolite would be expected to travel an average of 94 nm. The Webb calculation predicts the transit time to be of the order of 10^{-5} s. Enzyme catalytic-centre activities vary over a wide range $(1–10^7\,\mathrm{s^{-1}})$, but at this stage in our argument we may take $10^3\,\mathrm{s^{-1}}$ as typical (for an enzyme at saturating substrate concentration). For this particular string of approximations it seems clear that for many enzymes only a small part (1%) of the total lifetime of a metabolite is spent diffusing between enzyme molecules; a small but not negligible part (Fig. 5). We shall discuss fast enzymes in a later section.

Incidentally, the rotation time for an average protein in water is of the order of 10^{-7} s, which is short in comparison with both the inter-molecule diffusion time and the lifetime of the enzyme–substrate complex.

Fig. 4　　　　**Diffusion laws**

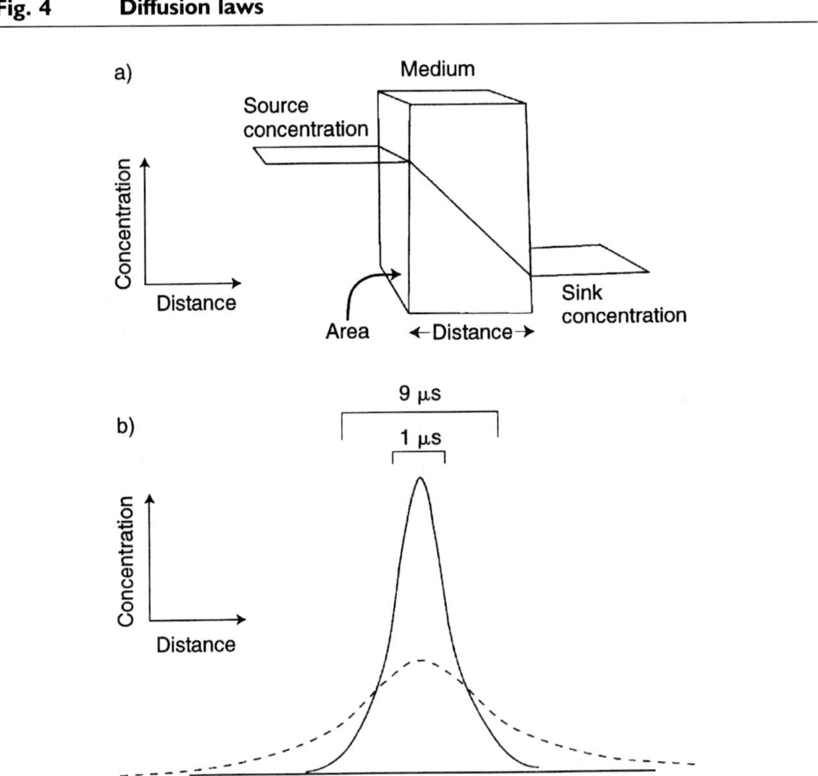

(a) Fick's law with a linear concentration gradient. (b) Einstein–Smoluchowski diffusion. The braces at $\pm$ d include 68% of the population, closely resembling a 'normal' distribution.

Table 2	The relationship between time and distance moved by a diffusing particle
d (nm)	τ (s)
5	2.5×10^{-8}
10	1.0×10^{-7}
100	1.0×10^{-5}
1000 (1 μm)	1.0×10^{-3}
10000 (10 μm)	1.0×10^{-1}

The root mean square distance (d) moved in time (τ) was calculated using the Einstein–Smoluchowski equation with a diffusion coefficient of 5×10^{-6} $cm^2 \cdot s^{-1}$, as might be appropriate for a molecule of M_r 500 diffusing in water [3].

This has some bearing on models in which adjacent proteins rotate to juxtapose their active sites.

The Fick's law approach gives an interestingly different slant on this. For a very crude application we could again take a pair of enzymes (b and c) each at 1 μM concentration, and identify a tiny cube containing (on average)

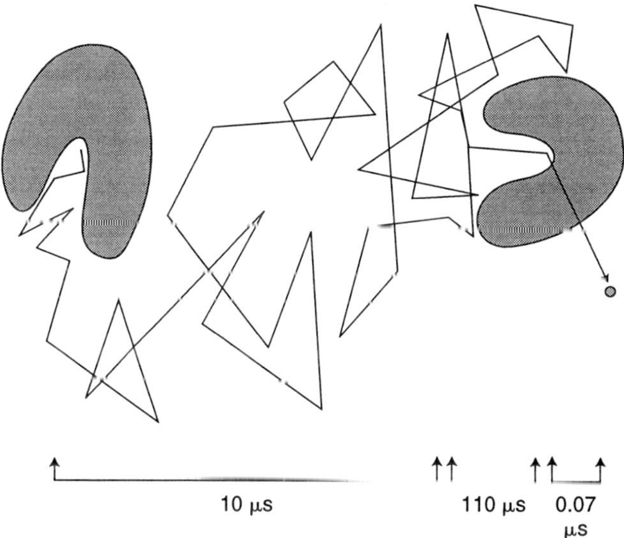

Fig. 5   Transition, docking and departure times

This figure (not to scale) represents the random walk of a small metabolite (e.g. O_2) between two protein molecules (e.g. myoglobin; see the text).

one molecule of each enzyme. We can again suppose c to be turning over at 10^3 s^{-1} and apply Fick's law to obtain the fall in concentration between the source face and the sink face of our little cube (see Fig. 4A). Assuming the same diffusion coefficient as before, there would be a steady-state concentration difference across the cube of 0.02 μM.

It is obvious that a fast enzyme ($k_{cat} > 10^4$ s^{-1}) will be significantly limited by the diffusional transit time, and that dilute enzymes (being further apart) will be more affected. Similarly, at dilute substrate concentrations, diffusion will be slower (see below) and gradients steeper, especially if diffusion is hindered appreciably by obstacles or 'viscosity'. However, for unhindered diffusion in water of single molecules dispersed at 10^{-6}–10^{-3} M, it will be accepted that diffusion is not expected to affect greatly the rate of enzymic reactions. This can be tested quite simply, perhaps by stirring, or more conventionally by adding viscogens to slow diffusion [9–11]. The viscosity of the cytoplasm and diffusion rates in cytoplasm will be discussed below.

Microscopic rates of binding and unbinding

Next we must ask what the substrate does when it reaches its enzyme. Might it perhaps dance away again without reacting? And we must enquire more deeply into the time scales of enzyme turnover. It will help to consider the uniquely well documented encounter between myoglobin and its small gaseous ligands, O_2 and CO.

Carbon monoxide (or oxygen), bound to the haem in the hydrophobic haem pocket of myoglobin, will occasionally break free by thermal dissociation, or it can be dislodged from the haem by a brief (10–20 ns) laser flash (photodissociation). The ligand and the excited protein can then relax back again in two fundamentally different ways: the ligand can simply return to the haem (with or without the protein first relaxing from its excited state; this is called geminate recombination), or the ligand can diffuse out of the pocket, mix with ligand molecules in the medium, re-enter the pocket and rebind (this can be called bimolecular recombination). This whole experiment can be done at any temperature between 4 and 320 K. At temperatures below 220 K, at which the protein freezes, the diffusion route is very slow, but at room temperature much of the photodissociated ligand will escape from the pocket rather than rebind directly to the haem; this fraction is called the quantum yield. When the ligand is CO, essentially all the ligand escapes; when the ligand is O_2, some 10% escapes while 90% rebinds (because of a much faster rebinding rate constant).

Absorbance spectroscopy can indicate, in the nanosecond to minute time domain, the liganding state of the haem; resonance Raman [12,13] and Fourier-transform infrared [14–16] spectroscopy can report not only on the protein but also on the ligand. In addition to these detailed kinetic data, there are the results of modelling; molecular dynamics simulations can produce trajectories that look, when compared with real data, very convincing. With these simulations it is possibly to ask what happens in the haem binding pocket on a femtosecond to picosecond time scale [17].

What, then, are the relative rates of the processes of diffusion up to the myoglobin molecule, diffusion into and out of the haem pocket, and binding and unbinding the haem? One of the most lucid accounts of this work is that of Gibson et al. [18]. (It is true, however, that their intelligible overall picture may hide or overlook genuine complexities to do with micro-states of the protein [14,15,19,20], 'open' and 'closed' diffusion pathways, etc. [12].) Gibson et al. analyse their data in terms of three states: A (or MbX) in which the ligand is co-ordinated to the haem; B, a geminate or contact-pair state in which the ligand is very close to the Fe^{2+}; and C, in which the ligand is separated from the haem but is still trapped in the protein. The fourth state (Mb + X) is with ligand free in solution.

$$A \underset{k_{BA}}{\overset{k_{AB}}{\rightleftharpoons}} B \underset{k_{CB}}{\overset{k_{BC}}{\rightleftharpoons}} C \underset{k_{XC}}{\overset{k_{CX}}{\rightleftharpoons}} Mb + X$$

Slow thermal release of CO from A is followed by almost complete loss of

Table 3	Fitted rate constants for proposed steps in the binding (and unbinding) of ligand to (or from) sperm whale myoglobin at pH 7 and 20°C [18]						
Ligand	k_{AB} (s^{-1})	k_{BA} (μs^{-1})	k_{BC} (μs^{-1})	k_{CB} (μs^{-1})	k_{CX} (μs^{-1})	k_{XC} $(M^{-1} \cdot \mu s^{-1})$	QY
CO	0.019	2.1	115	8.5	14.4	43.4	1
O_2	92	485	115	8.5	14.4	43.4	0.1

QY is quantum yield. k_{AB} describes the slow thermal release, not the rapid photodissociation.

CO to the medium (because $k_{BC} \gg k_{BA}$; see Table 3) while, for O_2, 90% is recaptured by the haem (because $k_{BC} < k_{BA}$). Association of these two ligands also follows different courses in its later stages. With both ligands the bimolecular formation of C, the loose state, is followed, more often than not, by loss of ligand back into the medium ($k_{CX} > k_{CB}$). (Note, incidentally that $k_{XC} = 8.68$ ms^{-1} at 0.2 mM ligand.) At the B state, however, the fates of O_2 and CO are different, for 80% of O_2 goes on to form the co-ordinated ligand (A), whereas 98% of CO returns to the C state.

By taking reciprocals, these rate constants can be converted into mean times, as follows (Fig. 5). If we extend the 'drunken sailor' metaphor deployed by most authors who discuss diffusion [7,8,21], we see dioxygen stumbling its random way through the cytoplasm to a myoglobin molecule. We wait 110 μs while it bumbles unsuccessfully around the myoglobin. Finally we see it go into the vestibule; but in 69.4 ns we see it flying out again (as though it had been trying to enter the Garrick Club without a necktie). On the third attempt (on average), instead of flying out of the vestibule, it flies on into the protein, where it latches on to the haem, and stays. The occupancy of the vestibule is therefore only 6×10^{-4}, and that low value greatly slows the otherwise rapid binding to the haem.

Hasinoff and Chishti [11] examined the effect of increasing the medium viscosity on the CO rebinding reaction. By adding glycerol to 80% (w/w) and cooling to 236 K they achieved viscosities of up to 46 000 times that of water. With viscosities of 10 cP (10 times that of water; 1 cP = 1 mPa·s) the medium viscosity was detectably slowing the association rate, while at 1000 cP diffusion was (essentially) totally rate-determining. This can be understood in terms of Fig. 5; the intermolecular transit time *in water* is small but is not negligible with respect to the subsequent processes of docking and binding.

The numbers above are, of course, specific to this system, but the problems faced by O_2 (or CO) docking on to myoglobin will be similar to those faced by most substrates and most enzymes. Except, of course, that enzymes destroy their substrates, and the whole process of loading must be endlessly repeated. They also create product, which must dissociate and diffuse away by a process that is kinetically similar to the above. If chemical transformation and release of product are slow with respect to loading, then any local deficit of substrate concentration will have time to recover; otherwise the second turnover will exacerbate the deficit.

A further complication arises when there are two (or more) substrates that must be bound per turnover. (Most enzymes are of this type.) The long delay in forming the loose complex between myoglobin and ligand followed by its rapid dissociation reminds us that termolecular collisions would be very rare. Ping-Pong enzymes (double-displacement or substituted-enzyme mechanisms) get over this problem by covalently tethering the transferred particle, and decreasing the overall reaction to two bimolecular reactions. Ternary-complex enzymes (single-displacement mechanisms), on the other hand, characteristically retain one of the substrates, for example NAD, in a long-lived binary complex pending the arrival of the second substrate.

Rates of diffusion of small and large molecules in hindered and unhindered media

Fick's law (eqn. 2) shows us that we must consider (a) concentration gradient, (b) area, and (c) diffusion coefficient.

Fick/Mitchell

The role of concentration in diffusion was analysed very clearly by Mitchell [22]. Mitchell started from the view that the force causing diffusional movement of molecules must be the potential difference, not the concentration gradient. If the concentration gradient in Fick's law (eqn. 2) is expressed in terms of chemical potentials (μ) by making the substitution:

$$c = e^{\mu/RT} \tag{4}$$

one obtains the expression:

$$\frac{\mathrm{d}n}{\mathrm{d}t} = \frac{-D \cdot A}{RT} \cdot c \cdot \frac{\mathrm{d}\mu}{\mathrm{d}x} \tag{5}$$

revealing that the rate of diffusion through a barrier is linearly dependent upon the concentration of molecules in the barrier (see also [23]). I (now) prefer the alternative view, that no force acts on the individual molecules undergoing diffusion, interpreting diffusion and Fick's law as a purely statistical result of having more molecules on one side of an imaginary plane than on the other [24,25].

Whichever way you care to look at it, however, the rate of diffusion through any medium is linearly dependent upon the concentration of molecules in that medium; a 10-fold lower substrate concentration will produce a 10-fold lower rate of diffusion. It is therefore at a low concentration of diffusant that we should expect diffusion to become limiting. This could be compensated by a steepening of the gradient (lowered concentration at the sink, which may slow the sink reaction) or by shortening the diffusion path, if the enzymes could be brought closer together.

The diffusion coefficient: Stokes–Einstein and non-Stokesian diffusion

For classical diffusion in a continuous fluid medium the diffusion coefficient is given by the well known Stokes–Einstein equation:

$$D = kT/6\pi\eta r \tag{6}$$

There are two variables in the denominator. The viscosity coefficient (η) describes the way momentum is transferred between molecules of the fluid matrix, and is a property of the fluid. (The viscosity of water is 1.002 cP or 1.002 mPa·s at 20 °C, and 0.678 mPa·s at 38 °C [26].) The radius (r), however, is that of the diffusant and shows how the rate of diffusion is related to the size of the diffusant. For a good Stokesian medium such as water the Stokes–Einstein equation holds good over an amazing range of sizes from protein molecules to marbles. However, structured media show a quite different relationship between rate of diffusion and size, with a much steeper dependence on size and a higher activation energy [27]. The (very plausible) interpretation is that diffusion requires the opening of holes in the structure. What then is the nature of diffusion in the cytoplasm?

Diffusion in cytoplasm

Diffusion in cytoplasm is indeed non-Stokesian. It may be that the concept of viscosity is confusing in this context; that is to say, motion through cytoplasm may not be determined primarily by momentum transfer between layers of flowing Newtonian solvent, but more by fibrous or globular obstacles [28].

Luby-Phelps et al. [29,30] showed that they could model the diffusion of microscopic particles through cytoplasm by adding 3.7% (w/v) actin filaments and 12.4% (w/v) globular protein to water. When not constrained by the tangled mesh of the fibrous proteins or by the volume-exclusion effect of the globular protein, small probes move almost as freely as they do in water. Thus cytoplasm presents little resistance to rotation, with rotational relaxation times and deduced viscosities close to those of water whether measured by NMR or picosecond fluorescence depolarization [28,31,32]. Adding increasing amounts of albumin to a fluorescent probe solution did not slow the rotating probes, but did steadily increase the proportion of bound probe that did not rotate [33]. On the other hand, lateral diffusion of small molecules suggests cytoplasmic viscosities around 3.7 times those in

Table 4 **Viscosity of cytoplasm relative to that of water at the same temperature, measured in different ways**

Test	Relative viscosity (η/η_0)	Refs.	Notes
Rotational diffusion	1.05–1.28	[28,32]	
	1.2–1.4	[33]	
Lateral diffusion			
of small molecules	3.7 (23)	[28]	1
of mRNA, proteins, ribosomes	6–∞	[30,35]	2,4
of 93 nm-diam. beads	?–∞	[34]	3,4
of Ca^{2+} in cytoplasm	3.2–32	[46,47]	4
Macroscopic viscosity			
of erythrocyte cytoplasm	7.1–9.9	[9]	

Notes: (1) Value in brackets obtained in cells shrunken to one-third volume; (2) no mobility outside restricted areas; (3) particles restricted to 250 nm cube but inside that too rapid to measure; (4) lower mobility may be due to barriers rather than viscosity.

water (Table 4). (Osmotically shrinking the cell by a mere 3-fold can drive this up to 23 times that of water [28], reminding us that the water of protein hydration is 10–100-fold less mobile than bulk water, and will seem to be essentially part of the protein to a small diffusing molecule.)

The lateral diffusion of larger probes shows that cytoplasm is markedly non-Stokesian, and diffusion constants may be 40 times those of water for particles as large as multienzyme complexes, ribosomes, polyribosomes or endosomes [34,35]. However, we are considering the diffusion of small metabolites with M_r ranging from 20–1000. On the other hand, the low viscosities measured by rotational techniques are equally irrelevant, for we are concerned with lateral diffusion past manifold macromolecular, but still sub-microscopic, obstacles. We may conclude that diffusion through cytoplasm may be 2.5–8.0 times slower than in water. If we are interested in longer-distance diffusion, e.g. from cell surface to cell centre, we must add on top of this the obstructing effects of the microscopically visible organelles found in eukaryotic cytoplasm, discussed above. Diffusion could then be slowed by a further factor of 2–4.

When is diffusion rate-limiting?

Are there well established cases where diffusion rates are indeed limiting, or are concentrations in cytoplasm essentially uniform? Where should we look? From the preceding discussion, we might expect diffusion limitation to show up for long-range diffusion, for diffusion through structural barriers, for rapid transients, rapid enzymes, and at low concentrations.

Particulate-catalyst reactors

Enzyme-catalysed reactions, do not, in general, speed up with stirring, yet such speeding up is well known in chemical engineering and has been thoroughly investigated. Similar, diffusion-limited, kinetics appear when enzymes are immobilized [36]. Presumably this is because soluble enzymes operate on a nanometre distance scale, whereas particles operate on a micrometre scale.

Bacterial outer membrane

Gram-negative bacteria, such as *E. coli*, are bounded by two hydrophobic membranes. The inner membrane is the typical cell membrane, highly impermeable to hydrophilic solutes and the site of specific transport carriers such as the lactose/proton symporter. The outer membrane appears to be a protection against larger molecules, for it is made moderately permeable to ions and solutes of up to M_r 700 by the presence of numerous water-filled pores. While transport through these porin pores follows Fick's law (first-order, i.e. a vertical line on Eadie–Hofstee plots, and an infinite V_{max} intercept), transport through the specific carriers shows saturation kinetics (Michaelis–Menten kinetics, i.e. an oblique line with negative slope on Eadie–Hofstee plots, and a finite V_{max}). Malcolm Page and I asked the question: are there conditions when the outer membrane becomes rate limiting for galactoside transport into *E. coli* [37]? The answer (Fig. 6) was that, as the medium sugar concentration fell below 1 mM, transport became progressively limited by a simple first-order diffusion barrier; presumably the outer membrane. We

Fig. 6   **Uptake kinetics of β-galactoside into _E. coli_**

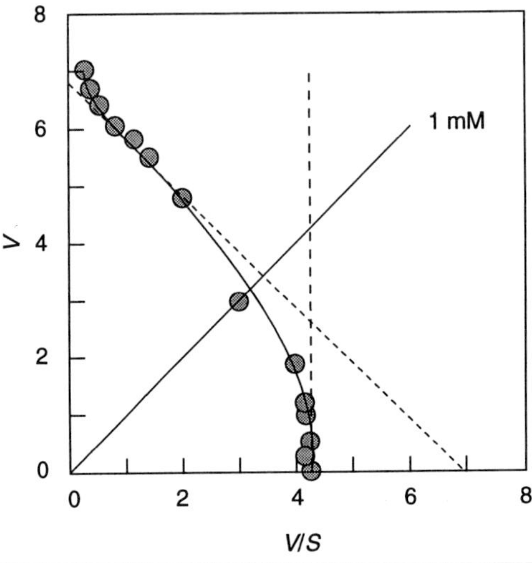

Eadie–Hofstee plot showing that saturation kinetics above a concentration of 1 mM galactoside tend towards first-order kinetics at infinite dilution. (From [37] with permission.)

went further; we used the lactose permease as a miniaturized, _in situ_, galactoside monitor to report the periplasmic galactoside concentration, and calculated the concentration drop across the outer membrane. This fitted surprisingly well the expected diffusion properties of the porin pores [37]. However, in this case there is a well defined physical barrier to diffusion, and the diffusion path might extend 10–100 nm across the outer membrane and the periplasm.

Unstirred layers: erythrocyte oxygen and glucose transport

Unstirred layers are a general problem in transport kinetics, particularly with fast transport processes. Their effects have been thoroughly analysed [38–41], though not very widely considered. Here a layer of stagnant medium is seen as forming a partial diffusion barrier between the membrane and the bulk medium (Fig. 7). In the absence of net flux this will have no effect (solid line); with flux (dashed line), the solute concentrations in the unstirred layers will be intermediate between the concentrations in the bulk phases; the effect increases with flux rate. This layer can be described by the quantity δ (Fig. 7). Increasing the viscosity will increase δ; stirring will lessen it. As it is not clear that cytoplasm is appreciably stirred, it may be confusing to talk of an 'unstirred' layer; yet there will be a 'depleted' layer wherever there is a supramolecular (albeit microscopic) sink.

It will be appreciated that O_2 movements into and out of the erythrocyte have to be extremely fast for they are confined to the 100–400 ms

Fig. 7　Unstirred layers in transmembrane transport

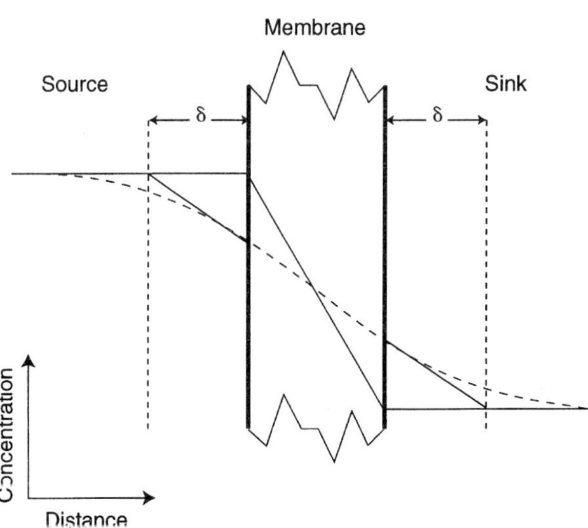

The thicknesses of the unstirred layers (δ) depend on the viscosity and bulk flow on each side of the membrane, but also on net flux rate. Solid line indicates slow transport; dashed line indicates rapid transport.

during which the corpuscle passes through the lung or tissue capillaries. Indeed, this will apply equally to glucose and CO_2 movements, considered below. Holland et al. [42] measured δ for the very fast entry of O_2 into erythrocytes to be 700 nm with maximum achievable stirring in a stopped-flow apparatus. The extracellular unstirred layer slowed O_2 entry 2-fold and provided at least 70% of the external resistance to O_2 uptake. This appreciable resistance (an underestimate, presumably, of the cytoplasmic value) shows us that there is a very considerable concentration gradient for O_2 from erythrocyte plasma membrane across the capillary wall to the inner membrane of a tissue mitochondrion. Indeed, it has been estimated that blood enters the tissue capillary with 100 mm Hg O_2 partial pressure (132 μM O_2 at 37 °C), leaves with 40 mm, while maintaining 1–5 mm O_2 partial pressure at the mitochondrion [43]. (However, this low concentration of O_2 at the mitochondrion is apparently not limiting for respiration. Only when the O_2 partial pressure in arterial blood falls to 12 mmHg, and the mitochondrial value to 0.1 mmHg, does the mitochondrial NAD^+ start to become dangerously reduced [44].)

As we saw above, placing a diffusion process in series with a carrier or enzymic process has the general effect of bending the linear plots (e.g. Lineweaver–Burk, Eadie–Hofstee, etc.) at low substrate concentrations, causing an overestimate of the true K_m, while leaving the V_{max} unaffected. In the intensely detailed kinetic analysis of the glucose carrier of the human erythrocyte, the question was raised as to whether, during rapid inflow of sugar, there might be a local build-up at the inner face of the plasma membrane, preventing equilibrium unloading of the carrier. Such an 'unstirred layer' would slow net inflow; the carrier would fail to unload (or would reload) before re-orientating. Kinetic tests were devised. With this moderately rapid carrier, a scant barrier was detectable outside the cell but an unstirred layer was demonstrated extending into the cytoplasm [38–40].

Ca^{2+} transients in animal cells

It is clear from the above examples that the cytoplasm cannot always be regarded as a uniformly mixed solution in which diffusion is so fast that concentration gradients are trivial; transient inhomogeneities in cytoplasmic concentrations can be significant. This is further exemplified in a highly visual way by the demonstration, in a wide variety of cell types, of waves of elevated cytoplasmic free Ca^{2+} concentration that can sweep across cells with a velocity of 10^{-5}–10^{-4} m·s^{-1} [45]. Cytosolic free Ca^{2+} can rise locally from 0.1–0.2 to about 1 μM. There is little doubt that there are spatial inhomogeneities of cytoplasmic free Ca^{2+} concentration, and that these can persist for 200 ms in restricted corners of the cell [46]. Modelling suggests that the movement of the wave (or wavefront) is largely determined by the diffusion constant for Ca^{2+}. (This, incidentally, has recently been measured in *Xenopus* oocyte cytoplasm to be 4×10^{-11} m^2·s^{-1} [47], which is 30-fold smaller than the limiting value in water [26].)

Fast enzymes: carbonic anhydrase

Erythrocyte carbonic anhydrase is an example of a very fast enzyme that operates at the diffusion limit [9]. This enzyme, concerned with CO_2 transport in the blood, has to work extremely rapidly for a very short time. By measuring the 'minimum association rate constant' (k_{min}; i.e. V_{max}/K_m, or the apparent rate constant for association of free enzyme with free substrate) for the HCO_3^- and CO_2 substrates at varying viscosity (using glycerol) and extrapolating to zero viscosity, Hasinoff [9] estimated that diffusion significantly affects association at 1 mPa·s (especially for the HCO_3^- substrate). At 6 mPa·s, close to the estimated viscosity of erythrocyte cytoplasm, diffusion dominates the process of association for both substrates. Similar results have been obtained with other enzymes.

Water activity in protein solutions

The colligative properties of aqueous solutions (osmotic pressure, vapour pressure, depression of the freezing point, etc.) are measures of the lowering of water activity by dissolved solutes, compared with the water activity of pure water (at the same temperature and pressure). Put very crudely, the solutes dilute the solvent. A small addition of an ideal solute will have a predictable effect; the same as any other ideal solute. However, protein solutions (including cytoplasm) are far from ideal; we shall have to consider carefully the mutually interacting thermodynamic properties of cellular components; solutes as well as solvent (water).

Molar, molal, and mole fraction scales

Biochemists are most familiar with the molar scale for expressing concentrations (mol per litre of solution). Physical chemists seem to prefer the molal scale (mol per 1000 g of solvent), while the most fundamental and thermodynamic scale is the mole fraction scale [mol of component A per total mol (A + B + C etc.)]. Each scale has its advantages. Ideal solutions are defined in terms of the mole fraction scale. Concentrations on the molal scale are easily weighed out, are precise and reproducible, and do not change with temperature (and the consequent changing density of water). Molar concentrations, on the other hand, represent volume concentrations and have a fundamental validity in their own right ([48]; and see below).

Changing the scale in which a quantity is expressed can make some surprising differences to the way in which those quantities appear and the way we feel about them. In erythrocyte cytoplasm, haemoglobin is present at $354 \, \text{g} \cdot (\text{l of cytoplasm})^{-1}$. Its concentration would be 5.3 mM on the molar scale familiar to biochemists. However, on the molal scale (mol per 1000 g of solvent), on the simplifying assumption that haemoglobin is the only solute present, its concentration would be 7.2 mmolal. This is because of the large volume fraction of (unhydrated) haemoglobin (0.265; leaving 0.735 as the volume fraction of water). If each haemoglobin molecule is regarded as carrying a hydration shell corresponding to 0.3 g of water/g of protein (see Fig. 1), the volume fraction of (hydrated) haemoglobin becomes 0.372, while the volume fraction of (free) water falls to 0.628. The concentration of (hydrated) haemoglobin remains the same in molar units, but in molal units it becomes 8.4 mmolal.

On the other hand, changing the scales obviously cannot change the thermodynamic properties of the system they describe, and in that sense is trivial.

The chemical potential of component B (μ_B), in an ideal solution, is defined as:

$$\mu_B = \mu_B^o + RT \ln x_B \tag{7}$$

where x_B is the mole fraction of B and μ_B^o is the chemical potential of B in some standard state [49]. Solutions that depart from this equation are therefore non-ideal, but they can be regarded as conforming to the following equation:

$$\mu_B = \mu_B^o + RT \ln \gamma_B x_B \tag{8}$$

where $\gamma_B x_B$ is known as the *activity* of B and γ_B as the *activity coefficient*. Clearly, changing from a mole fraction scale to molal or molar scales will necessitate appropriate numerical changes to both activity and activity coefficients.

Biochemists are familiar with the approximation that, in dilute aqueous solutions, the activity of a solute can be equated with its concentration; i.e. that our solutions are sufficiently dilute for ideal behaviour to apply. However, concentrated protein solutions, though dilute in molar terms, are far from ideal, as will be discussed in the next section. It is not immediately obvious which of our favourite simplifying concepts, such as the above, will hold for a solution as non-ideal as cytoplasm; and, if the protein behaves in a non-ideal way, what does this mean for the other components of the solution, i.e. small solutes and water molecules [50]?

Ideal and non-ideal solutions: excess entropy when solute molecules are much bigger than solvent molecules

A perfect gas can be defined as one for which there is a linear relationship between its chemical potential and the logarithm of its relative pressure. The molecules are visualized as having no mutual interactions, positive or negative, other than elastic collisions. The free energies of compression, dilution, mixing, etc. have no enthalpic component and are purely entropic, i.e. they depend on probability. Furthermore, in a perfect gas mixture the components will not differ in shape or size; they will differ only in what is called *configurational* entropy, calculable from the number of ways the components can be arranged or configured. However, even for many real gases it is a good approximation that the volume occupied by each molecule is very similar, because (at room temperature) this occupied volume is essentially independent of the size of the molecule and is a function only of the pressure and temperature (for a perfect gas at standard temperature and pressure the volume is $22.4 \, \text{l·mol}^{-1}$).

The thermodynamic description of liquid solutions is based (by analogy with the perfect gas mixture) on the hypothetical concept of an ideal solution, where there is no interaction between solute molecules or between solute and solvent. The chemical potential of each component is a linear function of the logarithm of its mole fraction. There is no enthalpy of dilution in ideal solutions, only an entropy change. Furthermore (by analogy with perfect gas mixtures), the solute and solvent molecules are conceived as occupying equal volumes (independently of their size).

Real solutions depart dramatically from the ideal; solute–solute and solute–solvent interaction energies are large, and the volumes occupied by real molecules of different sizes are not even remotely similar. (At 4 °C the volume per mol for water is 18 ml whereas for ethanol it is 57.38 ml, i.e. the molecular volumes are closely related to the molecular masses.) The mole fraction does not fully specify water activity. In an 11 mM solution of (say) methanol in water the mole fraction of methanol is about 1.98×10^{-4}, and the volume fraction will be rather similar. An 11 mM solution of haemoglobin, on the other hand, contains more than 70% protein (by volume); the molecules would be touching and solvent confined to the interstices. The discrepancy between the molecular masses of haemoglobin and water is 3700-fold. It is not surprising that, at moderate and high concentrations, the large size of protein molecules relative to solvent molecules causes a considerable departure from ideal behaviour.

Some aspects of ideal behaviour can be approached with progressive dilution. Molecular volumes remain discrepant, but solute–solvent interactions, though not removed, become constant, while solute–solute interactions can be brought essentially to zero as the molecules become more distant from each other. What about the size discrepancy? What effects does it have, and do these effects vanish with dilution?

Imagine a litre of pure water. The molecules are indistinguishable, so there is only one (distinguishable) configuration available to those 3.34×10^{25} molecules. Take out one molecule and replace it with a molecule of similar size, such as methanol. Clearly there are 3.34×10^{25} different ways we could do that. The change in entropy is considerable, but would not depend on the nature of the (ideal) substituent. If the replacement molecule were a large protein such as haemoglobin, displacing several thousand water molecules, there would still be only 3.34×10^{25} ways we could do the substitution, and (perhaps surprisingly) the entropic effect is the same as with methanol (provided that the protein is not infinitely flexible). We realize that this must be so from the fact that osmotic pressure measurements extrapolated to infinite dilution *do* give correct molecular masses. On the other hand, as we progressively replace water molecules with either methanol or haemoglobin, the size of the substituent becomes progressively important, in a way that is precisely calculable if the excluded volume is taken into account. The options available for placing the billionth haemoglobin molecule are restricted by the volume occupied by the foregoing molecules. This is a purely entropic effect; no enthalpic interactions are involved ([51–54]; see also Chapter 3 in the current volume). The entropic effect on pure solvent of adding a *macro*molecular solute is greater than that of adding an *ideal* solute; the effect has been called 'excess entropy'. This deviation from ideality resulting from excluded volume, though purely entropic, and derivable quantitatively by the methods of statistical mechanics, can also be viewed as a negative interaction, and derived with considerable accuracy by another route (see, e.g., [54]). (Other deviations from ideal behaviour may well occur in addition, due to enthalpic interactions, but these may be either positive or negative.)

Quite independently of whether the solute is ideal or non-ideal, the Gibbs–Duhem and Bjerrum relations ostensibly still hold [50]. Thus, if temperature and pressure are held constant but composition is varied (for this illustration let us consider a binary mixture), the chemical potentials of components A and B are interrelated, according to the Gibbs–Duhem relation. If the activity of one component increases, that of the other must decrease. (Neither the enthalpy nor the entropy of a solution belongs solely to component A or component B.) When there are three components (or more), one cannot predict even the sign, let alone the magnitude, of the changes in potential of components 2 and 3 that result from a change in the potential of component 1.

However, independently of the number of components in the solution, interacting components must interact reciprocally (according to the Gibbs–Bjerrum relation); if protein binds water, then water binds protein. To take and expand the example given by Edsall and Gutfreund [50], suppose that the addition of CO_2 to a solution of haemoglobin increases the chemical potential of O_2; we can then say: (a) that adding O_2 must reciprocally increase the potential of CO_2 (Bjerrum), and (b) that the potential of something else in the solution must go down (Duhem).

It would seem, therefore, that concentrated protein solutions such as the cytoplasm, in which the volume fraction of water might be as low as 0.8, could have the following non-ideal properties: (a) the activity of the protein might be higher than predicted from its mole fraction on the assumption of ideality; (b) the activity of the solvent water (displayed in measurements of osmotic pressure, freezing point, etc.) might be lower than predicted on that basis; and (c) the activity of other components might then go up or down.

Role of concentration and activity in the kinetics and thermodynamics of reaction pathways

Does reaction rate depend on concentration or activity?

For some 20 years, between the two World Wars, it was assumed that rates of chemical (and enzymic) reactions were governed not by concentrations, but by activities. Since the 1940s the opposite view has prevailed. Why is that?

The position of thermodynamic equilibria is indeed governed by the activities of the reactants. For reversible reactions there is usually good agreement between the (thermodynamic) equilibrium constant and the ratio of the forward and reverse rate (kinetic) constants. The neatness of this correlation led to a widespread assumption that rates should be expressed in terms of the activities of reactants and products (see, for example, [54], and our discussion of diffusion above).

However, for perfect gases and ideal solutions, it is clear that the frequency of collision is a simple geometrical function of volume concentration (e.g. on a molar scale). Furthermore, experimental results with near-perfect gases showed that rates were best described in terms of volume concentrations. [49]. It is true that, for non-ideal solutes, velocity constants expressed in terms of molarities are not strictly constant, but vary with concentration and ionic strength. However, the use of activities does not improve matters. Current practice is to express rates in terms of molarities, with correcting terms if necessary; and current understanding is that the initial collision of reacting molecules is indeed determined by volume concentration (not activity), while subsequent steps (progress towards, and eventually through, the transition state) are influenced by various non-idealities (intermolecular forces, dielectric constants, etc.).

It will be obvious by now that nothing is as clear-cut as we would like, and that alternative models are often equally valid. As an extreme illustration of both this and the roles of activity and concentration in determining rate, consider the activity and concentration of protons in water at pH 7.0 and in 100 mM aqueous potassium phosphate at pH 7.0. Visualize these two solutions separated by a thin glass membrane permeable only to dehydrated protons (H^+) as, for example, in a pH electrode. We note that no protons move across the membrane and conclude that proton activity is the same in each solution. But is the (molar) proton concentration in each phase 10^{-7} M, or are we talking about the hydronium ion OH_3^+? If being liganded to water does not worry us, then what about the protons liganded to phosphate? Do we therefore have 1.5×10^{-1} M protons in that phase? If activity determines the rates of reaction (diffusion etc.), then these should be the same in each solution, but experiment shows that this is by no means always the case (see, e.g., [55,56], and the concept of general acid catalysis).

Does binding raise or lower activity or concentration?

Binding of substrate to an enzyme surface presumably lowers activity, but may raise volume concentration, and hence reaction rate.

Tryptophan synthase

There is little doubt that channelling occurs in the case of the tryptophan synthase bienzyme complex. (Whereas the bacterial enzyme is isolated as an $\alpha\beta\beta\alpha$ tetramer, the $\alpha\beta$ subunits are covalently joined in the fungal enzyme into a multidomain peptide; cf. the AROM complex discussed in Chapter 9 in the current volume.) It has long been known that the two reactions (indole 3-glycerophosphate cleavage to indole and glyceraldehyde 3-phosphate on the one hand, and the formation of tryptophan and water from serine and indole on the other) are catalysed by different active sites (α and β respectively), and that indole is not released as a free intermediate into the medium [57]. X-ray crystallography of the bacterial complex [58] has resolved a cavity or tunnel extending 25–30 Å through the β subunit linking the two active sites which is wide enough to accommodate one, and long enough to accommodate four, indole molecules (Fig. 8). Furthermore, the results of inhibitor studies [59] make it very probable that indole passes down the tunnel during the physiological reaction (tryptophan synthesis from indole 3-glycerophosphate and serine). However, it is not so clear why the enzymes are arranged in this way.

It is true that the $\alpha\beta\beta\alpha$ tetramer is more kinetically efficient than the separated subunits, but this appears to be the result of reciprocal, long-range, protein–protein interactions [60]. Thus the binding of L-serine causes a 400-fold increase in association between the α and β subunits, while association reciprocally enhances the binding of serine by the same factor [61]. Association of the α subunit speeds the reaction of the β subunit some 30-fold [61], while the cleavage of indole 3-glycerophosphate by $\alpha\beta\beta\alpha$ is accelerated 150-fold when serine binds to the β subunit [62]. Even with this enhancement, cleavage, at $24\,s^{-1}$, is one of the slower steps in the overall reaction, limited to $8\,s^{-1}$ by the very slow release of tryptophan. It seems naive to assume that juxtaposition and channelling in this case are merely to speed the overall pathway.

Other factors to consider are: (a) unwanted side reactions, and (b) thermodynamics. The holoenzyme catalyses β-replacement of the serine hydroxy group by the rather poor nucleophile indole. Thiols are far better nucleophiles. The isolated β subunit will catalyse β-elimination and deamination of serine and the deamination of tryptophan (to indole, pyruvate and ammonia); these reactions are strongly inhibited by the α subunit [61]. It is tempting to see the channel (tunnel) as being able to restrict the nature of

---

Fig. 8   Tryptophan synthase bienzyme

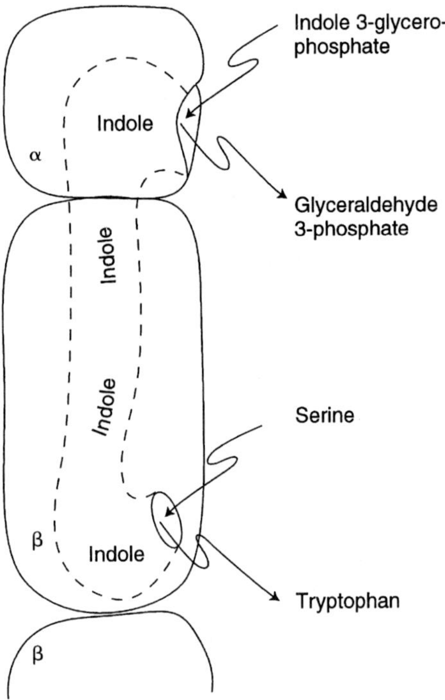

The figure shows half of the $\alpha\beta\beta\alpha$ tetramer, and the tunnel channelling indole from the α to the β active site. (After [59].)

the nucleophile offered to the activated, aminoacrylate, form of the serine–pyridoxal-phosphate complex; almost anything else might react faster than indole, but only indole is offered.

Peter Mitchell visualized, for isocitrate dehydrogenase ($NADP^+$-requiring), a bienzyme structure exactly as is now observed for tryptophan synthase; but he wanted one reaction to drive the other thermodynamically, a process he called micro-chemiosmosis [1,63]. That has yet to be demonstrated here; the question of thermodynamics has scarcely been touched upon. Wiesinger and Hinz [64] pointed this out, and presented some data on the enthalpies of the α and β reactions (α is endenthalpic; β is exenthalpic), but that is not enough; we need the free energies. If there turns out to be negligible or compensating entropic changes and the β reaction turns out to be exergonic, with an endergonic α reaction, we would have the spectacle of the β reaction pulling the α reaction, displacing an unfavourable equilibrium by removing one of the products.

Conclusions

Many different types of channelling undoubtedly exist, and doubtless serve a number of purposes; covalently tethered intermediates, multidomain peptides, multienzyme complexes, tunnelling bienzymes, etc., may have evolved to direct the pathways of metabolism, to couple energy-yielding to energy-requiring reactions. They may even have evolved to speed sluggish pathways or to minimize transients (lags and bursts). These last kinetic aspects are still the most nebulous and controversial.

From the considerations raised in this chapter, it seems likely that, in the prokaryotic cytoplasm, free diffusion between uniformly dispersed enzymes is seldom slow enough to limit enzymic pathways. Immediately we depart from uniform dispersion, however, we see concentration gradients forming. Thus even in *E. coli* there are appreciable gradients between medium and cytoplasm during galactoside uptake. Eukaryotic cytoplasm presents obstacles to diffusion which may be looked on as collectively lowering gross diffusion constants by a factor of between 10 and 40. At the same time specialization in these much larger cells first allows, and then demands, localization; as soon as enzymes are no longer uniformly dispersed, diffusion paths start to lengthen, and as they lengthen they slow up (with a square power dependence). Under these circumstances we could look for kinetic effects of diffusion, and kinetic benefits from juxtaposition.

I am grateful to Peter Nicholls and Phillip Jewsbury for helpful discussions and to Stanley Sherratt for stimulating my interest in this topic.

References

1. Mitchell, P. (1981) in Of Oxygen, Fuels, and Living Matter (Semenza, G., ed.), part 1, pp. 1–160, John Wiley and Sons Ltd., Chichester
2. Ovádi, J. (1991) J. Theor. Biol. **152**, 1–22
3. Webb, J.L. (1963) Enzyme and Metabolic Inhibitors, vol. 1, Academic Press, New York
4. Kuntz, I.D. and Kauzmann, W. (1974) Adv. Protein Chem. **28**, 239–345
5. Rupley, J.A. and Careri, G. (1991) Adv. Protein Chem. **41**, 38–172
6. Noyes, R.M. (1961) Prog. Reaction Kinetics **1**, 129–160
7. Bockris, J.O. and Reddy, A.K.N. (1970) Modern Electrochemistry, vol. 1, Plenum, New York
8. Feynman, R.P., Leighton, R.B. and Sands, M. (1963) The Feynman Lectures on Physics, Addison-Wesley Publishing Co., Reading, MA
9. Hasinoff, B.B. (1984) Arch. Biochem. Biophys. **233**, 676–681
10. Hasinoff, B.B. (1982) Biochim. Biophys. Acta **704**, 52–58
11. Hasinoff, B.B. and Chishti, S.B. (1982) Biochemistry **21**, 4275–4278
12. Tian, W.D., Sage, J.T. and Champion, P.M. (1993) J. Mol. Biol. **233**, 155–166
13. Sakan, Y., Kitagawa, T. and Frauenfelter, F.A. (1993) Biochemistry **32**, 5815–5824
14. Balasubramanian, S., Lambright, D.G., Simmons, J.H., Gill, S.J. and Boxer, S.G. (1994) Biochemistry **33**, 8355–8360
15. Hong, M.K., Braunstein, D., Cowen, B.R., Frauenfelder, H., Iben, I.E., Mourant, J.R., Ormos, P., Scholl, R., Schulte, A. and Steinbach, P.J. (1990) Biophys. J. **58**, 429–436
16. Ormos, P., Ansari, A., Braunstein, D., Cowen, B.R., Frauenfelder, H., Hong, M.K., Iben, I.E., Sauke, T.B., Steinbach, P.J. and Young, R.D. (1990) Biophys. J. **57**, 191–199
17. Jewsbury, P. and Kitagawa, T. (1994) Biophys. J. **67**, 2236–2250
18. Gibson, Q.H., Olson, J.S., McKinnie, R.E. and Rohlfs, R.J. (1986) J. Biol. Chem. **261**, 10228–10239
19. Frauenfelder, H., Sligar, S.G. and Wolynes, P.G. (1991) Science **254**, 1598–1603
20. Steinbach, P.J., Ansari, A., Berendzen, J., Braunstein, D., Chu, K., Cowen, B.R., Ehrenstein, D., Frauenfelder, H., Johnson, J.B. and Lamb, D.C. (1991) Biochemistry **30**, 3988–4001
21. Moore, W.J. (1962) Physical Chemistry, Longman, London
22. Mitchell, P. (1967) Adv. Enzymol. Relat. Areas Mol. Biol. **29**, 33–87
23. West, I.C. (1983) The Biochemistry of Membrane Transport, Chapman and Hall, London
24. West, I.C. (1991) J. Bioenerg. Biomembr. **23**, 703–714
25. West, I.C. (1995) in Biomembranes, vol. 1: General Principles (Lee, A.G., ed.), pp. 225–243, JAI Press, Greenwich, CT
26. Robinson, R.A. and Stokes, R.H. (1968) Electrolyte Solutions, Butterworth, London
27. Lieb, W.R. and Stein, W.D. (1986) in Transport and Diffusion Across Cell Membranes (Stein, W.D., ed.), pp. 69–112, Academic Press, San Diego
28. Kao, H.P., Abney, J.R. and Verkman, A.S. (1993) J. Cell Biol. **120**, 175–184
29. Hou, L., Lanni, F. and Luby-Phelps, K. (1990) Biophys. J. **58**, 31–43
30. Luby-Phelps, K. (1994) Curr. Opin. Cell Biol. **6**, 3–9
31. Bicknese, S., Periasamy, N., Shohet, S.B. and Verkman, A.S. (1993) Biophys. J. **65**, 1272–1282
32. Luby-Phelps, K., Mujumdar, S., Mujumdar, R.B., Ernst, L.A., Galbraith, W. and Waggoner, A.S. (1993) Biophys. J. **65**, 236–242
33. Fushimi, K. and Verkman, A.S. (1991) J. Cell Biol. **112**, 719–725
34. Kao, H.P. and Verkman, A.S. (1994) Biophys. J. **67**, 1291–1300
35. Luby-Phelps, K., Castle, P.E., Taylor, D.L. and Lanni, F. (1987) Proc. Natl. Acad. Sci. U.S.A. **84**, 4910–4913
36. Goldstein, L. (1976) Methods Enzymol. **44**, 397–450
37. West, I.C. and Page, M.G.P. (1984) J. Theor. Biol. **110**, 11–19
38. Edwards, P.A.W. (1974) Biochim. Biophys. Acta **345**, 373–386
39. Regen, D.M. and Tarpley, H.L. (1974) Biochim. Biophys. Acta **339**, 218–233
40. Lieb, W.R. and Stein, W.D. (1974) Biochim. Biophys. Acta **373**, 178–196
41. Berry, P.H. and Diamond, J.M. (1984) Physiol. Rev. **64**, 763–872

42. Holland, R.A., Shibata, H., Scheid, P. and Piiper, J. (1985) Respir. Physiol. **59**, 71–91
43. Berne, R.M. and Levy, M.N. (1993) Physiology, Mosby-Year Book, St. Louis, MO
44. Chance, B., Schoener, B. and Schindler, F. (1964) in Oxygen in the Animal Organism (Dickens, F. and Neil, E., eds.), pp. 367–388, Pergamon Press, Oxford
45. Berridge, M.J. (1990) J. Biol. Chem. **268**, 9583–9586
46. Kargacin, G.J. (1994) Biophys. J. **67**, 262–272
47. Allbritton, N., Meyer, T. and Stryer, L. (1992) Science **258**, 1812–1815
48. Ben-Naim, A. (1978) J. Phys. Chem. **82**, 792–803
49. Denbigh, K. (1971) The Principles of Chemical Equilibrium, Cambridge University Press, Cambridge
50. Edsall, J.T. and Gutfreund, H. (1983) Biothermodynamics: The Study of Biochemical Processes at Equilibrium, Wiley, Chichester
51. Flory, P.J. (1953) Principles of Polymer Chemistry, Cornell University Press, Ithaca
52. Tanford, C. (1961) Physical Chemistry of Macromolecules, Wiley, New York
53. Fast, J.D. (1962) Entropy, Philips Technical Library, Eindhoven
54. Minton, A.P. (1983) Mol. Cell. Biochem. **55**, 119–140
55. Engasser, J.M. and Horvath, C. (1974) Biochim. Biophys. Acta **358**, 178–192
56. Jonsson, B. and Wennerström, H. (1978) Biophys. Chem. **7**, 285–292
57. Yanofsky, C. (1989) Biochim. Biophys. Acta **1000**, 133–137
58. Hyde, C.C., Ahmed, S.A., Padlan, E.A., Miles, E.W. and Davies, D.R. (1988) J. Biol. Chem. **263**, 17857–17871
59. Dunn, M.F., Aguilar, V., Brzovic, P., Drewe, W.F., Jr., Houben, K.F., Leja, C.A. and Roy, M. (1990) Biochemistry **29**, 8598–8607
60. Kirschner, K., Lane, A.N. and Strasser, A.W. (1991) Biochemistry **30**, 472–478
61. Miles, E.W. (1991) Adv. Enzymol. Relat. Areas Mol. Biol. **64**, 93–172
62. Anderson, K.S., Miles, E.W. and Johnson, K.A. (1991) J. Biol. Chem. **266**, 8020–8033
63. West, I.C. (1992) Mol. Microbiol. **6**, 3623–3625
64. Wiesinger, H. and Hinz, H.J. (1985) Arch. Biochem. Biophys. **242**, 440–446
65. Fehrenbach, A., Einspanier, A., Nicksch, E. and Hodges, J.K. (1995) Tissue Cell **27**, 467–481

3

The consequences of macromolecular crowding for metabolic channelling

Mark M. Garner

Section on Macromolecular Analysis, Laboratory of Theoretical and Physical Biology, National Institute of Child Health and Human Development, National Institutes of Health, and FMC BioProducts, 191 Thomaston St., Rockland, ME 04841, U.S.A.

"There is a transcendence in biology which is essentially foreign to chemistry or physics. In these sciences we are allowed to play with stacked cards; and no harm will come from this, though the decks may have to be changed every thirty years. In biology, we do this at our own risk. The chemist presides over a comfortably closed universe, that of the biologist is wide open. Chemists do not have to bother about what could be called the sociology of molecules; the cell practices a form of togetherness for which the New York subway in the rush hour is a most inadequate model. But the cell is certainly more than a chemical slum. What is this 'more'?"

Erwin Chargaff [1]

Introduction

The ability of biological scientists to translate results obtained from studies performed on purified biological macromolecules in dilute, simple salt solutions to the behaviour of these same molecules inside living cells is remarkable. Even 'simple' bacterial cells have cytoplasmic protein concentrations of hundreds of milligrams/ml, phenomenal concentrations of DNA and RNA, with their associated ligands and counter-ions, as well as millimolar to molar concentrations of inorganic salts and charged and uncharged organic osmolytes [2,3]. Although these additional components are often thought of as being inert or, at most, exerting only non-specific effects on reactions of interest, it is now clear that such components can be an integral part of cellular regulation. Experiments with purified components in simple salt solutions are invaluable for elucidating the specificity of biological macromolecules. However, extrapolation from such data to behaviour inside a cell can be hazardous.

This review will concentrate on the effects which the very high total cellular protein concentration in cells can have on reactions involving enzymes which, themselves, are present at very low concentrations. It is this coupling between total macromolecular concentration and the activity (in the thermodynamic sense) of a particular species present at low concentration which gives rise to the phenomenon referred to as macromolecular *crowding*. Significant concentrations of small-molecule substances are also known to affect macromolecule equilibria [4], as does the reduced water activity presumably present inside cells [5], and these effects have been reviewed elsewhere. Several recent reviews of macromolecular crowding, considering the physical chemical phenomenon and the physiological consequences, have appeared [6–8]. Here, I will concentrate on describing the phenomenon of macromolecular crowding, and on some first attempts at applying these concepts to the behaviour of specific systems in the context of what consequences these effects will have on the formation of large, multienzyme complexes involved in the channelling of intermediates in metabolism.

Phenomenology

The clearest description of macromolecular crowding is simply to describe one way in which it can be measured. Let us suppose that one can, more or less directly, measure the thermodynamic activity of water in a solution of a single protein as a function of the concentration of that protein. Because of the Gibbs–Duhem relation, one can calculate the change in sol*ute* (protein) activity from the change in sol*vent* (water) activity, provided that any other activities remain constant. Since, in any real system, it is the thermodynamic activities (and not the concentrations) which are relevant, changes in the solute activity will affect any reaction (aggregation, ligand binding, enzyme catalysis) in which the protein in question participates.

Such experiments were done as long ago as 1927 using haemoglobin [9]. Adair measured the osmotic pressure (which directly relates to water activity) of haemoglobin solutions as a function of haemoglobin concentration. Fig. 1 shows the results, plotted with those expected if the system were behaving ideally. Clearly, at a physiological concentration of protein (approx. 300–400 mg/ml), the system behaves very non-ideally: the resulting osmotic pressure is almost six times that expected. Also, the data fit very well to the characteristic virial expansion, i.e. the osmotic pressure (π) increases as a power series with respect to protein concentration (c):

$$\pi = RTc + Ac^2 + Bc^3 + Cc^4 + \ldots \tag{1}$$

Ross and Minton [10] were able to calculate exactly the coefficients in this virial expansion, using the hard particle interaction coefficients of haemoglobin in solution (i.e. the two, three, four etc. body interactions) based on the known radius of a haemoglobin molecule and the concentration profile. From this, one can extract the dependence of the activity coefficient γ on the concentration of haemoglobin (the details of the calculation are discussed in [10]). The results of such a calculation are shown in Fig. 2. Two features readily emerge: at physiological concentration (>300 mg/ml) the non-ideality of the protein is enormous, and, in this concentration range, small changes in concentration lead to huge changes in the activity coefficient. The activity coefficient at 400 mg/ml is over 500, i.e. at 400 mg/ml the activity of haemoglobin is equivalent to a concentration of 200 000 mg/ml! Just as important is the dramatic sensitivity of the activity coefficient to concentration: a 33% change in protein concentration (300 to 400 mg/ml) results in a greater than 10-fold change in activity (Fig. 2, inset). It should be noted that the virial expansion method is not simply curve-fitting to the osmotic pressure data; the coefficients in the expansion were calculated assuming only a molecular size and concentration for haemoglobin, and these

Fig. 1 **Osmotic pressure of haemoglobin solutions as a function of concentration**

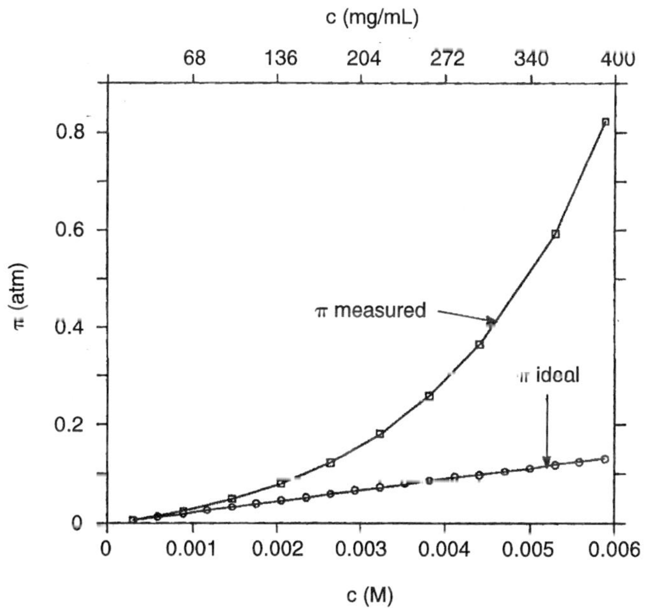

Osmotic pressure (π) measurements are from Adair [9]. π_{ideal} was calculated assuming a simple linear relationship between solute concentration and osmotic pressure: $\pi = RTc$. 1 atm = 101.3 kPa.

calculated coefficients were shown to precisely account for the available osmotic pressure versus concentration data [10].

In addition to virial expansion methods, one can adequately model concentration-dependence data such as those in Fig. 1 using a statistical mechanical method known as Scaled Particle Theory (SPT) [11,12]. SPT allows one to calculate the activity coefficient of the test molecule as a power series of its radius, the coefficients of which are determined by the number density (concentration) and sizes of all other molecules in solution. Thus the only inputs into the calculations are the concentrations and sizes of all macromolecules. The advantage of SPT is that it is applicable to mixtures of differently sized molecules, whereas this is not currently tractable using a virial expansion-type method. In addition, it is not necessary to assume that

---

Fig. 2   Activity coefficient of haemoglobin as a function of concentration

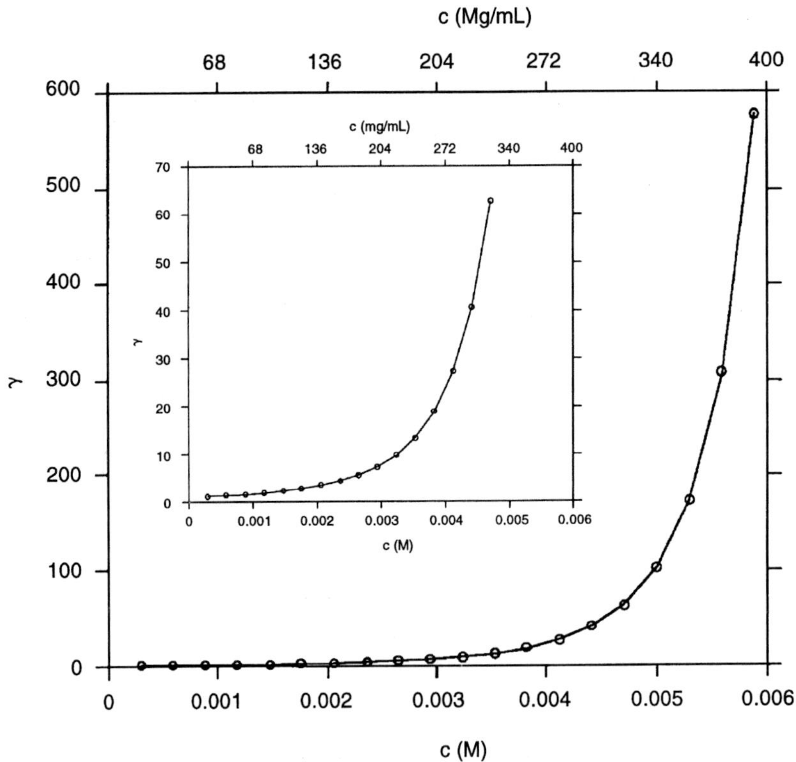

The activity coefficient (γ) was calculated using virial expansion. Data are taken from the calculations of Ross and Minton [6,10]. Inset: expansion of the figure to show the transition to a very steep change in γ as the concentration (c) approaches physiological.

the molecules are spherical; however, even using SPT it is not possible to do calculations for solutions containing mixtures of molecules of different shapes.

Molecular basis of crowding

Independent of any calculation of activity coefficients, it might be useful to develop a sense of the molecular origin of crowding, and the consequences it will have for proteins in solution. Protein molecules are crowded in solution because they exclude each other from occupying the same space. This is

---

Fig. 3   **Schematic illustration to show the source of non-ideality in crowded solutions**

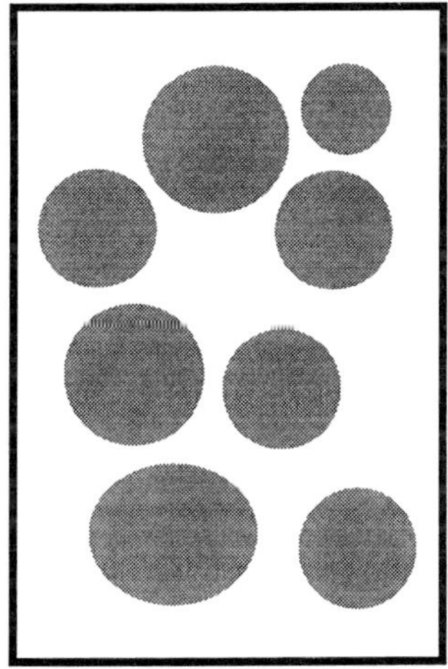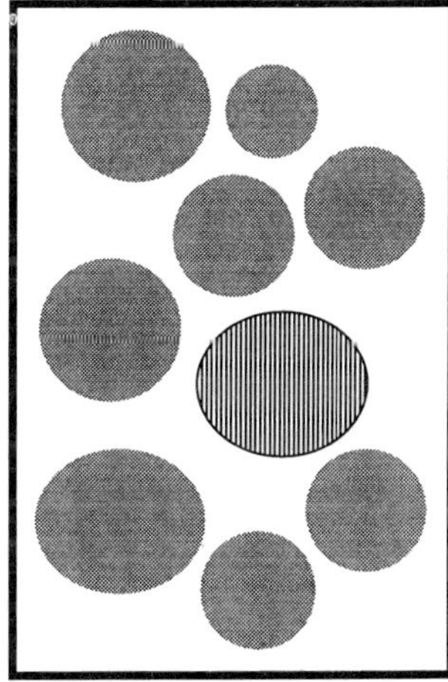

In both the left and right solutions the concentration and shape of the background (filled) molecules are the same. However, in the solution on the right the background molecules have been 'organized' to create a cavity to accommodate the test molecule (vertically shaded). The concomitant loss of configurational entropy is responsible for the increase in the activity coefficient. Reproduced from [5] with permission.

---

shown schematically in Fig. 3. In the left panel, it is impossible to fit the 'test' protein molecule into the solution because of the distribution of the other protein molecules in the solution. This is true even though there is sufficient room in the total solution to hold the test protein. By ordering the other protein molecules (Fig. 3, right panel), it is possible to fit the test protein into the solution. SPT essentially calculates the reversible work needed to create a hole in the solution big enough to fit the test protein into [12]. This ordering, of course, costs configurational entropy (or, equivalently, reversible work must be expended to create the cavity). As more and more of the solution volume is excluded to the test protein, either by increasing the present protein's concentration and/or by changing the sizes of the molecules, the non-ideality increases. This points to several of the most important qualitative features of macromolecular crowding.

1. The degree of non-ideality depends on the concentrations, sizes and shapes of all macromolecular species in a solution. All of these affect the way in which molecules can be packed into the solution, i.e. the volume that is inaccessible to the test protein.

2. Crowding is a *macromolecular* phenomenon. A small molecule can access essentially the entire volume of a solution, even one which has a very high protein concentration (by penetrating the interstices of the macromolecules). Attempts have been made [13] to account for the volume occupied by water in a crowded solution; the results of such calculations are qualitatively very similar to those which treat the solvent as a dielectric continuum, but they give slightly different (usually lower) activity coefficients. The high protein concentration does, of course, exert some effect on the activity of small solutes (for example, see [6]), but this is small compared with macromolecular excluded volume effects.

3. Theories of macromolecular crowding account only for non-ideality due to volume exclusion. All calculations assume that no through-space interactions (e.g. electrostatic repulsion) occur between the macromolecules in solution. In real solutions such effects are superimposed on volume-exclusion effects. Alternatively, one can account for these by assuming increased or decreased size of the molecules of interest (see [14]).

4. Crowding affects all macromolecular species in the solution. Although one can designate a given protein as the 'test' molecule, this is really only a *Gedankenexperiment*. All macromolecules in a given solution will be excluded from a significant volume, which will depend on the sizes, shapes and concentrations of all species in solution.

Calculation of crowding effects

Because it is primarily a volume-exclusion phenomenon, macromolecular crowding will exert predictable effects on reactions involving proteins or other macromolecules. Essentially, any association reaction or conformational change which lowers the total volume in solution occupied by the reactants will be favoured by macromolecular crowding. For example, if we take the well characterized binding reaction:

$$A + B \longleftrightarrow AB$$

the thermodynamic binding constant for this reaction would b ·

$$K_{eq} = \frac{[AB] \times \gamma_{AB}}{([A] \times \gamma_A)([B] \times \gamma_B)}$$

$$= \frac{[AB]}{[A][B]} \times \frac{\gamma_{AB}}{\gamma_A \times \gamma_B}$$

i.e.

$$K_{eq} = K_{app} \times \Gamma$$

where K_{app} is the phenomenological (measured) association constant, and:

$$\Gamma = \frac{\gamma_{AB}}{\gamma_A \times \gamma_B}$$

It can be seen from this that the ratio of activity coefficients of product and reactant macromolecules is the factor which determines the effects of crowding on equilibria involving macromolecules (hence the emphasis in the above discussion on activity coefficient calculation). Limiting cases of this include the following. (1) If species A is a small-molecule ligand, then any crowding effects on the equilibrium will be determined by the difference in volume occupied by macromolecule B in its liganded and unliganded states (i.e. if B undergoes a conformational change in which the bound state has a larger volume than the unbound state). (2) If species A is massive relative to everything else in solution (i.e. a membrane or large DNA molecule) the reaction can be treated as a phase transition ('squeezing' B out of solution). γ_A and γ_{AB} will cancel out, and the crowding effect will be determined by the activity coefficient of free B [3,15,16]. (3) If A and B are both macromolecules of comparable size, crowding effects will be determined by the difference in volume between AB and the sum of A and B [17].

Experimental measures of crowding phenomena

Volume-exclusion effects have been systematically measured in only a few cases. The most extensive studies have been carried out by Zimmerman and co-workers [7,16,18–20] on crowding effects on protein–nucleic acid interactions. These studies have shown that moderate to high concentrations of inert macromolecules have dramatic effects on the binding of gene-regulatory proteins to DNA. In all cases, crowding dramatically enhances the protein–DNA association, by factors up to three orders of magnitude. This effect is independent of the chemical nature of the added background macromolecule [poly(ethylene glycol), dextran and BSA all behave similarly], consistent with volume exclusion being the source of the enhancement. The apparent salt sensitivity of DNA polymerase I from *Escherichia coli* is dramatically affected by the presence of crowding agents, shifting complex stability to a salt concentration much closer to physiological [20]. This illustrates the importance of considering crowding effects when making predictions of *in vivo* behaviour based on *in vitro* studies.

In addition, the processivity of the multiprotein T4 DNA replication complex is greatly increased by crowding agents. The latter is due to stabilization of the multiprotein complex as well as enhanced binding of the complex to DNA [21].

In all of the above the volume-exclusion effects are quite large, and always act in the direction of driving protein–DNA association, presumably because both the ligand and substrate are macromolecules. Independent estimates of the magnitude of such effects on gene-regulatory proteins *in vivo* all predict an important role for macromolecular crowding in genetic regulation, via controlling the extent of protein–DNA complex-formation. Since, in *Escherichia coli* at least, the cytoplasmic protein concentration can vary by as much as 40% in response to changes in extracellular osmolarity, such effects have been invoked to explain the apparent *functional* homoeostasis of gene expression in the presence of changes in composition [3,15,16].

Similar modelling studies were carried out to attempt to explain the volume-regulatory response of canine erythrocytes [22,23]. In these cells the flux through ion transporters which control cellular volume appears to be tightly coupled to the cytoplasmic protein concentration. A plausible model based on crowding-controlled binding of a regulatory kinase to a membrane-associated regulatory protein has been presented.

The important conclusion from the *E. coli* and erythrocyte modelling studies is that complex biological phenomena cannot be adequately explained without identifying and accounting for all significant physiological effectors, even those which would appear to be innocuous or non-specific, such as cellular protein concentration.

Confinement versus crowding

Any mathematically tractable model for even a simple cell such as *E. coli* will be a gross oversimplification. This is even more true of eukaryotic cells, which have extensive subcellular structure(s), such as the microtrabecular lattice, microtubules, endoplasmic reticulum, etc. It has proven possible to make estimates of the non-ideality caused by confining a protein in an organized matrix [24]. Qualitatively, confinement behaves like crowding: as less space is available for the test protein to occupy (or, alternatively, as the matrix occupies more volume), non-ideality increases dramatically. However, confinement tends to drive the formation of complexes which 'fit' into the matrix rather than simply those which occupy the minimal volume. Furthermore, in a confined system the matrix presents numerous sites for association with the test protein. In addition to the cytoskeleton affecting soluble protein, the high concentration of soluble proteins will have pronounced effects on the formation of cytoskeletal elements. High background protein concentration has been shown to drive microfilament bundle formation [25]. Hence a combination of soluble and matrix-associated proteins may be involved in the 'organization' of metabolism on the cytoskeleton [26].

The importance of considering the effects of the cytoskeleton is illustrated by measurements of the restriction of translational motion for various macromolecular-sized probes. In these studies the translational diffusion of fluorescently labelled derivatives of Ficoll of various molecular masses was measured in mixtures of unlabelled Ficoll (a globular polymer) and F-actin filaments [27,28]. Similar measurements were also done on probes which were micro-injected into Swiss 3T3 cells. The F-actin/Ficoll mixture which gave a molecular-size-dependence of the restriction of diffusion most similar to that of the cells was 5 mg/ml F-actin filaments + 10% Ficoll; neither alone at any concentration was sufficient [29]. The conclusion from these studies is that both the cytoskeleton and globular proteins affect the transport (and presumably other properties) of proteins in the cell, and that models based on either alone will be inadequate.

Macromolecular crowding and metabolic channelling

From the foregoing, it is clear that the primary effect of macromolecular crowding on channelling will be to drive the formation of specific multi-enzyme complexes inside the cell [30]. Even though enzymes which may participate in such complexes in the cell can be purified free of any other 'contaminating' activities after cell lysis, *in vivo* they may be part of large non-covalent complexes which allow for the direct transfer of substrates between enzymes. Unambiguous demonstration of the existence of such functional complexes is difficult. Furthermore, the organization of metabolic enzymes on subcellular structures [25,26] or in membranes is unlikely to survive after lysis procedures. It is not difficult to imagine that, in the course of purification, removal of the background cellular proteins causes multi-enzyme complexes which are functional *in vivo* to dissociate, allowing the individual functional enzymes to be purified away from each other. Hence much of the evidence for metabolic channelling has relied on *in vivo* enzyme kinetic data (for examples, see [31] and other chapters in this book), rather than direct demonstration of enzyme–enzyme complexes. Studies have shown, for example, that swelling of hepatocytes changes their pattern of metabolism: glycogen synthesis is increased [32] and proteolysis inhibited [33] in proportion to cell volume. However, it is difficult to directly correlate such studies with changes in macromolecular crowding, since both cellular protein and small-molecule concentrations are changing simultaneously. Such studies show that cell volume, and therefore cytoplasmic protein concentration, does have an effect on metabolic processes.

Clearly, isolation of specific, functional multienzyme complexes is a necessary first step in the *in vitro* verification and characterization of metabolic channelling. However, unambiguous isolation of such complexes is precisely what is often lacking. In this regard, the example of sickle cell haemoglobin polymerization may prove instructive. Using purified, dilute haemoglobin S in *in vitro* studies, it was observed that the polymerization reaction believed to be the cause of erythrocyte sickling occurs only at oxygen tensions greatly exceeding physiological [34]. However, if the polymerization is studied at concentrations of haemoglobin which approximate to those seen in erythrocytes, polymerization occurs at physiological oxygen tensions [35]. These results can be explained by the greatly elevated thermodynamic activity of haemoglobin in the red blood cell, or in concentrated solutions of haemoglobin, due to crowding effects. Both the extent [35] and rate [36] of this very specific protein–protein assembly reaction are affected by total protein concentration: physiological behaviour only emerges under conditions which more nearly approximate physiological. Given that enzyme assays are usually carried out with vanishingly small concentrations of enzyme in simple buffered salt solutions, with no other added macromolecules, it should not be surprising that specific multienzyme complexes are difficult to isolate. Furthermore, when one considers that the formation of such complexes may be unlikely to be easily reversible, the difficulty in demonstrating their existence *in vitro* is unsurprising.

Summary

A few of the concepts enunciated above may be worth re-iterating.

A very high macromolecular concentration is an inherent property of any biological system. In the process of purification, this property is progressively lost as 'contaminating' enzyme activities are purified away. However, even though the other proteins in the cell may not directly participate in the catalytic reaction of interest, removing them alters the behaviour of those proteins(s) which do participate in the reaction, sometimes in unpredictable ways. To put it slightly differently, biology is inherently messy, and any attempt to clean up its act risks removing the biology.

Specific protein–protein interactions which are known (based on biological activities) to occur inside cells can be drastically stimulated *in vitro* by concentrations of background macromolecules similar to, or even much lower than, those found inside the cell. It is perhaps unsurprising that, at the vanishingly low concentrations often used in assays, such complexes cannot be detected. This would seem to be a promising direction to pursue in the study of metabolic channelling.

Although this review has concentrated on excluded-volume effects, there are, of course, numerous other elements of cellular systems which are probably lost in simple *in vitro* studies. For example, oncotic pressure effects, which would result from the reduced water activity inside cells, have been shown to drastically affect macromolecular interactions [37]. These 'hydration' effects can be a source of highly specific, stabilizing energies [38]. In real cells, of course, both crowding and hydration, and many other sources of non-ideality, are all present. Although it is convenient to (physically or intellectually) isolate the specific effect from all others, it must be remembered that:

> "…in the living tissue many events take place simultaneously; precursors, intermediates, and end products are formed in close propinquity; everything happens on top of each other, apparently without getting in each other's way; proteins and nucleic acids, lipids and polysaccharides are assembled and deposited where they belong: all presumably under the supervision of the genome, which is quite busy reproducing itself."
>
> Erwin Chargaff [1]

References

1. Chargaff, E. (1968) Prog. Nucleic Acids Res. Mol. Biol. **8**, 297–333
2. Garcia-Perez, A. and Burg, M.B. (1991) Physiol. Rev. **71**, 1081–1115
3. Cayley, S., Lewis, B.A., Guttman, H.J. and Record, M.T., Jr. (1991) J. Mol. Biol. **222**, 281–300
4. Timasheff, S. (1993) Annu. Rev. Biophys. Biomol. Struct. **22**, 67–97
5. Garner, M.M. and Burg, M.B. (1994) Am. J. Physiol. **266**, C877–C892
6. Minton, A.P. (1983) Mol. Cell. Biochem. **55**, 119–140
7. Zimmerman, S. B. and Minton, A. (1993) Annu. Rev. Biophys. Biomol. Struct. **22**, 27–65
8. Zimmerman, S.B. (1993) Biochim. Biophys. Acta **1216**, 175–185
9. Adair, G. (1928) Proc. R. Soc. London **A120**, 573–603
10. Ross, P. and Minton, A. (1977) J. Mol. Biol. **112**, 437–452
11. Ross, P. and Minton, A. (1979) Biochem. Biophys. Res. Commun. **88**, 1308–1314
12. Lebowitz, J., Helfand, E. and Praestgaard, E.J. (1965) Chem. Phys. **43**, 774–779
13. Berg, O. (1990) Biopolymers **30**, 1027–1037
14. Minton, A. and Edelhoch, H. (1979) Biopolymers **21**, 1308–1314
15. Garner, M., Cayley, D. and Record, M.T., Jr. (1990) Biophys. J. **57**, 62a
16. Zimmerman, S. and Trach, S. (1991) J. Mol. Biol. **222**, 599–620
17. Chatelier, R. and Minton, A. (1987) Biopolymers **26**, 507–524
18. Zimmerman, S. and Pheiffer, B. (1983) Proc. Natl. Acad. Sci. U.S.A. **80**, 5852–5856
19. Zimmerman, S.B. and Harrison, B. (1987) Proc. Natl. Acad. Sci. U.S.A. **84**, 1871–1875
20. Zimmerman, S.B. and Trach, S.O. (1988) Biochim. Biophys. Acta **949**, 297–304
21. Jarvis, T., Ring, D., Daube, S. and von Hippel, P.H. (1990) J. Biol. Chem. **265**, 15160–15167
22. Colclasure, G.C. and Parker, J.C. (1992) J. Gen. Physiol. **100**, 1–10
23. Minton, A.P., Colclasure, C.G. and Parker, J.C. (1992) Proc. Natl. Acad. Sci. U.S.A. **89**, 10504–10506
24. Minton, A.P. (1992) Biophys. J. **63**, 1090–1100
25. Madden, T. and Herzfeld, J. (1993) Biophys. J. **65**, 1147–1154
26. Clegg, J.S. (1992) Curr. Top. Cell. Regul. **33**, 3–14
27. Luby-Phelps, K., Castle, P.E., Taylor, D.L and Lanni, F. (1987) Proc. Natl. Acad. Sci. U.S.A. **84**, 4910–4913
28. Hou, L., Lanni, F. and Luby-Phelps, K. (1990) Biophys. J. **58**, 31–43

29. Luby-Phelps, K., Mujumdar, S., Ernst, L., Galbraith, W. and Waggoner, A. (1993) Biophys. J. **65**, 236–242
30. Srivastava, D.K. and Bernhard, S.A. (1986) Curr. Top. Cell. Regul. **28**, 1–68
31. Srivastava, D.K. and Bernhard, S.A. (1987) Annu. Rev. Biophys. Biophys. Chem. **16**, 175–204
32. Baquet, A., Hue, L., Meijer, A.J., Van Woerkom, G.M. and Plomp, P.J.A.M. (1990) J. Biol. Chem. **265**, 955–959
33. Haussinger, D. and Lang, F. (1991) Cell. Physiol. Biochem. **1**, 121–130
34. Eaton, W.A. and Hofrichter, J. (1990) Adv. Protein Chem. **40**, 63–279
35. Minton, A. (1977) J. Mol. Biol. **110**, 89–103
36. Noguchi, C. (1984) Biophys. J. **45**, 1153–1158
37. Leiken, S., Parsegian, V.A., Rau, D.C. and Rand, P. (1993) Annu. Rev. Phys. Chem. **44**, 369–395
38. Garner, M.M. and Rau, D.C. (1995) EMBO J. **14**, 1257–1263

Kinetic consequences of channelling

Athel Cornish-Bowden

Laboratoire de Chimie Bactérienne, Centre National de la Recherche Scientifique, 31 chemin Joseph-Aiguier, B.P. 71, 13402 Marseille Cedex 20, France

> "Il est vrai que certaines paroles et certaines cérémonies suffisent pour faire périr un troupeau de moutons, pourvu qu'on y ajoute de l'arsenic."
>
> Voltaire (1771)

> "Channeling can become a tremendously powerful tool of information gathering, self-growth and life enrichment. It can help you do everything from choosing a career path that's right for you to finding the right mate."
>
> Leaflet found in a laundromat (1989)

Introduction

Direct transfer of metabolites between consecutive enzymes, or channelling, has been a controversial topic at two different levels. The first is essentially chemical and kinetic, and concerns the strength of the evidence that is adduced in favour of channelling in numerous specific systems. The second is physiological, and concerns the effects, or lack of them, that channelling will have on metabolic systems if it occurs. These two controversies are, of course, independent: one can reasonably believe it to be established beyond doubt that channelling occurs without necessarily accepting that it has any significant physiological consequences; alternatively, one can believe channelling to be of potential physiological importance while still denying the reality of most of the specific examples. The former position is similar to my own, whereas the latter appears to be that of Gutfreund and Chock [1]. In this chapter I shall mainly be concerned with the kinetic consequences of channelling, i.e. with the second controversy, but first I shall briefly review some of the arguments about its existence.

The question of whether channelling actually occurs in the systems where it is reported [1–4] is especially controversial if the enzymes involved in the channel do not form a stable complex. In such a case the channelling is said to be "dynamic", and it implies that diffusional encounter between two macromolecules, an enzyme–substrate complex and a second enzyme, may be faster than diffusion of the free product released by the first enzyme–substrate complex to the second enzyme. This is not impossible, of course, if the concentration of enzyme-bound intermediate is so much higher than that of the free intermediate that collisions between enzyme and enzyme-bound intermediates occur more often than between enzyme and free intermediates despite the faster diffusion of each free intermediate molecule. The corresponding problem does not arise in "static" channelling, where the enzymes form a stable complex that exists throughout the chemical process, and so no diffusion of macromolecules is required.

There is good evidence that NADH, the most extensively studied candidate for channelling, can indeed be transferred directly from one enzyme active site to another. This evidence comes in particular from the *enzyme buffering* method designed by Srivastava and Bernhard [5], which is most easily explained by reference to an example. Suppose one is interested in testing the possibility of direct transfer of NADH from glyceraldehyde 3-phosphate dehydrogenase to lactate dehydrogenase. The first requirement is to measure the kinetic parameters for the lactate dehydrogenase-catalysed oxidation of NADH at some suitable concentration of the other substrate, pyruvate. This is done initially in the absence of glyceraldehyde 3-phosphate dehydrogenase. The parameters allow one to calculate what the rate ought to be at any low concentration of NADH. If such a low concentration is simply achieved by adding less NADH, then one can, of course, check the validity of the calculation directly, and in a properly carried out experiment there should be full agreement between the observed rate and the rate calculated from the kinetic parameters. Suppose, however, that the lower free concentration is achieved by adding enough glyceraldehyde 3-phosphate dehydrogenase to bind almost all of the NADH. In this case there are two possible results: if the complex of NADH with glyceraldehyde 3-phosphate dehydrogenase has no reactivity with lactate dehydrogenase the rate of oxidation should be exactly the rate calculated from the free NADH concentration, which can itself be easily calculated from the known dissociation constant of the complex; on the other hand, if the glyceraldehyde 3-phosphate dehydrogenase–NADH complex is a substrate for lactate dehydrogenase the rate will be higher.

In this example the measured rate turned out to be 5–6 times faster than the calculated rate [5], and corresponding results have now been obtained for 20 or more pairs of enzymes [6], in many cases with discrepancies of more than 20-fold. Even a 5–6-fold discrepancy is far outside the range of experimental error, which is known from "control" experiments with pairs of enzymes with the wrong stereochemistry (see below) for direct transfer.

Such results are normally taken to indicate that NADH can indeed be channelled from one member of each such pair to the other. Before accepting this conclusion uncritically, however, we should consider two other possible explanations that do not involve channelling. One is that addition of a very large excess of the buffering enzyme may result in artefactual effects due to its capacity to catalyse the other reaction. In the example considered, the concentration of glyceraldehyde 3-phosphate dehydrogenase was of the order of 10^6-fold higher than that of lactate dehydrogenase. As a result, even 0.0005% contamination of the glyceraldehyde 3-phosphate dehydrogenase with lactate dehydrogenase (or a contaminant capable of catalysing the lactate dehydrogenase reaction) would suffice to produce a 6-fold increase in rate over the calculated value. Srivastava and Bernhard [5] were well aware of this danger and took care to eliminate it, and later workers have been equally careful. Nonetheless, it is easy to overlook the problems of contamination that can arise when one enzyme is present in enormous excess over the other and it is important to be conscious of it in any enzyme buffering experiment, especially as it is quite normal for dehydrogenase preparations to be contaminated with other dehydrogenases.

The second possibility is that the glyceraldehyde 3-phosphate dehydrogenase had some activating effect on the lactate dehydrogenase unrelated to the presence of NADH. This type of effect is difficult to eliminate in any one example (because one cannot do kinetic experiments in the absence of substrate), but it stretches credulity to regard it as a general explanation once the enzymes concerned have been classified into pairs that give positive effects and pairs that do not, as I now discuss.

Enzymes that use NADH as a substrate show a remarkable stereospecificity that contrasts with the behaviour of most other classes of enzyme. NADH has two non-equivalent H atoms that yield the same NAD^+ molecule on oxidation, and any dehydrogenase can in principle show specificity for one or the other; in contrast to most other classes of enzymes, for which all that catalyse the same sort of reaction normally have the same stereospecificity, dehydrogenases are about evenly divided between ones that use the pro-S and ones that use the pro-R H atom of NADH [7]. Benner favoured an explanation in terms of chemistry and evolutionary optimization of the individual enzymes [7], but an alternative is to suppose that opposite stereospecificity in consecutive enzymes is a precondition for direct transfer of NADH from one active site to another without requiring the molecule to rotate during the transfer. This would imply evolutionary selection for enzymes catalysing consecutive reactions to have opposite stereospecificity as a way to permit the possibility of channelling.

It turns out that there is an excellent correlation between pairs of enzymes that give a positive result in the enzyme buffering test and enzymes with opposite stereospecificity; indeed, all pairs with the same stereospecificity give a null result in the enzyme buffering test. If all of the positive results in the enzyme buffering test were due to an NADH-independent activation of one enzyme by another, one would have to attribute this correlation to chance; it is more reasonable to interpret it as evidence that NADH can indeed be directly transferred between enzymes with opposite stereospecificity but not between enzymes with the same stereospecificity.

Physiological effects of channelling

It would be quite possible for channelling to occur quite widely even if it had no significant physiological effects, as it could reflect either chemical necessity or a frozen accident of evolutionary history. Srivastava and Bernhard [5], indeed, were careful to avoid any claim that their observations could be explained in terms of benefit to the organism: "At this time, we are unable to provide a convincing teleological argument for the phenomenon". Nonetheless, the level of passion aroused by discussions of metabolite channelling surely reflects a belief, not always explicitly stated, that if it occurs then it must be metabolically important [8]. One may even find authors who argue simultaneously that channelling does not exist but that if it did it would constitute the discovery of the century, a discovery that should be credited to one of themselves [1]! Even if this attributes an exaggerated importance to channelling it reinforces the relevance of examining its physiological effects.

There have been various suggestions, including several in other chapters of this book, that channelling can prevent accumulation of intermediates, which might strain the solvent capacity of the cell, or that it may prevent unwanted diversion of intermediates into competing pathways [8]. These two ideas are rather different from one another: if channelling occurred primarily to prevent accumulation of intermediates one should find it in long unbranched pathways; if it occurred primarily to restrict competition one should see it in highly branched pathways.

Srere [9] has estimated that around 80% of metabolites "have just one use in the cell", in the sense that they do not occur at branch points, and suggests that this is a reason to expect channelling in unbranched pathways. NADH, however, is about as far from a metabolite with just one use in the cell as one can imagine, and yet it is involved in many of the experimental examples. The idea that channelling of NADH exists to prevent competition and that, in effect, there are as many independent pools of NADH in any compartment as there are stereochemically compatible pairs of dehydrogenases is not one that everyone can easily entertain. This, indeed, may explain the reluctance of Srivastava and Bernhard [5] to propose a teleological explanation of NADH channelling.

On the other hand fatty acid metabolism offers what must surely be the longest unbranched pathways in metabolism, as Osmundsen and colleagues discuss in Chapter 15 of this book: in β-oxidation there are 28 steps between palmitoyl-CoA and acetyl-CoA, with 27 intermediates, none of which has any other major role in metabolism; fatty acid synthesis provides a similar picture. The organization of the enzymes of animal fatty acid synthesis into a well defined multienzyme complex ([10]; see also

Chapter 8 of the current volume) supports the idea that preventing intermediates from accumulating may be an important function. Corresponding complexes in β-oxidation were unknown in mammalian systems until the recent identification of a three-enzyme complex located in the mitochondrial inner membrane [11], but even so the possibility of channelling in β-oxidation has long been considered likely as an explanation for the low concentrations detected of the intermediates [12]. More sensitive techniques now allow many intermediates to be detected [13], but the concentrations are low enough for them still to be regarded as evidence for channelling [14].

The idea that channelling provides a means of lowering free concentrations of metabolic intermediates, thereby relieving the limiting solvent capacity of the cytoplasm, is often attributed, directly or indirectly, to Atkinson [15]. However, although the word "channeling" does occur in the passage referred to, it is clear from a careful reading that it is used in a very general sense and does not imply direct transfer of metabolites from one active site to another, i.e. there is no implication of metabolite channelling as the term is understood in this book; on the contrary, Atkinson's argument is that the need to conserve solvent capacity has necessitated the evolution of highly efficient enzymes capable of removing products as rapidly as they are released.[1] One of the aims of this chapter will be, in fact, to argue that Atkinson's own conclusion is the correct one, i.e. that efficient removal of products by enzymes with kinetic constants within the ranges observed for many enzymes is quite sufficient to explain the low concentrations of intermediates in long pathways such as β-oxidation. So although these low concentrations do not of course exclude the possibility of channelling, they do not require it either.

Are free concentrations smaller in channelled systems?

The supposed link between channelling and intermediate concentrations is actually less clear than it may appear from superficial study. Computer modelling studies [16] indicated that at a fixed net flux through a pathway the free concentrations of the intermediates in the steady state were independent of the degree of channelling. This work was open to an objection that can be applied to any computer simulation study, namely that it depended on the specific numerical values used in the simulation and that other values might have yielded concentrations that changed with the degree of channelling [17]. However, more recent analysis [18] used algebraic rather than numerical results, and showed, incidentally, how the apparent counter-examples [17] arose from misinterpretation of the data.

It is still possible to argue, of course, that the conditions applied in our analysis were too restrictive. Is it necessary to insist, for example, that effects on steady-state concentrations can only be linked with channelling if

---

[1] *I thank Dan Atkinson (personal communication) for confirming that I interpret his meaning as he intended.*

the parameter change (or combination of changes) that results in increased channelling is accompanied by no change in net flux through the pathway? Or that increasing channelling should be accompanied by no change in the total catalytic capacity of the enzymes between which the metabolite is transferred? Or that the catalytic activities of these enzymes should not change with respect to one another? Or that there should be no changes in the equilibrium constants relating the free concentration of the channelled metabolite to the free concentrations of other metabolites in the system?

The last of these is easily dealt with, as no change in a catalyst can alter an equilibrium constant unless it is acting in part as a reagent rather than a catalyst, and so any simulation purporting to represent the possibilities of enzyme evolution should leave equilibrium constants between free metabolites untouched.

The other restrictions are more arguable, but despite extensive discussion with others with different opinions, we continue to believe that they are necessary if one is to avoid the fallacy of *post hoc, ergo propter hoc* that Voltaire ridiculed long ago in the passage quoted at the beginning of this chapter. Our position is nicely summed up by the title of an article by Heinrich and Schuster [19]: "Is metabolic channelling the complicated solution to the easy problem of reducing transient times?". This applies as well to intermediate concentrations as to transient times, and it implies that we should be cautious about supposing that evolutionary pressure to solve particular problems will produce channelling if the same problems could easily be solved without channelling.

As an example, it has been known for many years that decreasing the activity of an enzyme in a pathway will tend to increase the concentration of its substrate and decrease that of its product, whereas increasing it will have the opposite effects [20]. If two consecutive enzymes in a pathway are modulated in opposite directions the effects on the common intermediate will reinforce one another even if their effects on the net flux cancel each other out. Even though indiscriminate misapplication of the "cross-over theorem" to numerous inappropriate systems led to serious confusion in the literature, as discussed by Heinrich and Rapoport [21], it remains quite valid in relation to linear pathways or linear segments of pathways if it is not complicated by regulatory loops. It follows that if one increases the degree of channelling in a model in a way that alters the relative activities of the enzymes involved in the channelling then one will certainly observe effects on the free concentration of the intermediate that are nothing to do with the channelling.

Mendes and co-workers (P. Mendes, D.B. Kell and H.V. Westerhoff, personal communication) have objected to this use of the term "cross-over", arguing that it properly refers to the effects on intermediate concentrations of inhibiting or activating a single enzyme in a pathway. They recognize that the increases in both the flux and the concentration of an intermediate that result from activating an enzyme upstream from the intermediate can be attributed to a cross-over effect, as can the decrease in flux and increase in the same concentration that result from inhibiting an enzyme downstream from the same intermediate. However, they object to attributing to cross-over effects the simultaneous changes (in the same direction) of the intermediate concentration that occur when both enzyme activities are changed simultaneously. Their opinion has some merit, especially in view of the earlier confusion noted above, but it takes the argument of Heinrich and Rapoport [21] further than they took it themselves, and it ought to be possible to avoid confusion without restricting the use of the term to this extent. It is certainly true, however, that the effects in the channelled system are not the simplest kind of cross-over effects, i.e. ones derived from inhibition or activation of a single enzyme.

In his chapter in this book (Chapter 5) Easterby argues that our analysis [18] is "conceptually flawed", and his earlier expression of the same view [22] is also quoted by Christopherson and Szabados who, however, do not give any further justification (see Chapter 16 in this volume). Easterby considers it easy to see that redistribution of flux between channelled and free-pool branches by varying rate constants in such a way as to maintain the total flux constant will leave free concentrations unchanged. With the wisdom that comes from analysing the actual behaviour, we agree, in retrospect, that our results ought to have been expected, but the fact that others believed that they had proved the opposite [17] suggests that they may have been less than obvious beforehand. Nonetheless, Easterby considers our analysis to be flawed, arguing that only second-order rate constants should be different in the channelled and non-channelled routes. This restriction seems at first sight arbitrary, but he qualifies it by arguing that not even the second-order rate constants are "really" different; they only appear to be different because of the higher concentration of intermediate in the local pool than in free solution. The problem in this model is to understand what prevents the pools of free and channelled intermediate from equilibrating during the infinite time required to establish a steady state. Easterby does not address this point, apart from stating that "no direct exchange of any significant extent occurs between channelled and free intermediate as this would essentially abolish the channel" [22]. This may be reasonable for a static channel in which the structure of the complex prevents diffusion into the bulk phase, as appears to be the case for tryptophan synthase. However, unless one explains what prevents such exchange in a dynamic channel in which each enzyme–enzyme complex has only a short lifetime, application of the model to such a channel is a return to the mysticism that characterized much earlier discussion of the supposed advantages of channelling.

All of this makes it difficult to justify offering channelling as the solution to the problem of conserving the solvent capacity of the cell in the steady state. The problem itself is nonetheless real: the solvent capacity is indeed limited, and so we need to consider what kinetic properties of the component enzymes in a highly repetitive pathway such as β-oxidation would allow the intermediate concentrations to remain very low even if channelling were not considered. This will be discussed next.

Low concentrations without channelling

The simplest reasonable kinetic model of β-oxidation that one can propose is one in which the four kinds of reactions are catalysed by four enzymes E_a (acyl-CoA dehydrogenase), E_b (enoyl-CoA hydratase), E_c (hydroxyacyl-CoA dehydrogenase) and E_d (thiolase) according to reversible Michaelis–Menten kinetics with competition between all possible substrates and products for each enzyme. If the concentrations of the various co-substrates and co-products are treated as constants they can be subsumed in the kinetic constants for the fatty acid intermediates. Such a model may seem almost hopelessly complicated to analyse, but with some plausible assumptions one can nonetheless arrive at useful conclusions. It is convenient to represent acyl-CoA, enoyl-CoA, 3-hydroxyacyl-CoA and 3-oxo-CoA with n carbon atoms in the acyl group as A_n, B_n, C_n and D_n respectively, and the corresponding concentrations as a_n, b_n, c_n and d_n respectively. It is then straightforward (albeit complicated) to write down an expression for the rate of any reaction, and a corresponding expression for the steady-state concentration of any intermediate in terms of those of the flanking intermediates is produced by setting equal the rates of its formation and consumption. For example, the concentration of $CH_3(CH_2)_8CH = CHCOSCoA$, or B_{12}, may be written as follows:

$$b_{12} = \frac{k_{12a}e_a a_{12}/S_a + k_{-12b}e_b c_{12}/S_b}{k_{-12a}e_a/S_a + k_{12b}e_b/S_b}$$

in which k_{12a} and k_{-12a} represent the forward and reverse specificity constants respectively for the reaction between A_{12} and B_{12} catalysed by E_a, k_{12b} and k_{-12b} are defined correspondingly, e_a and e_b are the concentrations of E_a and E_b respectively, and S_a and S_b are "saturation polynomials". Each of these is just a sum with one term for each form of the enzyme that exists: a term of 1 for the free enzyme, and for each enzyme–substrate complex a term equal to its concentration divided by that of the free enzyme. In the example considered, they are as follows for E_a and E_b respectively:

$$S_a = 1 + \frac{a_{16}}{K_{16a}} + \frac{a_{14}}{K_{14a}} + \ldots + \frac{a_2}{K_{2a}} + \frac{b_{16}}{K_{-16a}} + \frac{b_{14}}{K_{-14a}} + \ldots + \frac{b_4}{K_{-4a}}$$

$$S_b = 1 + \frac{b_{16}}{K_{16b}} + \frac{b_{14}}{K_{14b}} + \ldots + \frac{b_2}{K_{2b}} + \frac{c_{16}}{K_{-16b}} + \frac{c_{14}}{K_{-14b}} + \ldots + \frac{c_4}{K_{-4b}}$$

where each K represents a Michaelis constant for a forward or reverse reaction according to whether its index is positive or negative, and similarly for S_b. For example, K_{16a} is the Michaelis constant for the forward substrate (A_{16}) in step 16a, whereas K_{-16a} is the Michaelis constant for the reverse substrate (B_{16}) in the same step. This numbering is slightly different from that used in a previous discussion of this system [23], where the index letters in the subscripts for different Michaelis constants referred to the relevant substrate rather than to the relevant step. Although any system of indices is liable to be confusing in such a complex pathway, the one used here seems marginally less so than the one used previously, as it ensures consistency between subscripts for specificity constants (k) and Michaelis constants (K).

Similar expressions may be written for all of the 27 intermediates in the pathway. If we suppose that a set of conditions exists such that each intermediate concentration is low, not merely on some unspecified scale but in relation to the Michaelis constants for the forward and reverse reactions in which it participates, then each of the four saturation polynomials becomes approximately equal to unity. The apparent complication that many different molecules compete for each active site and each polynomial has in consequence many terms then becomes an irrelevance. Even if this is not accurately true the polynomials may nonetheless be similar enough in magnitude to one another for them to be cancelled from the concentration expressions with little error; the expression given above for b_{12}, for example, simplifies to

$$b_{12} = \frac{k_{12a}e_a a_{12} + k_{-12b}e_b c_{12}}{k_{-12a}e_a + k_{12b}e_b}$$

If we make the further reasonable assumption that all reactions have equilibria that sufficiently favour the forward reactions for all specificity constants for the reverse reactions to be negligible, then this further simplifies to $b_{12} = k_{12a}e_a a_{12}/k_{12b}e_b$. All of the other expressions for intermediate concentrations simplify similarly. If all of the forward catalytic activities (taken as products of enzyme concentrations and specificity constants) are similar in magnitude then all of the intermediate concentrations will be similar in magnitude also, though not necessarily small. If, however, all of the reactions in the pathway apart from the first are catalysed with similar activity, but the first is much more weakly catalysed, then all intermediate concentrations will be very small compared with the pool concentration of the initial reactant, and virtually all flux control will reside in the first step of the pathway.

The assumption that all equilibrium constants are very favourable is not strictly true in β-oxidation. For example, the equilibrium constant between decenoyl-CoA and 3-hydroxydecanoyl-CoA is about 2.3 [24]. This complicates the quantitative analysis given above, but it does not invalidate it qualitatively, because a highly active enzyme can always overcome an unfavourable equilibrium in the reaction that precedes it. In the metabolism of *trans*-ω-6-unsaturated fatty acids the corresponding equilibrium constant is much smaller, about 0.003 [24]: in such cases it is likely to be much more difficult to achieve low concentrations of intermediates with free-diffusion kinetics.

It does not follow, of course, that this is the only set of assumptions that could produce this result, but that has no importance. What matters is that a simple kinetic model, involving no implausible assumptions about the properties of any of the enzymes, is capable of predicting that all inter-mediate concentrations should be very small in the steady state and that all flux control should reside in the first step. There are thus no grounds for arguing that the low concentrations of intermediates by themselves require channelling or any other exotic hypothesis.

Nonetheless, as discussed already in the Introduction, the fact that channelling is not needed does not mean that it does not occur, and there may be other reasons for postulating it; for example, although a mixture of enoyl-CoA hydratase and 3-hydroxyacyl-CoA dehydrogenase from different sources gave exactly the time course expected [25] for a mixture of non-interacting enzymes, the complex having these two activities extracted from *Escherichia coli* did not, and completely lacked the expected lag in the build-up of final product [24]. This suggests that even if channelling may have no effect on the steady-state concentration of an intermediate [18] it may still have important effects during the approach to the steady state. This will now be examined, but in a model much simpler than the complete β-oxidation pathway, as the essential points can be established without the need for such a complex system.

Model

A model of a dynamic channel is shown in Fig. 1. It is structurally the same as that studied previously [16,18], but the kinetic equations have been modified from the original version [16] to give all steps equilibrium constants that favour the forward reactions, i.e. they have been modified in the direc-tion considered by Mendes et al. [17] to make the model more realistic and to favour the possibility of effects of channelling on the concentration of C. The behaviour of this model was studied using the program MetaModel [26], in a modified form that uses the 4th order Runge–Kutta method with adjust-able step size [27] to simulate the approach to the steady state. Note that although the free forms of E_2 and E_3 do not appear explicitly in the model as drawn (to avoid making it too complicated), they were fully taken into account in the simulations, i.e. there were no violations of conservation of the total concentrations of these enzymes.

Fig. I Model of a dynamic channel

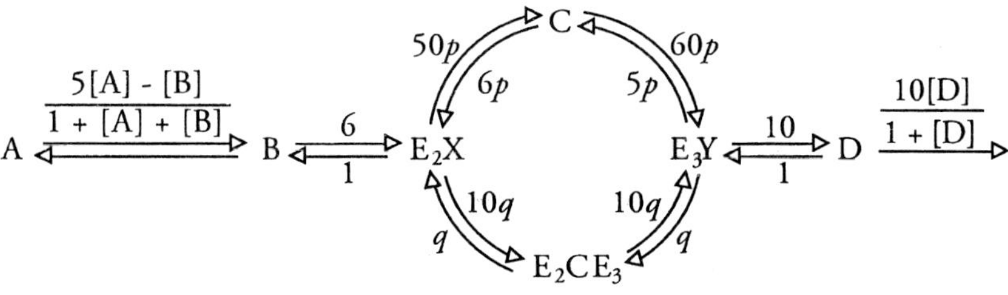

The by-pass via E_2CE_3 allows interconversion of the enzyme–substrate complexes E_2X and E_3Y without release of the channelled intermediate C into free solution. The proportion of the net flux from A passing through the channel was varied by varying the factors p and q in such a way as to maintain constant at 4.15 the steady-state flux from A. For discussion of the rate equations and rate constants shown above the reactions, see the Appendix. The intervention of free E_2 in three binding steps (to B or C to produce E_2X, and to E_3Y to form E_2CE_3) is not shown explicitly, nor is that of free E_3 in three similar steps, but both were fully taken into account in the simulations, i.e. both $[E_2] + [E_2X] + [E_2CE_3]$ and $[E_3] + [E_3Y] + [E_2CE_3]$ were held constant

Effect of channelling on the approach to the steady state

Fig. 2 shows the approach to steady state of the concentrations of the intermediates B, C and D in the model of Fig. 1 under conditions where the proportion of the steady-state flux passing through the channel is set to 1%, 50% or 99% by varying the factors p and q that determine the relative activities of the pool and channel steps respectively, with the total steady-state flux from A to products being maintained at a constant value of 4.15 throughout. Note that the time courses for B and D, the intermediates not involved in the channel, are virtually unaffected by the proportion of reaction that passes through the channel, and the same is true of the pre-steady-state fluxes (not shown) from A to B, from B to D, and from D.

Only the concentration of the channelled intermediate C has a time course that depends appreciably on the degree of channelling, so that, for example, if 99% of the flux is channelled, C remains far from its steady state at a time when the rest of the system is essentially in steady state. However, there are several features that are surprising enough to require some comment: (i) the effect is quite small, even at 99% channelling, so that the time taken to reach 50% of the steady-state concentration is increased only 5-fold with respect to the curve for 1% channelling; (ii) the curves for 50% and 1% differ very little from one another; (iii) the curves for 50% and 1% cross one another.

All of these points suggest the need to examine the time courses for C at a wider range of parameter values, and this is done in Fig. 3. Curves were also calculated for 2%, 5%, 10%, 20%, 30%, 40%, 50%, 60% and 70%

channelling, but these are not shown as they were not easy to distinguish from those at 1% and 80%. The essential point is that the behaviour changes rather little between 1% and 99% but substantially between 99% and 100%. Roughly speaking one can say that a 99% efficient channel is about half-way in behaviour between a perfect channel and no channel at all. However, this may be too rough for some purposes, and it may be better to make a more quantitative comparison, such as the time required for [C] to reach 50% of its steady-state value: this is plotted in Fig. 4 as a function of the proportion of the steady-state flux that is channelled (up to 99.8%). As expected from the curves shown in Fig. 3, this time changes very little until the channel flux exceeds 90%, but then rises very steeply, becoming infinite at 100% channelling.

Fig. 2   **Approach of metabolic intermediate concentrations to their steady-state values**

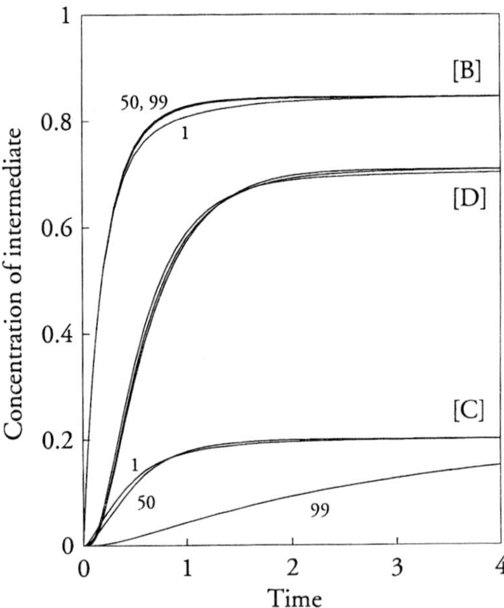

The model of Fig. 1 was simulated with p = 1.175, q = 0.1163, for which 1% of the steady-state flux passes through the channel, p = 0.5930, q = 5.8107 (50%), and p = 0.0118, q = 11.4983 (99%), in all cases with the same net steady-state flux of 4.15. The curves for the three intermediates B, C and D form three well separated families of three curves, as labelled. Within each family the curves are labelled, when sufficiently resolved, with the percentage of the net flux that passes through the channel in the steady state.

Fig. 3   Time courses for a channelled intermediate

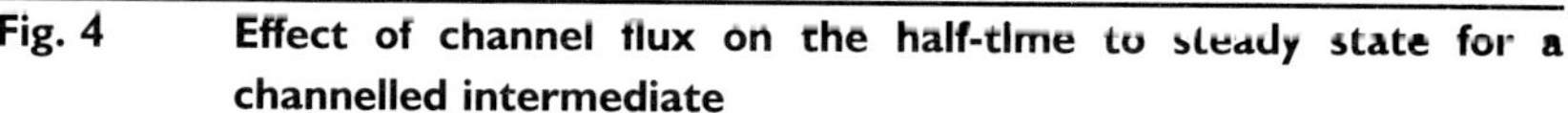
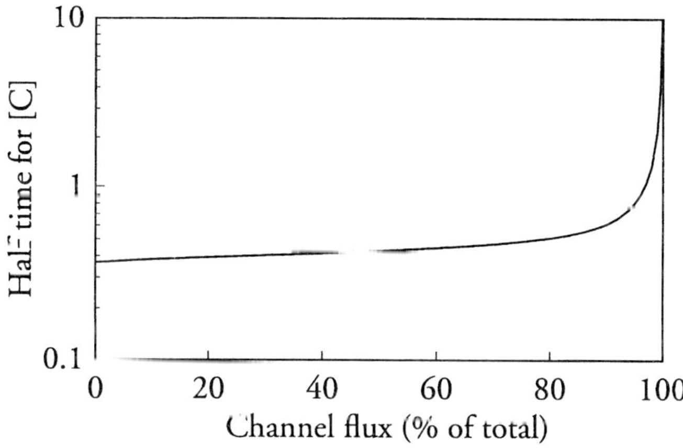

The factors p and q were varied as in Fig. 2 to vary the proportion passing through the channel from 0.1% to 99.9% while maintaining the net steady-state flux constant.

Fig. 4   Effect of channel flux on the half-time to steady state for a channelled intermediate

The factors p and q were varied as in Fig. 2 to vary the proportion passing through the channel from 0 to 99.8% while maintaining the net steady-state flux constant. Note that the half-time approaches infinity at 100% channelling: the highest ordinate value visible in the plot refers to 99.8%, not to 100%.

Slow approach to the steady state at low levels of channelling

The complication that the curves in Fig. 3 cross one another means, for example, that the curve for 0.1% channelling approaches the steady state more slowly than that for 1%, which may appear very surprising. It derives from the fact that even at very low channel fluxes the steady-state concentration of the complex E_2CE_3 is not negligible (accounting for about 7% of the total steady-state concentrations of E_2 and E_3 for the particular parameter values assumed). However, at low channel fluxes this steady-state concentration is reached extremely slowly compared with the decay of all the other transients in the system, and consequently it generates a slow drift in the concentration of C long after it appears to have reached its steady state. Fig. 5 illustrates this for the case where 0.2% of the steady-state flux is channelled: the general and pool fluxes are essentially in steady state after 1 or 2 time units, but the channel fluxes are still far from theirs at this time, one of them, indeed, being still negative even though its steady-state value is positive.

A consequence of this complication is that a totally unchannelled pathway in which the ternary complex E_2CE_3 cannot be formed at all is not just an extrapolation to zero channelling of the sort of model considered, because even at infinitesimal channelling this model leaves a non-negligible steady-state concentration of the ternary complex. (The discontinuity in Fig. 4 of ref. [17] can probably be explained in terms of this sort of effect.) However, in the limit this non-negligible concentration requires infinite time to be reached, and clearly in practice one would not consider it when defining the steady state. In the case of Fig. 3, one would probably consider in practice that the curve labelled 0.1 was approaching a steady-state level about 7% lower than that of the other curves, equivalent to deciding that channelling becomes "negligible" at some value between about 0.1% and 1%. Reasonable though this may be, it is important to realize that ultimately it is a matter of convenience rather than mathematics and that the analysis of the kinetic effects of channelling is full of complexities that make it dangerous to reach conclusions on the basis of what may appear "obvious".

Pre-steady-state advantages of channelling

It follows, then, that for channelling to be seen as a mechanism to prevent a build-up of free intermediates in the pre-steady-state period one must postulate either that virtually all the flux passes through the channel (because a 90% channel is only trivially different from no channel at all), or that the pathway is in operation for such a short time that even the net flux does not reach its steady state. The latter condition seems most unlikely to be met in β-oxidation, and the former would likewise be very unlikely in the absence of clear evidence for static organization of all the enzymes involved. The recent discovery of a three-enzyme complex [11] is thus a useful step, but it is insufficient: unless all of the enzymes constitute a static complex, a channelling explanation for the lack of intermediates must inevitably involve some degree of dynamic channelling. Models of static and dynamic channels behave

---

Fig. 5   Approach of fluxes to the steady state

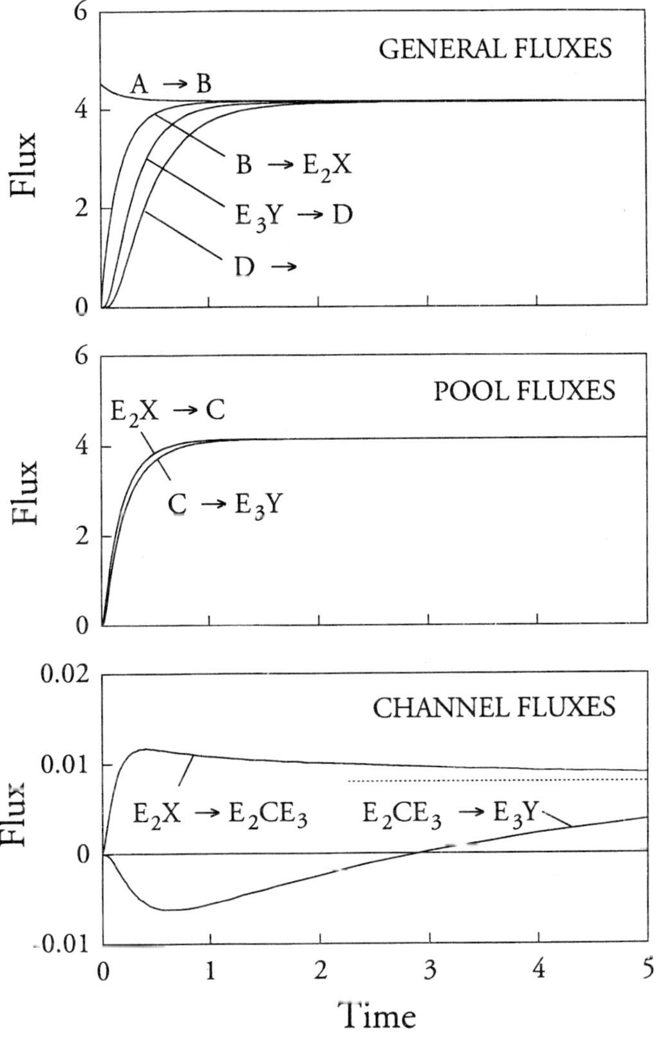

The model of Fig. 1 was simulated with p = 1.185, q = 0.0233, which corresponds to 0.2% channelling of a net steady-state flux of 4.15. Note that the channel fluxes approach their steady states much more slowly than the other fluxes. This sort of effect accounts for the flattening of the curves in Fig. 3 for low channelling proportions long before the true steady states are approached.

rather similarly, but they are very different at the level of mechanistic plausibility, because a dynamic channel requires assumptions about diffusion rates for macromolecules [18,28] that are difficult or impossible to reconcile with the known effects of molecular "crowding" on the diffusion behaviour of large and small molecules [29,30]. The high viscosity of the cytoplasm has often been referred to in discussions of channelling, but its effects are by no means straightforward, and are in general much more evident in the diffusion of macromolecules than in that of small metabolic intermediates. Elsewhere in this book (Chapter 2) West discusses this question in some detail.

Most of the intermediates in β-oxidation contain large hydrophobic groups, and their release into free solution is by no means as favourable as it is for most of the disputed examples of channelling in other areas of metabolism. Two-dimensional diffusion on the surface of a static complex could thus be a much faster process than diffusion through the aqueous solution. However, whether this would be metabolite channelling as it is usually understood is another matter.

I thank John Easterby, Olin Spivey and Hans Westerhoff for useful comments on parts of this chapter.

References

1. Gutfreund, H. and Chock, P.B. (1991) J. Theor. Biol. **152**, 117–121
2. Kvassman, J., Pettersson, G. and Ryde-Pettersson, U. (1988) Eur. J. Biochem. **172**, 427–431
3. Chock, P.B. and Gutfreund, H. (1988) Proc. Natl. Acad. Sci. U.S.A. **85**, 8870–8874
4. Srivastava, D.K., Smolen, P., Betts, G.F., Fukushima, T., Spivey, H.O. and Bernhard, S.A. (1989) Proc. Natl. Acad. Sci. U.S.A. **86**, 6464–6468
5. Srivastava, D.K. and Bernhard, S.A. (1985) Biochemistry **24**, 623–628
6. Spivey, H.O. (1991) J. Theor. Biol. **152**, 103–107
7. Benner, S.A. (1982) Experientia **38**, 633–637
8. Ovádi, J. (1991) J. Theor. Biol. **152**, 1–22 (with commentaries from numerous authors)
9. Srere, P.A. (1987) Annu. Rev. Biochem. **56**, 89–124
10. Walkin, S.J. (1989) Biochemistry **28**, 4523–4530
11. Uchida, Y., Izai, K., Orii, T. and Hashimoto, T. (1992) J. Biol. Chem. **267**, 1034–1041
12. Stanley, K.K. and Tubbs, P.K. (1975) Biochem. J. **150**, 77–88
13. Eaton, S., Bhuiyan, A.K.M.J., Kler, R.S., Turnbull, D.M. and Bartlett, K. (1993) Biochem. J. **289**, 161–168
14. Sumegi, B., Porpaczy, Z. and Alkonyi, I. (1991) Biochim. Biophys. Acta **1081**, 121–128
15. Atkinson, D.E. (1977) Cellular Energy Metabolism and its Regulation, pp. 16–17, Academic Press, New York
16. Cornish-Bowden, A. (1991) Eur. J. Biochem. **195**, 103–108
17. Mendes, P., Kell, D.B. and Westerhoff, H.V. (1992) Eur. J. Biochem. **204**, 257–266
18. Cornish-Bowden, A. and Cárdenas, M.L. (1993) Eur. J. Biochem. **213**, 87–92
19. Heinrich, R. and Schuster, S. (1991) J. Theor. Biol. **152**, 57–61
20. Chance, B., Williams, G.R., Holmes, W.F. and Higgins, J. (1955) J. Biol. Chem. **217**, 439–451
21. Heinrich, R. and Rapoport, T.A. (1974) Eur. J. Biochem. **42**, 97–105
22. Easterby, J.S. (1993) J. Mol. Recognition **6**, 179–185
23. Cornish-Bowden, A. (1994) Biochem. Soc. Trans. **22**, 451–452

24. Yang, S.-Y., Cuebas, D. and Schulz, H. (1986) J. Biol. Chem. **261**, 15390–15395
25. Storer, A.C. and Cornish-Bowden, A. (1974) Biochem. J. **141**, 205–209
26. Cornish-Bowden, A. and Hofmeyr, J.-H.S. (1991) Comput. Appl. Biosci. **7**, 89–93
27. Press, W.H., Flannery, B.P., Teukolsky, S.A. and Vetterling, W.T. (1986) Numerical Recipes, pp. 550–560, Cambridge University Press, Cambridge
28. Pettersson, G. (1991) J. Theor. Biol. **152**, 65–69
29. Knowles, J.R. (1991) J. Theor. Biol. **152**, 53–55
30. Cárdenas, M.L. (1991) J. Theor. Biol. **152**, 111–113

Appendix: Kinetic equations in metabolic models

In any metabolic simulation in the computer it is important to use reversible rate equations for all or nearly all of the steps. Reactions that represent flow out of the system into an external reservoir (such as the arrow out of D in Fig. 1) can be made irreversible without greatly affecting the qualitative behaviour of the system, and hence can be expressed as in Fig. 1 by the familiar irreversible Michaelis–Menten equation. However, all internal steps need to be reversible or the simulated system will behave in ways that are not at all characteristic of living organisms. (In the language of metabolic control analysis, the root of the problem is that substrate elasticities in irreversible reactions normally have small finite values in the range 0–1, whereas for reversible reactions the corresponding range is infinite, and the qualitative types of possible behaviour are completely different [1].)

For reactions that are not involved in channelling, such as the interconversion of A and B in Fig. 1, it is enough to use the reversible form of the Michaelis–Menten equation. As discussed in textbooks on enzyme kinetics [2], this takes the form:

$$ v = \frac{k_A e_0 a - k_B e_0 b}{1 + \dfrac{a}{K_{mA}} + \dfrac{b}{K_{mB}}} $$

in which e_0 is the total enzyme concentration, a and b are the concentrations of substrate and product respectively, k_A and K_{mA} are the specificity constant and Michaelis constant respectively for the forward reaction, and k_B and K_{mB} are the corresponding parameters for the reverse reaction. Note that this simplifies to the ordinary irreversible Michaelis–Menten equation if either a or b is zero. In the simplest case of a two-step reaction with rate constants k_1 and k_{-1} for the first step and k_2 and k_{-2} for the second: $k_A = k_1 k_2 / (k_{-1} + k_2)$; $K_{mA} = (k_{-1} + k_2)/k_1$; $k_B = k_{-1} k_{-2}/(k_{-1} + k_2)$; $K_{mB} = (k_{-1} + k_2)/k_{-2}$ [2].

To model enzymes involved in channelling the kinetics of the individual steps of the mechanism need to be shown explicitly. However, it should be clear from the preceding paragraph that the forward and reverse rate constants of 6 and 1 respectively shown for the step $E_2 + B = E_2X$ in Fig. 1, together with those of $50p$ and $6p$ for the step $E_2X = E_2 + C$, correspond to the reversible Michaelis–Menten equation for the two steps together (ignoring the channel steps via E_2CE_3) with the following numerical form:

$$v = \frac{\dfrac{6 \times 50p}{1 + 50p}\,b - \dfrac{1 \times 6p}{1 + 50p}\,c}{1 + \dfrac{6b}{1 + 50p} + \dfrac{6pc}{1 + 50p}}$$

The advantage of using the individual rate constants instead of this composite form is that one can then add channelling steps such as the pathway via E_2CE_3 without disturbing the ones already considered.

References

1. Cornish-Bowden, A. (1995) Adv. Mol. Cell. Biol. **11**, 21–64
2. Cornish-Bowden, A. (1995) Fundamentals of Enzyme Kinetics (2nd edn.), pp. 37–43, Portland Press, London

5

Pathway dynamics and the analysis of metabolite channelling

John S. Easterby

Department of Biochemistry, The University of Liverpool, P.O. Box 147,
Liverpool L69 3BX, U.K.

Introduction

It has been recognized for many years that some pathways or consecutive enzyme sequences within the cell may be present in multienzyme complexes or multifunctional proteins [1–5]. Such complexes could confer a kinetic advantage by the direct transfer of pathway intermediates between enzymes, without the need for release and dilution into the bulk phase of the cell and subsequent diffusion to the next enzyme of the sequence. In general, no flux advantage would result from this mechanism [6,7], except in the limited case where the direct transfer of substrate between two isolated and transiently interacting enzymes is being considered [8]. In the more extended complex, the flux will generally be determined outside of any individual step in the pathway and the kinetic advantage results from the reduction in the size of intermediate pools. In the most extreme case the transfer of metabolite between consecutive enzymes may be considered to be direct, with no intervening intermediate pool. In general, however, one may imagine that an intermediate pool exists within the complex and that the direct transfer mechanism would be a limiting case. The consequence of this is that the internal pool can be of reduced size compared with the situation in which the enzymes and intermediates are freely diffusing, and the enzymes of the complex will see a higher, localized, concentration of the metabolite. Consequently the transient time of the sequence is also reduced and hence so is the time it takes to approach a new steady state. The flux remains unaltered, merely being achieved at a lower metabolite concentration. It should be understood from the outset that the metabolite concentration is lower as it is the practice to refer concentrations to the system volume. In fact the enzyme active centre would see a smaller pool of greatly elevated concentration.

Despite the recognition that channelling may confer these advantages, there has been little attempt to make a quantitative kinetic analysis of the advantage in transient decreases. This is partly due to the perceived difficulty and complexity of such an analysis. Ovádi et al. [9] have analysed the situation in a two-enzyme complex or in the case of two transiently interacting enzymes. However, their elegant analysis in terms of mean lifetimes of channelled and free intermediate was of limited general applicability, as it assumed pseudo-first-order kinetic behaviour of the enzymes involved and is not easily extended to larger complexes and more complex kinetic behaviour.

It has been tacitly assumed that the channel is the result of the underlying physical structure of the enzyme complex and that the metabolite is restricted to the complex by a physical barrier to its free diffusion into the surrounding milieu. Indeed, in the most thoroughly documented example of channelling, namely in tryptophan synthase, this physical restriction is markedly evident [10]. More recently, some authors have criticized the whole concept of channelling and have proposed that it cannot result in reduced pool sizes or transient times. Whether channelling actually occurs or not, I believe their analyses to be conceptually flawed. Their treatment of rate coefficients does not take into account the physical restriction placed on metabolites. The approach adopted cannot result in pool decreases as it is based on a misconceived manipulation of rate coefficients.

Pathway dynamics and temporal response, and their relationship to metabolite channelling

Metabolic regulation is usually assumed to imply the control of pathway flux and its determinants. In particular, the control of enzyme activity and homoeostasis in the maintenance of steady states has been a focus of attention. In the cell many changes involve relatively large changes of flux and require a finite time to occur. The time scale of such changes is important and can be directly affected by channelling. The transient behaviour is therefore both a consequence and an indicator of the occurrence of channelling. A full description of regulation of a system must include temporal analysis. It is insufficient to ask what pathway flux will be; it is also necessary to know how long it takes the system to adapt from one steady state to another. This temporal responsiveness sets the time scale on which metabolism operates and is described by the pathway transition or transient time, τ. A potential difficulty in the study of pathway dynamics arises from the need to make real-time measurements or to have a detailed knowledge of pathway kinetics in order to model the system. Such experimentation is difficult but may not always be necessary.

The theoretical study of pathway transient behaviour developed out of a related interest in the optimization of coupled or consecutive enzyme reactions, and has resulted in a remarkably useful and simple approach to the analysis of temporal responses. This area of investigation was initiated by McClure [11] with a description of the kinetic behaviour of a two-enzyme system in which the first enzyme was severely rate-limiting and the single intermediate was converted irreversibly into a measurable product by a single coupling or auxiliary enzyme. The two-enzyme system was extended to three

[12] and finally developed to describe a system containing an unlimited number of coupling enzymes [13]. In all of these studies the rate-limiting nature of the first enzyme of the series, and the irreversibility of the intervening steps between substrate and pathway end-product, ensured that the intermediate concentrations in the sequence were low and that the coupling enzymes followed pseudo-first-order kinetics with respect to the intermediates. This in turn meant that the differential equations describing the system were linear and amenable to analytical solution. In all cases the steady-state production of end-product by the system was preceded, as expected, by a lag period during which the intermediates of the sequence were accumulating to their steady-state levels. If the steady-state asymptote to the progress curve in product formation was projected to the time axis, it intercepted at the lag or transient time. In the case of a two-enzyme system, at least 4.6 transient times must elapse before the intermediate concentration and the rate of product formation approach their steady-state values to within 1% [13]. For progressively longer sequences this time is proportionately decreased until, in the case of very long sequences, the system obeys a step function and enters the steady state immediately on reaching the transient time [14].

These simple analyses were never intended to represent the behaviour of metabolic pathways, but were sometimes applied to more complex reaction sequences than they were intended for. They did, however, indicate some principles which might apply more generally to pathways. Firstly, the transient time for the sequence was found, rather surprisingly, to be independent of the initial rate-limiting enzyme. Secondly, each secondary or coupling enzyme in the sequence had a transient time corresponding to the reciprocal of the pseudo-first-order rate constant for the reaction catalysed. In irreversible first-order systems the reciprocal of the rate constant also corresponds to the mean lifetime or turnover time of the intermediate associated with the enzyme. Thirdly, the transient times of the system were additive and the total system transient was their sum. Fourthly, the intercept on the ordinate axis of a plot of sequence end-product versus time corresponded to the negative sum of the steady state intermediate concentrations of the sequence. These observations, derived from a very simple system, provided pointers to the physical interpretation of transience in more complicated pathways.

The transient times associated with individual enzymes in the sequence were given by the K_m/V_{max} ratios. Therefore not only enzymes with low activity, but also those with low affinity for their substrates, could generate appreciable transient times, and the term 'time-limiting enzyme' was adopted to describe them [13,15]. Such enzymes could determine the distribution of flux between branches of a pathway if they followed the branch point, as the branch would only enter a steady state if the feeder pathway were sustained for a sufficient length of time. An enzyme of this type was soon discovered in the *arom* complex of *Neurospora*. This was shikimate kinase and was a member of what was thought to be a multienzyme complex but is now known to be a multifunctional protein [3]. From the *arom* system also came the first indications of the possibility of metabolite channelling, manifested in a considerable decrease in transient time compared with the simulated behaviour of free-solution systems of enzymes of comparable kinetic parameters. The conclusions drawn from the first-order, linear-enzymic-chain model system were subsequently applied to several other pathways and multienzyme complexes, but always with a certain danger in view of the very restricted original model.

The coupled-enzyme model is, in fact, a special case of a much more general model of pathway transient behaviour. If the rate of input of substrate to a pathway through the feeder enzyme or barrier is maintained constant, then certain consequences derive which are based simply on mass conservation principles and are unaffected by the prevailing kinetic mechanisms within the pathway. Fig. 1 represents the accumulation of product with time in such a sequence. If there were no intermediates present in the pathway, then the progress curve for product formation would follow a straight line with slope equal to the steady-state rate and passing through the origin. This line would correspond to the steady rate of substrate input. The difference between this line and the actual progress curve in product formation is clearly equal to the concentration of accumulated intermediates, irrespective of the kinetic description of the system. Thus the transient time can be deduced from a consideration of mass conservation without the need to model the system. This can be represented mathematically as:

$$[P] = Jt - \Sigma_i [S_i]_{ss} \tag{1}$$

where [P] represents the concentration of accumulated pathway product, $[S_i]_{ss}$ the steady-state concentration of intermediate and J the steady-state flux corresponding to the rate of substrate input. Eqn. (1) may be rewritten as:

$$[P] = J \left(t - \Sigma_i [S_i]_{ss}/J \right) \tag{2}$$

The second term in parentheses on the right-hand side of the equation clearly has the dimensions of time and perturbs the actual system time. It is, in fact, the pathway transient time.

As a result, associated with each intermediate in a metabolic system is a transient given by:

$$\tau_i = [S_i]_{ss}/J \tag{3}$$

where τ_i represents the pool lifetime or turnover time of intermediate S_i. The total, system, transient time is simply the sum of the individual intermediate transients. Thus the same basic interpretation of transience applied to the first-order linear-enzymic-chain model is shown to obtain and indicates the value of even a simple kinetic model in the development of a general approach. The general theory was first stated by Easterby [16] but had also been recognized in a more limited form by Bartha and Keleti [17]. The important thing to note about the transient is that it is associated with the intermediate pools and not with individual enzymes. The transient time is the time required to generate the steady-state pools of intermediates and is only associated with individual enzymes in systems in which the interconversion of intermediates is directional and irreversible. To eqn. (3) may be added the following result:

$$\tau = \Sigma_i [S_i]_{ss}/J = \Sigma_i \tau_i \tag{4}$$

where τ represents the system transient.

This approach to the analysis of pathway transient times has the advantage for the experimentalist of being independent of any prior assump-

---

Fig. I   **Relationship between product concentration and time in a system of consecutive enzymes**

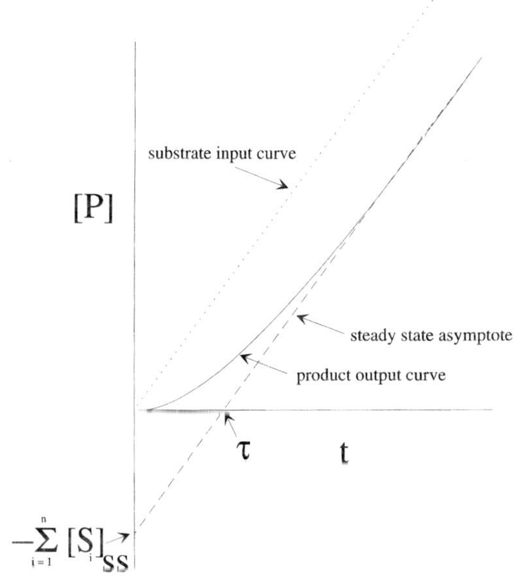

Substrate S is converted into end-product P through several intermediates S_i. The initial enzyme of the sequence is assumed to determine the flux. The steady-state asymptote to the progress curve intersects the time axis at the transient or transition time, τ. The ordinate axis is intersected at the negative sum of the intermediate concentrations. The line drawn parallel to the steady-state asymptote and passing through the origin represents the input of material to the pathway. The displacement of this line from the asymptote, along the product axis, is equal to the sum of steady-state intermediate concentrations, irrespective of the kinetic mechanisms of the enzymes involved.

tion of a kinetic model to describe the pathway. Nor is it necessary to make dynamic measurements in order to assess the temporal response. Simple measurements of intermediate concentrations and fluxes in the steady state suffice to identify the time scale on which the pathway operates and the contributions of individual steps to that time scale. It is also obvious that a direct consequence of metabolite channelling, which is reputed to decrease pool sizes, will be to decrease the pathway transient. Not only will this decrease occur but, as we shall see later on, the extent of the decrease can be used to gauge the extent and efficiency of channelling of intermediates within a complex.

A pathway, as represented in the above analyses, may be defined as follows. The flux across the initial boundary must be constant with time, and the final boundary may be placed anywhere along the path to the end-product. The end-product itself constitutes the integrated sum of all material crossing the final boundary. In measuring the transient time it is assumed that initially no intermediate is present and the flux is zero; thus the transient time is associated with the establishment of the pathway from rest. This is an unrealistic view of what happens in the cell, where passage between steady states is much more common. Such transitions are accommodated easily by the approach [16]. Transient times are functions of state and are independent of the route by which the steady state was reached. The time required for a transition between steady states may therefore be described in terms of the transient times associated with the establishment of each steady state from rest. Thus the transient time for a transition from steady state A to steady state B is given by:

$$\tau_{A \to B} = \tau_B - (J_A/J_B) \cdot \tau_A \tag{5}$$

where τ_A and τ_B represent the transients associated with the establishment of each steady state from rest and J_A and J_B are the respective fluxes.

The description of the pathway given assumes that the initial reaction or boundary involves a constant rate of input of substrate. In general this will mean that the initial step is flux-generating. This restriction may be lifted if allowance is made for variation in the rate of input [18]. This generates an additional transient time given by the definite integral:

$$\tau = \frac{1}{J_{ss}} \int_0^{J_{ss}} t \cdot dJ \tag{6}$$

where J is the rate of input, J_{ss} represents the steady-state input rate (i.e. the steady-state flux) and the integral extends from a flux of zero to the steady-state value. Variation in J may arise from either substrate depletion or feedback on the initial boundary of the system. Substrate depletion is easily overcome experimentally but feedback is more of a problem. However, in practice the magnitude of this transient is likely to be small compared with the total pathway transient time. Where it is necessary to consider it, the only answer may be to resort to computer simulation [18]. Even if it is necessary to consider variation in the rate of input, eqn. (5) still holds. In the case of negative feedback the transient of eqn. (6) will be negative and will reduce the overall transient time. One function of negative feedback may therefore be to accelerate the attainment of the steady state. Apparent overcapacity of some enzymes may be necessary in order to ensure a rapid transition between steady states, with the final flux being determined by feedback. If both substrate depletion and feedback on the initial boundary are absent then this transient reduces to the characteristic time of the initial enzyme and again will usually be correspondingly small and negligible. Therefore the pool lifetimes remain the most important single determinant of the temporal response.

The above discussion centres on how transient times are measured experimentally, namely from fluxes and pool sizes, and the theory does not constitute a model of pathway behaviour. It is sometimes useful to have in mind a kinetic model to describe the steady-state pool sizes and fluxes. Given such models, it is possible to compare theory with experiment. A model in this context merely means some function which will adequately represent the transformation/removal of an intermediate within the pathway during the steady state. The approach is therefore almost phenomenological in the sense that the function does not require great generality but must merely represent the enzyme's rate adequately under the restricted steady-state conditions being considered. Functions are of the form:

$$\mathrm{d}[S_i]/\mathrm{d}t - J_{ss} - f\,([S_i],\mathrm{x,y,z}\dots) - 0 \tag{7}$$

where x,y,z ... etc. are any modulators of enzyme activity. These functions are generally fairly simple where irreversible conversion of the intermediate is involved. They become complex where reversible processes are involved [14,16]. Some common cases are as follows.

(a) Conversion of intermediate follows pseudo-first-order kinetics:

$$\tau_i = {}^iK_\mathrm{m}/V_i \tag{8}$$

where ${}^iK_\mathrm{m}$ is the Michaelis constant and V_i the maximum velocity of the converting enzyme.

(b) Conversion follows Michaelis–Menten kinetics.

$$\tau_i = {}^iK_\mathrm{m}/(V_i - J) \tag{9}$$

A closer examination of systems of this sort shows that if enzyme capacity exceeds flux by a factor of more than 2, then first-order behaviour gives a reasonable representation of transient responses [16].

In all of these analyses it has been assumed that the transient time is due to the accumulation of free intermediate pools within the pathway. In practice enzyme-bound intermediates also contribute to the transient and will be of prime importance when considering channelling processes. τ for a Michaelis–Menten enzyme is then given by:

$$\tau_i = [E_T]/V_i + {}^iK_m/(V_i - J) \tag{10}$$

$$\tau_i = 1/k_{cat} + {}^iK_m/(V_i - J) \tag{11}$$

where $[E_T]$ represents the total enzyme concentration and the first term represents the contribution of the enzyme-bound intermediate. The conclusion is that the contribution of enzyme-bound intermediate to the transient is only significant when the enzyme concentration approaches the K_m [16]. In other words it will generally be insignificant except in the channelling situation. A complete description of the transient would, of course, have to take into account variation in the rate of input to the pathway. The complete description of τ therefore becomes:

$$\tau = \frac{1}{J_{SS}} \int_0^{J_{SS}} t \cdot dJ + \sum_i \left(\frac{1}{k_{cat_i}} + \frac{{}^iK_m}{V_i - J_{SS}} \right) \tag{12}$$

The first term represents the variation in input flux, the second the mean lifetimes of enzyme–substrate complexes and the third the lifetimes of the pools of free intermediates.

One use of modelling of this sort is to identify diffusional restrictions or substrate channelling within experimental systems. The transients described were derived on the assumption that both enzymes and substrates are present in a system where free diffusion can occur. If measured transients correspond to theoretical values then one may conclude that this is a valid assumption. If transients are greater than those expected on the basis of theory then some form of diffusional restriction, owing perhaps to high intracellular viscosity, may be occurring. Conversely, if the transient times are smaller than expected, substrate or intermediate channelling is indicated.

The theory of transience described relies heavily on the knowledge of pool sizes and fluxes within the steady state. The transient is determined largely by the pool sizes, and the control exerted by any particular enzyme on the transient response will depend on its ability to modify any or all of the metabolite pools and pathway flux. The analysis of regulation of the transient time by specific component enzymes of the system is therefore analogous to the analysis of flux regulation set out in the theory of Metabolic Control Analysis as defined principally by Kacser and Burns [19] but also by Heinrich and Rapoport [20]. Temporal control coefficients may be defined [21–23] in terms of the common flux and concentration control coefficients:

$$C_{e_i}^{\tau_j} = \frac{d\tau_i}{de_i} \cdot \frac{e_i}{\tau_i} = C_{e_i}^{[S_j]} - C_{e_i}^{J} \tag{13}$$

$$C_{e_i}^{\tau} = \frac{d\tau}{de_i} \cdot \frac{e_i}{\tau_i} = C_{e_i}^{\Sigma[S_j]} - C_{e_i}^{J} \tag{14}$$

where τ_j represents an individual pool lifetime and τ represents the system transient. e_i is the concentration or activity of the ith enzyme of the system. A summation property applies to both control coefficients similar to that seen for flux control coefficients:

$$\sum_i C_{e_i}^{\tau_j} = -1 \tag{15}$$

$$\sum_i C_{e_i}^{\tau} = -1 \tag{16}$$

Thus control coefficients and summation properties apply both to individual metabolite pool lifetimes and to the system transient.

The sums of control coefficients here are negative, as increasing an enzyme concentration will generally increase flux and reduce pool sizes, thus reducing the transient time. The analysis of transience has therefore been incorporated into the general field of Metabolic Control Analysis, and much of the data required to obtain temporal control coefficients for specific systems will already exist. Again it should be emphasized that this analysis applies to free-solution behaviour and may be expected to be modified in channelling systems.

The analysis of metabolite channelling and its consequences for pathway transient behaviour

Substrate channelling may either occur within multienzyme complexes and multifunctional proteins (static channels) or between dynamically interacting consecutive enzymes of a pathway. By this process, intermediates in the reaction chain can be transferred directly between enzymes without the need for diffusion into the bulk medium. It might be envisaged that at least three pools of intermediate exist within the pathway. One would occupy the bulk medium, a second would correspond to enzyme-bound intermediate and a third to intermediate trapped or channelled within the complex but not directly associated with enzyme active sites. When the free-solution pool and the channelled pool are reduced to a minimum, direct transfer of intermediate between enzyme active centres occurs. The system described is a 'leaky' one in which some intermediate is retained within the complex and some enters the bulk phase and must diffuse back to the complex to be converted through to product. Such a system has three possible advantages. Firstly, the existence of the multienzyme complex may serve to isolate the reactions and intermediates of a pathway. Secondly, co-ordinated regulation of enzymes within the complex may be possible [3,4]. Thirdly, a minimization of the transient time for the pathway may occur, thus obviating the need for the accumulation of intermediates. The concentration of intermediate encountered by enzymes of the complex is greater than if free diffusion were allowed and, therefore, according to the mass conservation principle, less material and time is wasted in generating unwanted intermediate pools.

Channelling offers no flux advantage, providing that enzyme capacities are generally adequate, as flux is still determined by the initial rate of input to the pathway or at least outside of any particular reaction step [6,7,24,25].

It is clear that channelling can be analysed in terms of the transient times involved. Channelling leads to a reduction in the sizes of pools and therefore in the associated transient times. At an empirical level the advantage gained from channelling can be assessed by comparing the measured transient time for the complex with that derived from a consideration of free-solution kinetics. Having established that the temporal behaviour of metabolic systems may be analysed in rather simple terms, the aim is now to see what further insight can be gained into the channelling of intermediate metabolites by the analysis of transient response.

Fig. 2   **Model of substrate channelling within multienzyme complexes and multifunctional proteins**

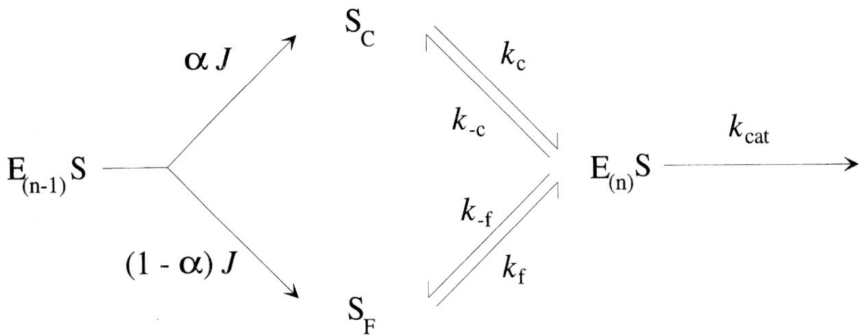

S_c represents channelled intermediate, S_F intermediate released into free solution and J the steady-state flux. $E_{(n-1)}$ and $E_{(n)}$ represent the $(n-1)$th and (n)th enzymes of the series. k_c and k_{-c} are the rate coefficients for the formation and dissociation of the $E_{(n)}S$ complex via the channelled route; k_f and k_{-f} are the corresponding rate coefficients via the free-solution route. k_{cat} is the rate coefficient for the formation of product from the $E_{(n)}S$ complex and corresponds to the catalytic-centre activity of the enzyme; it represents the number of substrate molecules processed by each active centre per unit time. It is equal to $V/[E_T]$, where V is the maximum velocity of the nth enzyme and $[E_T]$ its total concentration. α represents the fraction of flux passing through the channelled route, and it is envisaged that α will be determined by the structure of the complex and reflects the relative magnitudes of the rate coefficients for release by the alternative routes.

Fig. 2 describes a minimum model compatible with channelling of intermediates within a multienzyme complex or multifunctional protein. According to the scheme an enzyme releases its product, the intermediate S, either into an internalized pool within the complex (S_c) or into free solution in the bulk medium (S_F). The channelling process is 'leaky', with fraction α of the steady-state flux entering the internal pool and fraction $(1 - \alpha)$ being released into the bulk phase. α is termed the channelling efficiency at this stage in the enzyme sequence [9,24]. The next enzyme in the sequence can receive intermediate either from the internal pool or from the external pool and convert it into the next intermediate of the pathway with rate constant k_{cat}. Release of product from the enzymes is considered irreversible in this model in order to reduce the mathematical complexity, but in principle reversibility could be included at these stages. No direct exchange has been included between the internal and external pools as this, if significant, would effectively destroy the channelling advantage. It should be stressed here that the extent of channelling is determined by α, which is in turn a function of the relative magnitude of the rate constants for release of the intermediate into the bulk phase and the internal pool. It will be predetermined by the structure of the complex and the physical constraints placed upon the free diffusion of the metabolite.

Simple analysis of the steady-state kinetic behaviour of the system described in Fig. 2, without solution of differential equations, allows comparison of the transient times for the channelled and non-channelled routes. Associated with each metabolite pool is a transient time which is the lifetime of the pool or the time required for the pool to turn over in the steady state. These transients are additive in determining the total transient response of the system, as indicated previously. Variation or fluctuation in the rate of input of material to the pathway, during the approach to the steady state, adds an additional term to the description of the pathway transient. This will alter the pathway transient but will not alter the transient times associated with the intermediate pools or the kinetic advantage conferred by channelling [18].

In the present system, rate equations for each of the metabolite pools are written and set equal to zero in the steady state. In this way the pool sizes are determined and the associated transient times are defined. In the scheme of Fig. 2, the total transient time associated with intermediate S at the nth step in the sequence is given by:

$$\tau = ([S_c] + [S_F] + [E_{(n)}S])/J \tag{17}$$

where steady-state concentrations are implied and J represents the steady-state flux through the pathway. In this analysis, intermediate concentrations are averaged over the total system volume. Therefore $[S_c]$ in eqn. (17) represents the mean concentration of channelled intermediate averaged over the total volume and not the local concentration within the enzyme complex. In the steady state, the pool sizes may be estimated by solution of the appropriate rate equations:

$$d[S_c]/dt = d[S_F]/dt = d[E_{(n)}S]/dt = 0 \tag{18}$$

The result of this analysis is:

$$\tau = 1/k_{cat} + [\alpha k_{cat}/k_c + (1 - \alpha)k_{cat}/k_f + k_{-c}/k_c + k_{-f}/k_f]/(V - J) \tag{19}$$

Eqn. (19) may be expressed in an alternative form:

$$\tau = \alpha \cdot \tau_c + (1 - \alpha) \cdot \tau_f \tag{20}$$

where τ is the total transient associated with this stage in the sequence and τ_c and τ_f represent the transient times associated with the wholly channelled (upper) and free solution (lower) routes respectively of Fig. 2. τ_c is the value of τ obtained from eqns. (19) and (20) when α is unity; τ_f is the value of τ when α is zero. It should be noted that, even by the channelled route, intermediate will still be able to enter the free solution pool by dissociation of the $E_{(n)}S$ complex. This is necessary as free-solution intermediate must be able to find its way back into the complex for further metabolism if it is not to accumulate. In the very restricted case where there is an alternative fate possible for the free-solution metabolite, re-entry into the complex may not be essential. Similarly, even by the free-solution route, intermediate can enter the internalized pool by dissociation of the $E_{(n)}S$ complex.

The transient times for the free solution (τ_f) and channelled (τ_c) routes are given by:

$$\tau_f = 1/k_{cat} + K_m/(V - J) + {}^cK_s/(V - J) \tag{21}$$

$$\tau_c = 1/k_{cat} + {}^cK_m/(V - J) + K_s/(V - J) \tag{22}$$

where ${}^cK_s$ is the dissociation constant of intermediate from the ES complex into the channelled pool, K_s is the dissociation constant into the bulk phase and ${}^cK_m$ is the Michaelis constant of the channelled intermediate.

The definitions of the Michaelis and dissociation constants are as follows:

$$K_m = (k_{-f} + k_{cat})/k_f \tag{23}$$

$${}^cK_m = (k_{-c} + k_{cat})/k_c \tag{24}$$

$$K_s = k_{-f}/k_f \tag{25}$$

$${}^cK_s = k_{-c}/k_c \tag{26}$$

It can be seen that eqns. (21) and (22) each comprise three terms. The first is the lifetime or turnover time of the enzyme–substrate complex. The second is the time associated with the generation of the pool of intermediate either in free solution (eqn. 21) or within the complex (eqn. 22). The third term represents the time associated with the establishment of an intermediate pool either within the complex (eqn. 21) or in the bulk phase (eqn. 22) by simple dissociation of the enzyme–substrate complex on a branch to the main pathway flux.

The kinetic constants either superscripted or subscripted with c in eqns. (21)–(26) refer to processes involving channelled intermediate; those superscripted or subscripted with f or without a superscript or subscript refer to processes involving intermediate in the bulk phase. The expression for the overall transient time τ, derived from eqns. (19) or (20), may be expressed as follows:

$$\tau = 1/k_{cat} + [K_m + {}^cK_s + \alpha({}^cK_m - {}^cK_s + K_s - K_m)]/(V - J) \tag{27}$$

This equation represents the transient time associated with a single intermediate in the pathway. An analogous transient will be associated with each intermediate.

If any improvement in the transient response is due to the channelling process rather than to conformational and consequent kinetic changes in the enzymes on forming the complex, then eqn. (27) may be simplified. The advantage due to channelling will be the result of the higher local intermediate concentration within the complex and will result in an apparent increase in the 'on-constant' for the formation of the enzyme–intermediate complex relative to the free-solution behaviour, without any change in the 'off-constant'. The increase in on-constant results from the greater probability of an encounter between the enzyme active centre and the intermediate within the complex, and should therefore affect the Michaelis and dissociation constants equally. The off-constant is unaffected, and therefore k_{-c} and k_{-f} are identical. The factor by which the on-constant k_c is increased is termed the channelling advantage and is represented by the symbol β. β is given by:

$$\beta = k_c/k_f = K_m/{}^cK_m = K_s/{}^cK_s \tag{28}$$

The transient time may now be written in terms of the free-solution kinetic constants, the channelling efficiency α and the channelling advantage β:

$$\tau = 1/k_{cat} + [K_m + K_s/\beta + \alpha(K_m/\beta - K_s/\beta + K_s - K_m)]/(V - J) \tag{29}$$

Similarly the definitions of τ_f and τ_c become:

$$\tau_f = 1/k_{cat} + K_m/(V - J) + (K_s/\beta)/(V - J) \tag{30}$$

$$\tau_c = 1/k_{cat} + (K_m/\beta)/(V - J) + K_s/(V - J) \tag{31}$$

An alternative interpretation of the channelling advantage β can be given in terms of the volumes of the metabolite pools internal to and external to the complex. If the kinetic model is analysed in terms of local rather than average concentration of intermediate, then k_c and k_f can also be considered identical and β represents the ratio of internal to external metabolite concentrations. This is equivalent to the ratio of system volume to internal pool volume.

For a significant difference to exist between the transient times for the free-solution and channelled routes, and for channelling to represent a kinetic advantage, τ_c must be much less than τ_f. From eqns. (21), (22), (30) and (31), the following inequalities must obtain:

$$K_s \ll K_m \tag{32}$$

and:

$$k_{cat} \gg k_{-f} \tag{33}$$

This means that K_m must be greater than the dissociation constant of the enzyme–substrate complex and implies that enzymes exhibiting rapid-equilibrium kinetic mechanisms are unlikely to obtain a kinetic advantage through channelling. This condition may also be expressed as the need for k_{cat} to be much greater than the off-constant of the enzyme–substrate complex, and means that the intermediate will be removed along the enzyme sequence before it can dissociate from the enzyme–substrate complex into free solution. Eqns. (21) and (22) indicate a further constraint on kinetic advantage due to channelling. If the enzyme concentration is increased at constant flux, V increases and the transients associated with free-solution and channelled pools decrease (i.e. the second and third terms of the equations decrease). Both τ_f and τ_c then reach the same limiting value, namely $1/k_{cat}$, the lifetime of the enzyme–substrate complex [16], and a direct transfer mechanism prevails. Thus at high protein concentration the free and channelled pools are minimized and no kinetic advantage is obtained from channelling. Examination of eqns. (21) and (22) reveals that by high enzyme concentration we mean an enzyme concentration comparable with K_m or K_s, whichever is the greater. Eqn. (32) suggests that this will generally mean that enzyme concentration must be comparable with or greater than K_m.

To summarize, there is no kinetic advantage or reduction of transient time due to the channelling process if either of the following conditions obtain: (a) the enzyme has a rapid-equilibrium kinetic mechanism (this restriction only obtains for channelling efficiencies less than unity, where exchange between free-solution intermediate and the enzyme–substrate complex is necessary); and (b) the enzyme concentration is high (i.e. $[E_T] \geq K_m$).

Eqns. (27) and (29) also allow the determination of α and β. Eqn. (27) may be expressed as:

$$\alpha = [(\tau - 1/k_{cat})(V - J) - {}^cK_s - K_m]/({}^cK_m - {}^cK_s + K_s - K_m) \tag{34}$$

The alternative form using eqn. (29) is:

$$\alpha = [(\tau - 1/k_{cat})(V - J) - K_s/\beta - K_m]/(K_m/\beta - K_s/\beta + K_s - K_m) \tag{35}$$

In practice β is likely to be large and therefore ${}^cK_s$ and ${}^cK_m$ are likely to be very small. Eqns. (34) and (35) then reduce to:

$$\alpha = [(\tau - 1/k_{cat})(V - J) - K_m]/(K_s - K_m) \tag{36}$$

This is a more convenient form, as ${}^cK_s$ and ${}^cK_m$ are likely to be difficult to determine. It represents the direct transfer of intermediate between enzyme active centres. This has been the starting point for most previous analyses. Under these conditions the pool of channelled intermediate vanishes. Eqn. (36) can be further simplified if K_m is greater than K_s. The expression becomes:

$$\alpha = 1 - (\tau - 1/k_{cat})(V - J)/K_m \tag{37}$$

Here there is no dissociation of the enzyme–substrate complex into the free-solution pool and the transient time for the channelled intermediate is simply the lifetime of the enzyme–substrate complex. All quantities in eqns. (36)

and (37) refer to free-solution behaviour of the enzyme and should be more readily measurable.

An alternative use for the equations might be to estimate the channelling advantage, β. This may be done using eqn. (35) if an independent method is available for the determination of α. One such method would be to measure the isotopic dilution of exogenously added labelled intermediate [26–29].

Channelling advantage in relation to metabolic and evolutionary strategies

Cornish-Bowden and Cárdenas [30] have claimed to have shown that channelling of a metabolite within a dynamic enzyme complex, and by implication also within static channels, cannot lead to a reduction in the size of the pool of free intermediate. This of course implies that no kinetic advantage results from channelling and contradicts what has been demonstrated here. I consider their elegant analysis using flux and concentration control coefficients to be conceptually flawed. They start with a pre-existing channel in which part of the flux is directed through the channel and part through the free solution. They then ask what happens to the pool sizes if the flux is redistributed. To effect this redistribution they increase all of the rate constants along a particular branch by the same factor without altering the total flux. Without applying Control Analysis it is easy to see that this will not result in a change in pool sizes. If all rate constants change by the same factor then all equilibrium constants remain unchanged and, as a consequence, so do the equilibrium and steady-state pool sizes. The authors are aware of this and also of the fact that the flux and concentration summation properties of Control Analysis were first derived making this assumption.

What one needs to do is not to analyse changes to the pre-exisiting channel, but to contrast the situation in which no channel exists with that in which it is active. To do this, the rate constants cannot all be changed by the same factor. Indeed it makes no sense to do so, as only second-order rate constants can be affected by the channelling process. What has been done here is as follows. Firstly the distribution of flux has been arranged so that the total flux J is kept constant, as suggested by Cornish-Bowden and Cárdenas [30]. Indeed the flux is seen as being determined outside the step in the pathway under scrutiny. The 'leakiness' of the channel, and hence the distribution of flux, is accounted for by the channelling efficiency, α. This in turn reflects the rate coefficients for the release of intermediate into the respective pools and is determined by the structure of the complex. All rate constants along the channelled route are unaffected by the channelling process except the rate constant associated with the formation of the enzyme–substrate complex (the on-constant). In other words, no special kinetic advantages or 'tricks' are associated with channelling. The on-constant changes for the reason always intuitively understood and assumed to be the advantage of channelling. Namely, if the intermediate of the pathway is restricted within the complex and not free to diffuse throughout the system, then its concentration as seen by the enzyme will be higher; thus the likelihood of an encounter resulting in complex-formation will be greater and therefore the rate attained will be reached at a lower concentration. This all results from the fact that there is a greater probability of enzyme and intermediate meeting each other and forming a complex. It is due to the fact that the binding process is second-order and involves diffusion and encounter, while all other processes are first-order and are unaffected by channelling. There are no changes to the enzyme or to the energetics of the reaction along the channelled route. The enzyme is merely force-fed with substrate as a result of the structural properties of the complex.

It is necessary to increase the on-constant because of the way in which concentrations are defined. Although the intermediate may be retained within a very restricted volume within the complex, or even transferred directly from one enzyme to the next, its concentration is referred to the total system volume. If one could imagine oneself sitting inside the complex, then the local concentration of intermediate would be much higher and the on-constant would appear to be unchanged from that in the free-solution, unchannelled situation. In other words, channelling has conferred a purely statistical advantage, and influence on the binding process and the thermodynamics of binding (binding energy) are essentially unaffected. The ratio of the on-constant in the channel to that in free solution is no more than the ratio of the total system volume to the volume occupied by the internalized pool of intermediate. It is equivalent to the channelling advantage, β. Once a channel is established, as in the present model, a simultaneous increase in all rate constants along the channelled route or free-solution routes by a constant factor would not alter the pool sizes, in agreement with Cornish-Bowden and Cárdenas [30]. These pool sizes are effectively set by the values given to the rate constants when the channel is established, and in the present instance are the result of the values assigned to α and β. It is the small internal volume of the channel and the correspondingly large value of β which decide the relative sizes of the channelled and free-solution pools. In the case of the analysis of Cornish-Bowden and Cárdenas [30], it is their initial choice of relative rate constants along the channelled and free-solution routes which decides the relative sizes of the pools, and no redistribution of flux by altering all rate constants in proportion can alter the relative pool sizes initially set. In the present context, such an alteration would constitute altering α to change the distribution of flux, but then changing all other rate constants similarly to annul the effect on pool sizes. A change in α in the present model constitutes an alteration to only one of the rate constants on each route, namely that rate constant which decides the efficiency or leakiness of the channel. In this way it is possible to ask what happens when the channel leaks or does not leak, while the channelling advantage remains constant. Cornish-Bowden and Cárdenas [30] have been careful to point out that distribution of flux is not the same as distribution of pool sizes. This point has been made here in the definition of α and was recognized earlier [22,24]. A critique of the analysis of Cornish-Bowden and Cárdenas [30] has been presented previously [25].

It is now appropriate to ask: what are the real benefits of channelling? [6]. There is no reason, given adequate enzyme capacities, why flux limitation should be a problem in a steady-state system. The required flux can always be reached by increasing pool sizes. This applies to normal kinetic limitation and also to diffusion-controlled processes. Problems associated with large transit times, owing to diffusional restriction, can be overcome by increasing the size of the metabolite pool. The penalty for this is an increased transition time, but it represents a shifting of the 'temporal burden' to the transition period (approach to the steady state) and away from the steady state. The primary restriction may, therefore, be on the pool size rather than on the flux.

Pool sizes may need to be restricted because of the limited solvent capacity of the cell, as suggested by Atkinson [31], but a further restriction may be the need for a rapid system response. Large pools act as a buffer against change where a transition between steady states may be required. This is due to the dependence of the system transition time on the pool lifetimes, specifically on the ratios of pool sizes to metabolic flux [16]. The existence of large pools therefore acts as a homoeostatic mechanism and there is a conflict between the need for homoeostasis and the need for a rapid system response.

A rapid system response may be achieved either through minimization of pools or by increasing enzyme capacities. It is tempting to speculate that the apparent overcapacity of glycolytic enzymes in yeast [32] and many other cells is required to allow the cell to adapt rapidly rather than to compensate for suboptimal conditions or diffusional restrictions encountered *in vivo*. Negative feedback also contributes to the rapid response. Enzyme capacities may be high during the transitional period and then limited by feedback in the steady state [18]. This, of course, has a considerable energy cost in terms of enzyme synthesis. A more energy-efficient solution may be the reduction of pool sizes through channelling. It is likely that the same pathway will respond differently in different tissues depending on the physiological requirement for either homoeostasis or flexibility of response. In instances where a rapid response is required, channelling would be appropriate; where the demand for the pathway is relatively constant and homoeostasis is more important, large pools of intermediates might be expected. The channelling process may therefore incur a penalty; namely the decrease in homoeostasis and a reduction in the temporal stability of the system. The actual pool sizes encountered *in vivo* probably represent a compromise between these conflicting needs for stability and flexibility.

There is a further problem relating to pool sizes when flux control is considered. If the flux through a pathway is stimulated by activating a rate-limiting or control enzyme through covalent modification or some other stimulus external to the system, then the flux increase can be considerable. The enzymes downstream from the control point respond to this initial activation by increasing their activities. These increases are usually considered to be the result of changes in the pool sizes. However, it will be obvious that the changes in pool sizes must be correspondingly large to generate the increased flux if single point control is in operation. An alternative strategy would be to stimulate both ends of the pathway and arrange for intermediate steps to be both reversible and near equilibrium. In this way, with over-capacity of intervening enzymes, relatively small changes in pool size could produce large changes in *net* flux. This may be the mechanism obtaining in glycolysis. It is clear that such problems would be obviated by channelling and the presence of small, internalized pools. Indeed, with direct transfer mechanisms the intermediate pools would be totally absent, except in the sense of enzyme–substrate complexes, and no problems of escalating pool size would occur.

References

1. Reed, L.J. and Cox, D.J. (1966) Annu. Rev. Biochem. **35**, 57–84
2. Yanofsky, C. and Crawford, I.P. (1972) Enzymes 3rd Edn. **7**, 1–31
3. Welch, G.R and Gaertner, F. (1976) Arch. Biochem. Biophys. **172**, 476–489
4. Nicholson, S., Easterby, J.S. and Powls, R. (1987) Eur. J. Biochem. **162**, 423–431
5. Gontero, B., Cárdenas, L. and Ricard, J. (1988) Eur. J. Biochem. **173**, 437–443
6. Easterby, J.S. (1991) J. Theor. Biol. **152**, 47–48
7. Knowles, J.R. (1991) J. Theor. Biol. **152**, 53–55
8. Srivastava, D.K. and Bernhard, S. (1986) Curr. Top. Cell. Regul. **28**, 1–68
9. Ovádi, J., Tompa, P., Vértessy, B., Orosz, F., Keleti, T. and Welch, G.R. (1989) Biochem. J. **257**, 187–190
10. Hyde, C.C., Ahmed, A.A., Padlan, E.A., Miles, E.W. and Davies, D.R. (1988) J. Biol. Chem. **263**, 17857–17871
11. McClure, W.R. (1969) Biochemistry **8**, 2782–2786
12. Barwell, C.J. and Hess, B.(1970) Hoppe-Seyler's Z. Physiol. Chem. **351**, 1531–1536
13. Easterby, J.S. (1973) Biochim. Biophys. Acta **293**, 552–558
14. Easterby, J.S. (1984) Biochem. J. **219**, 843–847
15. Heinrich, R. and Rapoport, T.A. (1975) BioSystems **7**, 130–136
16. Easterby, J.S. (1981) Biochem. J. **199**, 155–161
17. Bartha, F. and Keleti, T. (1979) Oxid. Commun. **1**, 75–84
18. Easterby, J.S. (1986) Biochem. J. **233**, 871–875
19. Kacser, H. and Burns, J.A. (1973) Symp. Soc. Exp. Biol. **27**, 65–104
20. Heinrich, R. and Rapoport, T.A. (1974) Eur. J. Biochem. **42**, 89–95
21. Easterby, J.S. (1990) Biochem. J. **269**, 255–259
22. Easterby, J.S. (1990) in Control of Metabolic Processes (Cornish-Bowden, A. and Cárdenas, M.L., eds.), pp. 281–290, Plenum, New York
23. Meléndez-Hevia, E., Torres, N.V., Sicilia, J. and Kacser, H. (1990) Biochem. J. **265**, 195–202
24. Easterby, J.S. (1989) Biochem. J. **264**, 605–607
25. Easterby, J.S. (1993) J. Mol. Recognit. **6**, 179–187
26. Lue, P.F. and Kaplan, J.G. (1970) Biochim. Biophys. Acta **220**, 365–372
27. Matchett, W.H. (1974) J. Biol. Chem. **249**, 4041–4049

28. Christopherson, R.I. and Jones, M.E. (1980) J. Biol. Chem. **255**, 11381–11395
29. Christopherson, R.I., Traut, T.W. and Jones, M.E. (1981) Curr. Top. Cell. Regul. **18**, 59–77
30. Cornish-Bowden, A. and Cárdenas, M.L. (1993) Eur. J. Biochem. **213**, 87–92
31. Atkinson, D.E. (1969) Curr. Top. Cell. Regul. **1**, 29–43
32. Boiteux, A. and Hess, B. (1981) Philos. Trans. R. Soc. London B **293**, 5–22

6

Control and regulation of channelled versus ideal pathways

Boris N. Kholodenko*†, Marta Cascante† and Hans V. Westerhoff‡

*A.N. Belozersky Institute of Physico-Chemical Biology, Moscow State University, 119899 Moscow, Russia, †Department de Bioquimica i Fisiologia, Universitat de Barcelona, Marti i Franques 1, Barcelona, Spain, and ‡E.C. Slater Institute, Biocentrum, University of Amsterdam, Plantage Muidergracht 12, and Department of Microbial Physiology, Free University, De Boelelaan 1087, NL-1081 HV Amsterdam, The Netherlands

Introduction

The notion that intracellular metabolism takes place in highly organized cellular structures is probably older than the notion that metabolism takes place in an essentially homogeneous aqueous phase [1,2]. Indeed, in some cells the concentration of polymers is comparable with that in our laboratory gels, and in early experiments a cytogel rather than a cytosol appeared upon removal of the plasma membrane. In some minds this notion has led to the inference that metabolism must also be highly organized, in the sense that metabolites must be handed over directly by the enzyme that produces them to the enzyme that consumes them (see, e.g., [3–7]). Accordingly, enzymes belonging to a metabolic pathway would have to be organized in supercomplexes.

None of this appears to be necessary, however. Apart from a fraction of water that is bound, most intracellular water appears to have a diffusion coefficient that is comparable with that of water from the tap, when measured over small distances [3]. Also, the NMR relaxation times of most metabolites measured inside the 'cytogel' are not too different from those measured in test tubes. Only a few enzymes can be isolated as multienzyme complexes. These range from well known examples such as the pyruvate dehydrogenase complex (where the metabolite that is handed over remains covalently bound), the tryptophan synthase complex [8,9] (where an internal tunnel has been observed by X-ray diffraction) and the AROM protein {which, in higher fungi, contains five enzyme activities on a single polypeptide chain and behaves as a leaky channel ([10,11]; see also Chapter 9 in the present volume)} to the phosphotransferase system, which hands over protein-bound phosphate ultimately from phosphoenolpyruvate to glucose [12]. For some enzyme couples there is evidence that there may be a complex *in vivo* which does not survive isolation [13], whereas for other proteins the evidence is defective or there is even evidence to the contrary [14].

If one assumes (1) that the intracellular medium allows diffusion of small molecules to proceed only somewhat more slowly than in pure water, and (2) a random distribution of enzymes, then one can calculate that for mainstream metabolic pathways the enzyme molecules are more than close enough together for the diffusion transit times to be much shorter than the catalytic turnover times. In this scenario metabolic pathways are not limited by diffusion [15,16]. Indeed, most molecules should delocalize over much of the volume of the compartment they are in before they are metabolized. In addition, many metabolic pathways have been reconstituted *in vitro*, and it has been shown that the dissociation rates of metabolites from the enzymes are not so slow that they preclude the free-diffusion mechanism, and that enzymes do not release their metabolite only when the subsequent enzyme in the pathway is there to receive it. Clearly, metabolism based on the free diffusion of metabolites is feasible. If diffusion is free, it is kinetically competent. If the enzymes release their products sufficiently rapidly, then the concentrations of most metabolites should be essentially similar throughout the cell, unless the producer and consumer enzymes are located at opposite sides of the cell or are present at extremely low concentrations, or the free metabolite concentrations are below 1 μM. It is noteworthy that, to reach these conclusions, it is not necessary that the enzymes themselves diffuse rapidly; diffusion of the metabolite suffices. This is important, as there is reason to suspect that diffusion of proteins and nucleic acids is decreased inside cells, for example due to binding to structural elements.

The concept that intracellular metabolism proceeds essentially as if in a well stirred reactor has been of great benefit to the development of biochemistry and cell biology. It has promoted the isolation and characterization of individual enzymes from metabolic pathways, which has been crucial for the delineation of the metabolic map. In the particular example of membrane-linked free-energy transduction it has led to co-reconstitution of proton pumps from different organisms, leading to the detection of proton-gradient-mediated free-energy transduction between chemical reactions and hence proving the essence of the chemiosmotic coupling hypothesis (for review and further analysis see [17]).

The fact that the chemical essence of metabolism can be understood if one assumes a random-diffusion mechanism induced in 'men who shave with an Occams razor', is to assume that metabolism indeed behaves in this manner. This assumption is risky, however. First, especially in the biological sciences, there is no epistemological reason for simplicity to be more likely than complexity [18]. The second reason is that not only the tools, but also the concepts, used to analyse metabolism have been too crude to elucidate the extent of organization of metabolism if that organization exhibits any of the subtlety that we are getting used to in biology.

For ourselves, much inspiration for the quantitative analysis of metabolic channelling stemmed from the history of the analysis of a related issue, i.e. which enzyme limits the flux through a pathway. In this case also, in the very early years it was thought that this issue was impossible to address because it would require too much interference with the metabolic pathway. Subsequently there was a period in which enzymes that catalyse irreversible reactions and are near the beginning of metabolic pathways (e.g. phosphofructokinase) were identified as the rate-limiting steps. This led to significant progress in the understanding of how these enzymes were themselves regulated and to the identification of many allosteric interactions. Only in later years, however, starting with the pioneering papers [19–23], was it realized that the common assumption that metabolic pathways have a single such rate-limiting step was unfounded. For example, the ornithine carbamoyltransferase of *Neurospora* [24], the adenine nucleotide translocator and cytochrome oxidase of mitochondria [25], the H^+-ATPase of *Escherichia coli* [26], the phosphofructokinase of *Saccharomyces cerevisiae* [27] and many other assumed rate-limiting steps were shown to be only partly involved in the control of the flux through their respective pathways. It was found that metabolic control is much more subtle than to have single rate-limiting steps. The development that was essential for this progress was conceptual: a definition of the extent to which an enzyme is rate-limiting that allowed that extent to be not only 1 or 0, but also anything in between. Since it was also proved mathematically that the sum of the extent of rate limitation by all the enzymes must equal 1 (but see below), this made it clear that the only way to test the validity of the concept of 'a single rate-limiting step' is to measure rate limitation quantitatively. In these and related analyses it also became clear that the extent to which an enzyme controls the flux through its pathway depends on the conditions under which that pathway operates. In addition, when an enzyme exerts a lot of control on flux, it does not necessarily exert much control on metabolite concentrations. Thus there are apparently many aspects to control.

We also believe that the question of the organization of metabolism requires a quantitative approach for its ultimate resolution. The question should not be whether or not metabolism is channelled, but which part of metabolism is channelled, to what extent and under what conditions. It is likely that metabolic organization also depends subtly on conditions, and differs between pathways.

Significant progress has been made in the quantitative definition of what channelling is. Important aspects have been the distinctions between static and dynamic channelling, transient time analysis, and non-thermodynamics and kinetics of channelling [13,28]. What has been a significant limitation, however, is the uncertainty in defining the control exerted by channelling on pathway flux and on metabolite concentrations in the channelled pathway. In this chapter we review the recent developments of concepts that should now allow unequivocal definition of the control of metabolite channelling. We describe the laws that relate the extent to which enzymes control channelling to enzyme properties. Finally, we apply the new methods to address an issue that has been controversial in the recent literature, i.e. whether increasing metabolite channelling may have the effect of decreasing the concentrations of free metabolites.

Metabolic Control Analysis of ideal pathways

We begin with 'classical' definitions of special indicators of the control exerted by any enzyme on flux [19–23]. These suffice for a complete description of the control and regulation in a so-called 'ideal' metabolic pathway (i.e. an enzymologist's test tube). In such pathways: (a) the enzymes are independent catalysts, and (b) the concentrations of enzyme-bound metabolites can be neglected compared with their free concentrations (for a recent review see [29]).

Classical definitions of the control exerted by enzymes, and the summation theorem

The loose question of whether a particular enzyme i does or does not control flux can be made both operational and quantitative by rephrasing it as follows: if we change the activity of enzyme i by, say, 1%, what will be the percentage change in flux at the steady state? A strict mathematical definition extrapolates the percentage variation to an infinitesimal one and relates a fractional change $(\mathrm{d}J/J)$ in the steady-state flux to the fractional modulation $(\mathrm{d}e_i/e_i)$ of the enzyme concentration [20]:

$$C_{e_i}^J = \left(\frac{\mathrm{d}J}{J}\right)\bigg/\left(\frac{\mathrm{d}e_i}{e_i}\right)_{\mathrm{sys}} = \left(\frac{\mathrm{d}\ln|J|}{\mathrm{d}\ln e_i}\right)_{\mathrm{sys}} \tag{1}$$

The subscript 'sys' signifies that differentiation conditions require the steady state of the system.

The dimensionless coefficient $C_{e_i}^J$ is called the flux control coefficient of enzyme i. If the control coefficient equals zero, the enzyme (i) does not control the flux at all (is not rate-limiting); if it equals 1, then i is rate limiting. Thus these two categories of the older qualitative analysis are retained in the new terminology. More importantly, however, in any intermediate case the control coefficient can assume any value and it can be considered as a quantitative indicator of the relative degree to which the enzyme controls (or limits) the overall flux.

In the case when the maximal catalytic activity is not proportional to the enzyme concentration, a more general definition of control is helpful [20,30]. The latter compares a relative change in the local reaction rate $(\mathrm{d}v_i/v_i)$ with the resulting change in the system's flux at steady state [21]. Its explicit expression considers changes in an enzyme rate as caused by a variation in any parameter (p_i) which affects only that rate v_i ($\partial v_i/\partial p_i \neq 0$; $\partial v_j/\partial p_i = 0$ for any $j \neq i$):

$$C_{v_i}^{J} = \frac{(\mathrm{d}\ln|J|/\mathrm{d}p_i)_{\mathrm{sys}}}{(\partial\ln|v_i|/\partial p_i)_{\mathrm{enz}}} = \frac{v_i}{J}\cdot\frac{(\mathrm{d}J/\mathrm{d}p_i)_{\mathrm{sys}}}{(\partial v_i/\partial p_i)_{\mathrm{enz}}} \tag{2}$$

The subscript 'enz' signifies that a perturbation in the local rate $(\partial v_i/v_i)$ is considered as though the reaction of enzyme i were in isolation from the pathway (when taking the derivative $\partial v_i/\partial p_i$, all the concentrations of metabolites should be kept at the values of the initial steady state of the pathway).

This control coefficient designated $C_{v_i}^{J}$ is called the control coefficient with respect to the enzyme catalytic activity (V_{max}) rather than to the enzyme concentration. An attractive property of this rate-linked control coefficient is that, in ideal pathways, it does not depend on the particular choice of a parameter (p_i) as long as that parameter affects only the rate v_i [31–33]. Moreover, in ideal pathways the rate-linked control coefficients $(C_{v_i}^{J})$ are identical with the control coefficients referring to the enzyme concentration $(C_{e_i}^{J})$ (cf. [34]). However, in non-ideal pathways the coefficients $C_{v_i}^{J}$ and $C_{e_i}^{J}$ may differ significantly [34–38]. Moreover, in many non-ideal pathways, the control coefficient $(C_{v_i}^{J})$ as defined according to eqn. (2) depends on the choice of parameter p_i [36–39]. This dependence appears to be due to direct or indirect (i.e. via moiety conservation involving different enzymes bound to the same substrate moiety) interactions between enzymes.

In an analogous manner (see eqns. 1 and 2) the concentration control coefficients can be defined. They measure the response of the concentration of a particular metabolite to changes in a specific parameter (e.g. e_i or p_i):

$$C_{e_i}^{x_k} = (\mathrm{d}\ln x_k/\mathrm{d}\ln e_i)_{\mathrm{sys}} \tag{3}$$

$$C_{v_i}^{x_k} = \frac{(\mathrm{d}\ln x_k/\mathrm{d}p_i)_{\mathrm{sys}}}{(\partial\ln|v_i|/\partial p_i)_{\mathrm{enz}}} = \frac{v_i}{x_k}\cdot\frac{(\mathrm{d}x_k/\mathrm{d}p_i)_{\mathrm{sys}}}{(\partial v_i/\partial p_i)_{\mathrm{enz}}} \tag{4}$$

where x_k is the concentration of an intermediate.

One of the best known and intuitively most understandable properties of flux control coefficients is that, when summing over all enzymes of a system, they add up to unity:

$$\sum_i C_{e_i}^{J} = 1 \tag{5}$$

In ideal pathways this property, called the summation theorem, is valid independent of the structure of a pathway and the local kinetic properties of the enzymes. Indeed, in such pathways any steady-state flux is a homogeneous first-order function of the enzyme concentrations (i.e. if the enzyme concentrations change simultaneously by a factor α, then all fluxes in the system will change by the same factor α), and the summation theorem (eqn. 5) is a simple consequence of Euler's theorem [32,40]. When direct interactions between different enzymes are absent, the summation theorem (see eqn. 5) continues to apply after substitution of coefficients $C_{v_i}^J$ for coefficients $C_{e_i}^J$ [35,36]. However, in channelled pathways the sum in eqn. (5) may be not equal to unity for either of the enzyme control coefficients [39,41]. The behaviour of the sum of the flux control coefficients in different systems will be analysed below. We shall see that measuring this sum can give a deeper insight into the regulatory properties and mechanistic aspects of real cellular pathways.

The real cell: what is non-ideal?

In the traditional view cellular metabolism is considered as a number of enzymes in an aqueous solution that obtain their substrates from a well stirred bulk phase and return their products back to that phase. However, as mentioned in the Introduction, various features of real metabolic pathways do not conform to this simple concept. In highly organized cellular pathways, direct enzyme–enzyme interactions and enzyme associations take place which can lead to a direct transfer of intermediates [4,42–44]. In some pathways such a direct transfer is even standard, for example in the electron-transfer chains of free-energy-transducing membranes and in the bacterial phosphotransferase systems for sugar uptake [12].

The term 'channelling' has been coined to refer to a sequence of chemical conversions taking place by a direct transfer mechanism (reviewed in [13]). The reaction sequence in a channelled phase may involve various types of enzyme associations. In the case of so called 'static' channelling the enzyme–enzyme complex is assumed to be at thermodynamic equilibrium with its constituent enzymes. The latter may be tightly bound, i.e. complexes may exist for longer than the mean passage time of metabolites through that part of the pathway [8,9]. In an extreme case the linkage is covalent, for example in the pyruvate dehydrogenase complex. Obviously, in the latter case the concentrations of different 'domains' of the complex cannot be varied independently, so that the question of how variations in the concentrations of different enzymes (domains) affect the flux becomes irrelevant.

Much of the current debate in the literature is more concerned with 'dynamic' enzyme associations, involving metabolic intermediates. A simple scheme of such a dynamic channel [44–47] is depicted in Fig. 1. A feature of this dynamic channel is that the ternary complex (E_1XE_2) has to be formed and broken down at each cycle in the conversion of a substrate molecule into the product of the reaction pair (Fig. 1). The concentration of the ternary complex depends (dynamically) on the concentrations of the other enzymes and metabolite intermediates and on the flux through the system. It may (or

Fig. I   **A dynamic channel**

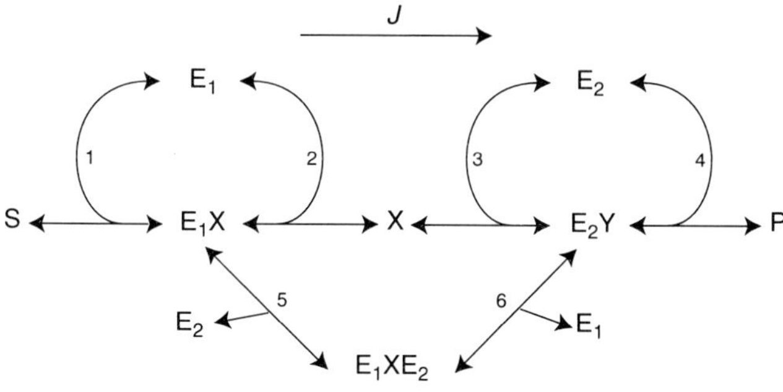

The concentrations of the initial substrate S and of the end-product P are constants. The positive direction of the flux J is from S to P. The enzyme–enzyme complex E_1XE_2 is formed after binding of the substrate S to E_1. The upper route represents the usual reaction pathway through the bulk-phase intermediate (X), catalysed by free enzymes, and the lower route represents dynamic channelling. The numbering of the elemental steps is shown.

may not) be negligible compared with the concentrations of monomeric enzymes.

Fig. 2 shows a possible scheme of a static channel. Here the enzyme–enzyme complex E_1E_2 catalyses the direct transfer of substrate (S) to product (P) that occurs in the channelled phase (corresponding to the lower route in the scheme of Fig. 2). At any steady state the complex E_1E_2 is at thermodynamic equilibrium with the enzyme intermediates E_1 and E_2.

In general, an important distinction between static and dynamic channelling is that the conversion of substrate into product that occurs in the channelled route requires association and subsequent dissociation of an enzyme–enzyme complex in a dynamic channel, but not in a static channel. Note that the same scheme may harbour both dynamic and static channelling routes (different schemes that are possible in general have been described in detail in [13,48]). For instance, the channelled routes in the scheme of Fig. 3 are: (i) steps 6, 7 and 8 (static), (ii) steps 9, 7 and 10 (dynamic), (iii) steps 9, 7, 8 and 5 (dynamic), and their combinations. Note that in the scheme of Fig. 3, step 5 of the formation of the complex E_1E_2 is no longer at thermodynamic equilibrium with the enzyme intermediates E_1 and E_2 (as in the scheme of Fig. 2). Below we shall develop a general control theory that is applicable to an arbitrary physical-chemical mechanism of channelling, whether static or dynamic.

Control theory of channelling

Early approaches to understanding control in channelled pathways include [49–53]. It has been realized that the summation property (eqn. 5) is not

Fig. 2　　**A static channel**

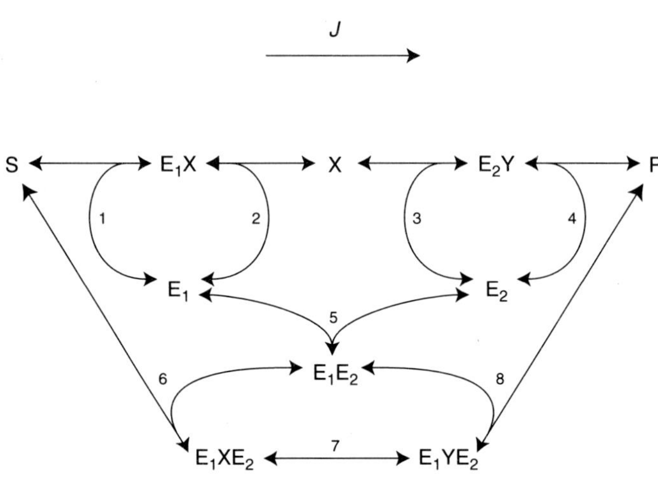

In this case only the free ('empty') forms of enzymes 1 and 2, i.e. E_1 and E_2, can associate to form a complex.

valid for channelled pathways, and it has been suggested that the sum of the control coefficients should be measured in order to diagnose channelling [30,49,50,52–54]. However, these early approaches were not able to relate the control exerted by enzymes to the particular kinetic properties of the processes involved, nor to analyse the general case of partially channelled pathways.

Sauro and Kacser [52] tried to relate the global control properties of a static channel, i.e. the control coefficients of enzymes, to the underlying local kinetic properties of enzyme reactions 'in isolation'. Assuming thermodynamic equilibrium between the separate enzymes and the complex, they calculated the elasticities of partial reactions (proceeding in the bulk phase and in the channelled phase) with respect to the total enzyme concentrations. It has been assumed that these elasticities, which are referred to as protein (π)-elasticities, depend only on the equilibrium constant and the total amounts of the enzymes. This is true, however, only under special conditions, in particular for what can be called a 'frozen channel'. In a frozen channel the distribution of the enzyme between monomers and the enzyme–enzyme complex changes over a much longer time scale than that over which catalytic conversions take place. Another example where approximation of π-elasticities can be used is a static channel, in which not only the association/dissociation of different enzyme–enzyme complexes, but also all the different forms of each enzyme monomer, are at equilibrium [52]. In this case, in order to fulfil the conditions necessary for the calculation of

π-elasticities via equilibrium parameters, one would have to assume that: (i) all possible enzyme–enzyme complexes exist (cf. Fig. 3), and (ii) the corresponding association/dissociation steps of the complexes and the conversions of the different monomeric forms of the same enzyme are very fast [20,37]. Below we show that, in most cases, the approximate method of implementing π-elasticities cannot be applied and, moreover, that these elasticities cannot be considered as local properties of partial reactions [41].

The approach of π-elasticities is most readily illustrated for a static channel (see Fig. 2). The reaction scheme of Fig. 2 can be viewed as a set of three partial reactions, catalysed by e_1^*, e_2^* and e_3^* respectively, where the first two enzymes refer to the monomeric forms and e_3^* refers to the E_1E_2 complex. Control coefficients with respect to e_1^*, e_2^* and e_3^* can be defined (eqn. 1) and expressed into well defined elasticity coefficients. The matrix of π-elasticities, which comprises the dependence of the concentrations of e_1^*,

---

Fig. 3   **Scheme involving both dynamic and static channelled routes**

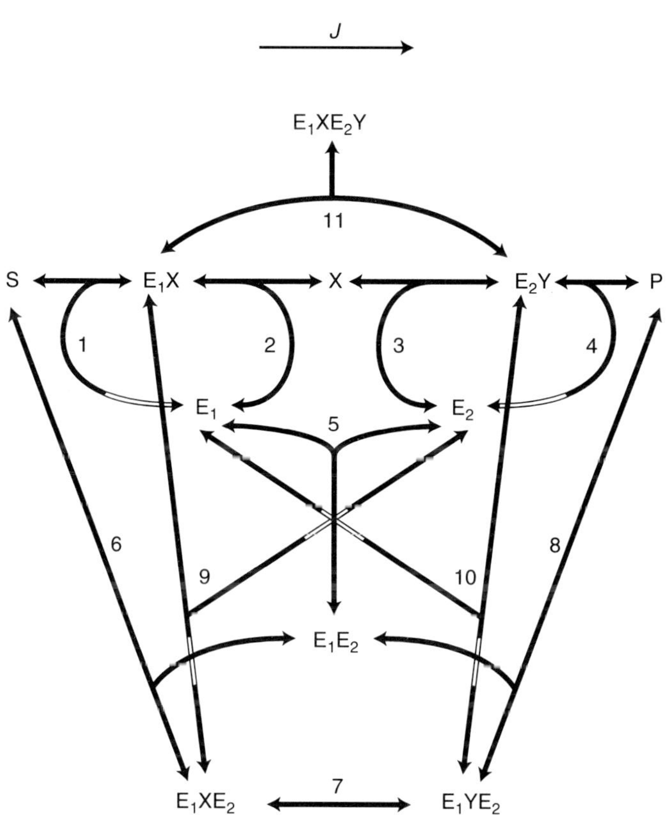

e_2^* and e_3^* on the total concentrations (e_1 and e_2) of the enzymes of the channel, allows one to quantify the control exerted by these enzymes, e.g. for enzyme 1 [52]:

$$C_{e_1}^J = C_{e_1^*}^J \cdot \pi_{11} + C_{e_2^*}^J \cdot \pi_{21} + C_{e_3^*}^J \cdot \pi_{31}; \qquad \pi_{i1} = \partial \ln e_i^* / \partial \ln e_1 \qquad (6)$$

However, closer inspection shows that unless step 5 (which is at thermodynamic equilibrium) is much slower than the other steps, the π-elasticities of partial reactions should vary with the flux and the concentrations of intermediates. Indeed, even at fixed concentration of the intermediate X, a parameter change in, for example, the partial reaction catalysed by e_1^* will affect the concentration of the enzyme forms E_1X and E_1, and hence the concentration of E_1E_2. Therefore the reaction catalysed by e_3^* would obtain an apparent elasticity with respect to the parameter (p_1) of the partial reaction catalysed by e_1^*. Moreover, at a fixed concentration of X the elasticities π_{31} and π_{32} would also depend on that parameter (p_1). This contradicts the very meaning of elasticities as the local properties of a step, since at fixed concentrations of metabolic intermediates the elasticities depend only on the parameters of the particular step. We conclude that, in general, π-elasticities cannot be calculated only in terms of parameters of partial reactions (or in terms of the equilibrium constant and the total amounts of the enzymes, as has been suggested [52]).

Fig. 1 may serve to illustrate the additional problem of defining the control exerted by channelling enzymes. For instance, enzyme 1 participates in two reactions rather than in one (the channelled reaction from S to P as well as the reaction from S to X), and both enzymes 1 and 2 participate in the same channelled reactions. Hence, applied to a dynamic channel, the classical control theory breaks down. Also, the approach of π-elasticities cannot be applied for a dynamic channel like that in Fig. 1.

A study of control in non-ideal pathways: descending to the elemental processes and remounting to the enzyme reactions

A method for determining the enzyme control coefficients for a general case of (partially) channelled pathways has been proposed recently [41,55]. The enzyme control coefficients were expressed in terms of the control coefficients of the elemental steps of the reaction network and the relative concentrations of enzyme–enzyme complexes (the ratios of mean lifetimes of the monomeric and complexed enzyme forms). The control coefficients of the enzymes in channelled pathways have been also expressed directly into the elasticity coefficients of the elemental steps, and a simple algorithm for such calculations has been suggested [56,57]. Here this new approach of Metabolic Control Analysis will be illustrated in a simple example of the dynamic channel in Fig. 1.

To deal with this problem, we return for a moment to a simple metabolic pathway of two sequential enzymes where channelling is absent (Fig. 4). In terms of the traditional (macro) description, the control coeffi-

Fig. 4   **An 'ideal' pathway for comprising enzymes**

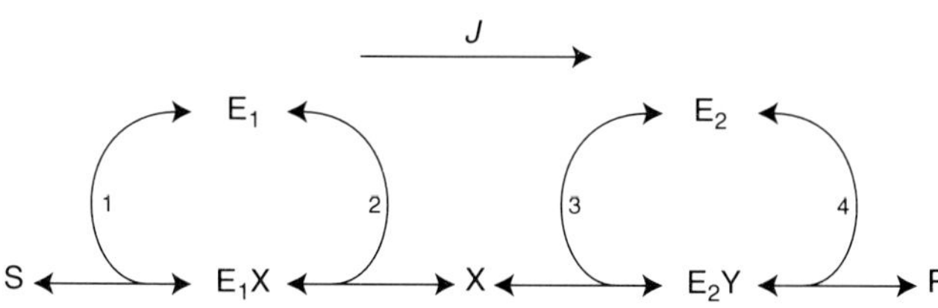

cient of either enzyme, e.g. enzyme 1, over the pathway flux can be estimated by considering a small increase in the total concentration of that enzyme (e_1). Here we note that, at the level of elemental steps within enzyme mechanisms, i.e. in the terms of a 'microdescription', such an increase in e_1 corresponds to a simultaneous proportional increase in the forward and reverse rate constants of all the steps of the enzyme 1-catalysed reaction. To make this statement exact, we need to define the control coefficients of the elemental processes (steps) of enzyme 1 with respect to the overall steady-state flux through the pathway (C_i^J):

$$C_i^J = (\mathrm{dln}\,|J|/\mathrm{dln}k_i^{+})_{\mathrm{sys}}; \qquad k_i^{-}/k_i^{+} = \mathrm{const.}; \qquad i = 1, 2 \tag{7}$$

Since the forward (k_i^{+}) and the reverse (k_i^{-}) rate constants of the elemental process i are changed by the same factor, this definition does not affect microscopic reversibility. An equivalent, but more general, definition of the elemental control coefficient (C_i^J) can be given in a manner similar to eqn. (2). In this case, however, the rate (v_i) becomes the rate of the ith elemental process rather than the rate of the entire enzyme i reaction. Most importantly, when addressing the elemental processes, eqn. (2) defines the control coefficient, C_i^J, as a general quantity, independent of a special choice of a parameter p_i for both ideal and non-ideal cellular pathways [39,58]:

$$C_i^J = \frac{(\mathrm{dln}\,|J|/\mathrm{d}p_i)_{\mathrm{sys}}}{(\partial\mathrm{ln}\,|v_i|/\partial p_i)_{\mathrm{proc}}} \tag{8}$$

The analogous definition for the elemental control coefficient over any concentration (x_k) reads:

$$C_i^{x_k} = \frac{(\mathrm{dln}\,x_k/\mathrm{d}p_i)_{\mathrm{sys}}}{(\partial\mathrm{ln}\,|v_i|/\partial p_i)_{\mathrm{proc}}} \tag{9}$$

Now, for the ideal pathway of Fig. 4, the control coefficients relative to both the concentration ($C_{e_1}^J$) and the activity ($C_{ve_1}^J$) of enzyme 1 can be written as the sum of the elemental control coefficients of the two steps in which this enzyme is involved:

$$C_{e_1}^{J} = C_{ve_1}^{J} = C_1^{J} + C_2^{J}$$

Here ve_1 is used to emphasize that the control coefficient is related to the entire enzyme e_1 rate rather than to the rate of the elemental step.

Importantly, the summation theorem can be written in terms of both the elemental control coefficients (sum of $C_1^{J} + C_2^{J} + C_3^{J} + C_4^{J}$) and the enzyme control coefficients:

$$C_{e_1}^{J} + C_{e_2}^{J} = C_1^{J} + C_2^{J} + C_3^{J} + C_4^{J} = 1$$

This re-formulation of the control analysis of ideal pathways at the micro level preludes the control treatment of the channelled systems: one should recognize also that channelled pathways are networks of chemical conversions and that they may be treated in terms of control coefficients of the elemental processes. For instance, for the dynamic channel shown in Fig. 1 there are six elemental processes and six elemental flux control coefficients. The reaction sequence in the channelled phase corresponds to steps 5 and 6 (the lower route in Fig. 1), and the control coefficients over flux are defined by eqn. (7), with $i = 5$ and 6. Because the steady-state flux is a homogeneous function of all the elemental rate constants, the following summation theorem holds for this channelled system (cf. [59]):

$$C_1^{J} + C_2^{J} + C_3^{J} + C_4^{J} + C_5^{J} + C_6^{J} = 1 \tag{10}$$

i.e. the sum of the flux control coefficients continues to equal 1 provided that the sum is taken over all the elemental processes.

Now, from the level of the elemental processes of a pathway (the 'microdescription' level), we return to the level of enzyme reactions. The concept of elemental control coefficients allows us to assign an analogue of the control coefficient with respect to the enzyme activity ($C_{v_i}^{J}$) to the individual enzymes of a channel. Suppose we simultaneously change the elemental rate constants of all processes in which the enzyme i is involved by the same factor. Considering the corresponding change in the steady-state flux J, we define the 'impact' control coefficient, $^{\text{imp}}C_{e_i}^{J}$, as the sum of the elemental control coefficients over the processes in which any of the forms of enzyme i are involved (E_i-dependent processes):

$$^{\text{imp}}C_{e_i}^{J} = \sum_{\substack{\text{all } E_i\text{-dependent} \\ \text{processes } k}} C_k^{J} \tag{11}$$

This coefficient evaluates the total impact enzyme i may have on the flux J (the term 'E_i-dependent' refers to any form of enzyme i, monomeric or complexed, that contains an E_i moiety) [29,41].

Central to the special control properties of channelled pathways is the fact that, when the two enzymes form a complex, the corresponding elemental steps involved in the protein interaction are dependent on both enzymes. For example, in the dynamic channel of Fig. 1 the channel steps 5 and 6 both contribute to the control exerted by either enzyme:

$$^{\mathrm{imp}}C_{e_1}^J = C_1^J + C_2^J + C_5^J + C_6^J; \qquad ^{\mathrm{imp}}C_{e_2}^J = C_2^J + C_4^J + C_5^J + C_6^J \tag{12}$$

We note that the definition of the impact control coefficient $^{\mathrm{imp}}C_{e_1}^J$ (by modulation of the activities of all E_1-dependent processes) does not correspond to the effect of just a change in the total concentration of enzyme 1 at a constant concentration of enzyme 2, which was the definition of the traditional control coefficient (with respect to enzyme concentration; $C_{e_1}^J$). Indeed, the concomitant change in the form E_1XE_2 caused by changes in activities of the elemental steps interferes with the conservation of the total concentration of enzyme 2. So, in cases of enzyme–enzyme interactions, as well as in other non-ideal pathways, there is a difference between the control coefficients defined in terms of modulation of activity and those defined in terms of modulation of the enzyme concentration.

Most importantly, for any given channelling scheme the classical enzyme control coefficients can be expressed in terms of the elemental control coefficients [41,55,60]. For the dynamic channel of Fig. 1 this expression reads (see eqn. 10 in [41]):

$$C_{e_1}^J = \left({}^{\mathrm{imp}}C_{e_1}^J - {}^{\mathrm{imp}}C_{e_2}^J \cdot [E_1XE_2]/e_2 \right) \Big/ \left(1 - \frac{[E_1XE_2]^2}{e_1 \cdot e_2} \right)$$

$$C_{e_2}^J = \left({}^{\mathrm{imp}}C_{e_2}^J - {}^{\mathrm{imp}}C_{e_1}^J \cdot [E_1XE_2]/e_1 \right) \Big/ \left(1 - \frac{[E_1XE_2]^2}{e_1 \cdot e_2} \right) \tag{13}$$

Here $[E_1XE_2]$ is the concentration of the enzyme–enzyme complex, e_1 and e_2 are the total concentrations of the enzymes, and the impact control coefficients $^{\mathrm{imp}}C_{e_1}^J$ and $^{\mathrm{imp}}C_{e_2}^J$ are expressed via elemental control coefficients by eqn. (12).

Consequences of channelling for regulation and control

The theory reviewed above provides formal tools and concepts for analysis of the implications of channelling for regulation and control (cf. [29,58]). Important information from this theory is that an enzyme in a channel controls flux and metabolite concentrations in more than one mode. For instance, a decrease in enzyme concentration and inhibition of the enzyme at constant concentration will result in different effects on both pathway flux and metabolite concentrations [38,39,61].

Control of flux

Evaluation of the sum of enzymes' control coefficients can be useful for the experimental diagnosis of channelling [34,50,52,53]. Early conjectures concerning the control behaviour of channelled metabolism included the statement that when all flux runs through a channel pathway consisting of n

enzymes, the control of each of the n enzymes should equal 1; each enzyme should behave as if it were the rate-limiting step. This should lead to a total control of n [53].

For a dynamic channel formed by the two coupled enzyme reactions (Fig. 1) the estimation of the sum of the enzymes' control coefficients is straightforward from eqns. (10)–(13). Here we present results for the case where the total concentrations of the two enzymes are equal ($e_1 = e_2 = e$) [41]:

$$C_{e_1}^J + C_{e_2}^J = (1 + C_5^J + C_6^J)/(1 + [E_1XE_2]/e)$$

$$= \{1 + (J_{chan}/J)\cdot[1 - (C_1^J + C_4^J)]\}/(1 + [E_1XE_2]/e) \tag{14}$$

J is the total flux through the pathway, and J_{chan} denotes the flux through the channel.

Eqn. (14) partly confirms the conjecture in [53]. This is the situation in which J_{chan}/J is close to 1, and the prediction of the equation is that the sum of the control coefficients equals the number of enzymes (two), but only if a small fraction of the enzymes exists as the enzyme–enzyme complex (i.e. $[E_1XE_2] \ll e$) and there is little control in steps 1 and 4 (e.g. if the binding of S and P is near equilibrium). In general, the magnitude of the sum of the flux control coefficients can vary from less than unity to two, depending on the ratio of the channelled and bulk-phase fluxes and on the amount of the complexed enzymes. This is illustrated by Fig. 5, which shows the dependence of the sum of the enzyme control coefficients on the total concentration of the enzymes of the dynamic channel. The sum ($C_{e_1}^J + C_{e_2}^J$) assumes the classical value of 1 at very low concentrations of the enzymes where the channelled flux fraction is negligible. With an increase in the enzyme concentrations, the channelled flux fraction (J_{chan}/J) increases as the rate of step 5 increases. This is accompanied by an increase in the control exerted by the channelled steps. As a result the sum of the control coefficients increases, attaining a value much greater than unity. With a further increase in the concentrations of the enzymes this sum decreases again. The latter effect reflects enzyme sequestration; enzyme 1 is sequestered by enzyme 2 in the complex E_1XE_2. At such high enzyme concentrations the sum of the enzyme control coefficients falls below unity, eventually down to or below 0.5. This is because of the term $[E_1XE_2]/e$ in the denominator of eqn. (14) (the value of 0.5 occurs if control by steps 1 and 4 is negligible). These entirely new phenomena cannot occur in pathways lacking the channel.

Extension of the theoretical development to a pathway of n enzymes with dynamic channels formed by bimolecular complexes between adjacent enzymes leads to a maximum sum of control coefficients of 2 [56,59]. In a dynamically channelled pathway consisting of, say, five enzymes, it is unlikely that the association of enzymes 4 and 5 is required for the combined catalytic action of enzymes 1 and 2. However, if several enzymes can assemble in a single channel (e.g. a static channel), the sum of the control coefficients may increase to equal the number of enzymes, especially when the protein–protein complexes that do not contain all pathway enzymes are ineffective in the channelled transfer of metabolism [53]. This may result in a very sharp increase in flux with increasing concentrations of pathway enzymes. This feature of channelling may be advantageous and may therefore have been selected during evolution.

Concentration control

The consequences of metabolic channelling for the concentrations of bulk-phase metabolites (pool sizes) have been the subject of intensive discussion and a recent controversy [13,62–65]. To answer the question of whether channelling can specifically affect pool size, we shall compare the effect of a parameter change enhancing the direct transfer flux in the channelled pathway of Fig. 1 with the effect of the same parameter change in the pathway of Fig. 4, which is identical to the former except that the enzymes cannot associate into a complex.

At very low enzyme concentrations, when the fraction of the flux running through a channel is almost zero, the pathways in Figs. 1 and 4 pass

---

Fig. 5 **Dependence of the sum $(C^J_{e_1} + C^J_{e_2})$ of flux control coefficients and the fraction of the flux going through the channel (J_{chan}/J) on the total concentration of the enzymes of the pathway of Fig. 1.**

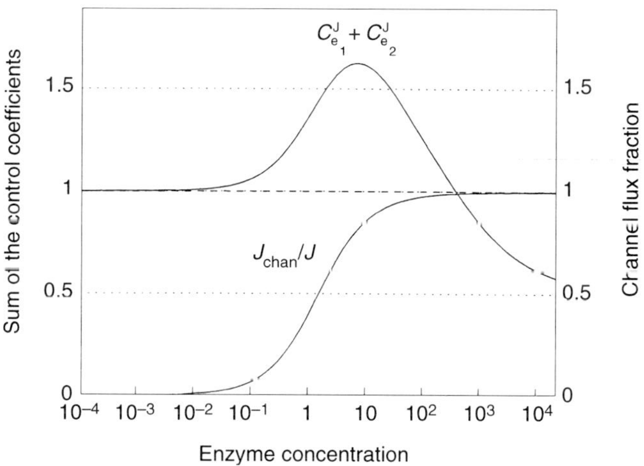

See eqn. (14). The concentrations of the two enzymes were taken to be equal, and are given in dimensionless units. The parameter values were (dimensionless units): $S = 1$, $P = 0$, $k_1^+ = 100$, $k_1^- = 50$, $k_2^+ = 1$, $k_2^- = 1$, $k_5^+ = 1$, $k_3^+ = 1$, $k_3^- = 1$, $k_4^+ = 200$, $k_4^- = 100$, $k_5^- = 20$, $k_6^+ = 20$, $k_6^- = 1$.

almost the same amount of flux and sustain the same concentration of the bulk-phase metabolite (X). A natural way of enhancing the channelling is to increase the concentrations of the two directly interacting enzymes, and hence the concentration of their complex ($[E_1XE_2]$). An equal relative change in both enzyme concentrations is a type of parameter adjustment that does not affect at all the pool of intermediate X in the pathway lacking the channel (Fig. 4). However, these changes do affect the free-metabolite pool in the dynamic channel of Fig. 1. [34,37].

To investigate how pool size is affected by such a proportional increase in the enzyme concentrations, we will rephrase this question in terms of Metabolic Control Analysis: what is the sum of the enzyme control coefficients with respect to pool size? In ideal pathways the sum of the enzyme control coefficients over this pool equals zero (the summation theorem [20,21]). This is in line with the lack of effect of a proportional increase in the enzyme concentrations on the intermediate pool in these pathways. For channelled pathways new summation theorems have been derived ([41,55,66]; cf. [60]). When the concentrations of the two enzymes in Fig. 1 are equal ($e_1 = e_2 = e$), the sum of the enzyme control coefficients with respect to the intermediate pool (X) is proportional to the sum of the elemental control coefficients of steps 2 and 3 (cf. eqn. 14):

$$C_{e_1}^X + C_{e_2}^X = (C_5^X + C_6^X)/(1 + [E_1XE_2]/e)$$

$$= (C_2^X + C_3^X) \cdot [J_{\text{chan}}/(J - J_{\text{chan}})]/(1 + [E_1XE_2]/e) \tag{15}$$

In the pathways of Figs. 1 and 4 the total flux will increase with the proportional increase in enzyme concentrations. Eqn. (15) now shows that whether the pool size increases, remains constant or decreases depends on whether the sum of the elemental control coefficients of steps 2 and 3 is greater than, equal to or smaller than zero. Step 2 supplies, whereas step 3 consumes, the bulk-phase intermediate X. Therefore, normally, C_2^X is positive and C_3^X is negative. As a consequence, the sign of their sum ($C_2^X + C_3^X$) depends on whether step 2 or step 3 exerts more control on X. Hence whether the pool concentration X increases or decreases as cytosolic enzymes increase in concentration depends on the magnitudes of the kinetic constants within enzyme mechanisms, as these ultimately determine the control coefficients C_2^X and C_3^X.

Steps 1 and 3 involve substrate binding and may also include some catalytic transformations. When the activation barriers of these steps are substantially higher than such barriers of the product-release steps (2 and 4), one may conjecture that the control exerted by steps 1 and 3 is substantial, whereas the control exerted by steps 2 and 4 is small. From eqn. (15) one can conclude that in such cases the pool size falls while the channel flux rises with the increase in enzyme concentrations. To illustrate this point analytically we simplify the dynamic channel in Fig. 1 to a 'hit-and-run' channel (Fig. 6) in which the concentration of the ternary complex E_1XE_2 is negli-

Fig. 6   **Hit-and-run channel**

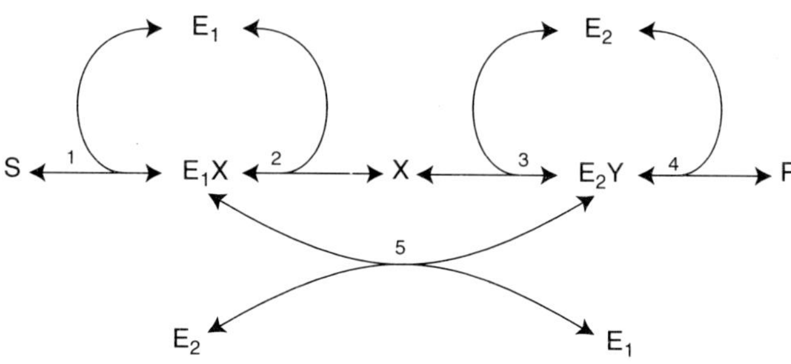

This case differs from the more general case of Fig. 1 in that the conversion of E$_1$X into E$_2$Y is a single step, as the steady-state concentration of the complex E$_1$XE$_2$ is assumed to be negligible.

gible (cf. [64]). In such a simplified channel the conversion of E$_1$X into E$_2$Y occurs via a single step (step 5 in Fig. 6). Similar thermodynamic restrictions apply to both models of a dynamic channel, i.e. $K_2^{eq} \cdot K_3^{eq} = K_5^{eq} \cdot K_6^{eq}$ for the channel in Fig. 1 and $K_2^{eq} \cdot K_3^{eq} = K_5^{eq}$ for the hit-and-run channel in Fig. 6 (K_i^{eq} is the equilibrium constant of step i). These restrictions on the possible magnitude of the rate constants reflect the fact that for any channel the Gibbs energy changes for each branch must be identical. Note that the hit-and-run channel of Fig. 6 can be considered as the limiting case of the dynamic channel of Fig. 1 when the rate constants k_5^- and k_6^+ are increased by the same factor (leaving the product $K_5^{eq} \cdot K_6^{eq}$ unaffected). Increases in these rate constants result in decreases in the concentration of the ternary complex E$_1$XE$_2$ to negligible values.

Let us consider the channelled pathway (Fig. 6) for the case when the activation barrier for step 2 is so low (and hence its rate constants are so high) compared with other steps that step 2 is near equilibrium, whereas steps 1, 3, 4 and 5 are further away from equilibrium. Clearly, under such conditions step 2 will not exert any significant control. In thermodynamic terms the quasi-equilibrium state of step 2 corresponds to very low values of the Gibbs energy difference across this step:

$$\Delta G_2 = RT \left\{ \ln\left(\frac{[E_1X]}{E_1 \cdot X}\right) - \ln K_2^{eq} \right\} \ll RT$$

Hence the ratio of the concentrations (thermodynamic activities) approaches the equilibrium constant:

$$\frac{E_1 \cdot X}{[E_1X]} = K_2^{eq} \tag{16}$$

The sum of the concentrations E_1 and $[E_1X]$ equals the total concentration of the enzyme (e). As a consequence, the equilibrium ratio (see eqn. 16) fixes these concentrations as follows:

$$E_1 = e/(1 + X/K_2^{\mathrm{eq}}); \qquad [E_1X] = e \cdot (X/K_2^{\mathrm{eq}})/(1 + X/K_2^{\mathrm{eq}}) \tag{17}$$

Now we use eqn. (17) to express the total flux (J), which is equal to the steady-state rate of step 1 (v_1), in terms of X and e:

$$(v_1)_{\mathrm{ss}} = J = e(k_1^{+}S - k_1^{-}X/K^{\mathrm{eq}}{}_2)/(1 + X/K_2^{\mathrm{eq}}) \tag{18}$$

where ss denotes steady-state conditions. Differentiating eqn. (18) with respect to $\ln e$ and taking into account that, under conditions of equal concentrations of the pathway enzymes this gives the sum of the enzyme control coefficients, one arrives at:

$$\frac{\mathrm{d}\ln J}{\mathrm{d}\ln e} = C_{e_1}^J + C_{e_2}^J = 1 - f \cdot (C_{e_1}^X + C_{e_2}^X);$$

$$f = e(k_1^{+}S + k_1^{-}) \cdot (X/K_2^{\mathrm{eq}})/[J \cdot (1 + X/K_2^{\mathrm{eq}})^2]$$
$$= (k_1^{+}S + k_1^{-}) \cdot E_1[E_1X]/(J \cdot e) \tag{19}$$

The factor f is positive provided that the flux J (i.e. from S to P) is positive. Therefore eqn. (19) shows that the sum of the enzyme control coefficients over the pool concentration (X) is negative if and only if the sum of the enzyme control coefficients over the total flux (J) is greater than 1. As has been shown in the previous section, for the general case of dynamic channelling the latter is true for a wide range of rate constants [41,58].

For the hit-and-run channel (Fig. 6) we shall now show that, if step 2 can be considered as a near-equilibrium step, the sum of the enzyme control coefficients over J exceeds 1. Using eqn. (14) for the sum of the enzyme control coefficients with respect to the flux J, one obtains (cf. [67]):

$$C_{e_1}^J + C_{e_2}^J = 1 + C_5^J \tag{20}$$

C_5^J is the (elemental) control coefficient of channel step 5. In a hit-and-run channel the sequestration of enzymes by the formation of the enzyme–enzyme complex (E_1XE_2) is negligible compared with the amounts of the monomeric forms (E_1, E_1X, E_2, E_2Y). From this it is already intuitively clear that the total flux will always increase with the activity of the channel step, i.e. $C_5^J > 0$. One can also prove the latter inequality by applying the summation and connectivity theorems to the elemental control coefficients [29,60,68]. Taking into account the fact that the control coefficient of the near-equilibrium step 2 can be neglected in comparison with the control coefficients of the other steps and using the branch (summation) theorem [69], one can write:

$$C_3^J/C_5^J = (J - J_{\mathrm{chan}})/J_{\mathrm{chan}}$$

For thermodynamic reasons the fluxes through the branches should flow in the same direction. As a consequence, C_5^J and C_3^J must have the same sign (i.e. both are positive or both are negative). Furthermore, from the connectivity theorem with regard to $[E_2Y]$ it follows that C_4^J must have the same sign as C_5^J and C_3^J, and from the connectivity theorem with regard to X it follows that C_1^J also has the same sign. Since the sum of all the (elemental) control coefficients over the flux J is equal to 1, all these signs must be positive. Hence C_5^J is greater than 0, and the sum in eqn. (20) is greater than 1. Therefore (see eqn. 19) the sum of the enzyme control coefficients over the pool concentration (X) is negative under the conditions considered. Thus we have shown that, for some kinetic properties of the enzymes forming the channel, the pool concentration X decreases with an increase in the concentrations of proteins; hence with channelling.

Numerical illustrations

For the dynamic channel of Fig. 1, Fig. 7 shows the sums of the control coefficients of the enzymes (solid line) and of steps 2 and 3 (broken line) with respect to the pool concentration X for a case in which step 3 was more limiting. One can see that the sum of the enzyme control coefficients with respect to X approaches zero at very low enzyme concentrations. In line with eqn. (15), it assumes negative values if and only if the sum of the elemental control coefficients of steps 2 and 3 does the same. For the same case, Fig. 8 compares the behaviour of the bulk-phase intermediate (X) for the two pathways of Figs. 1 and 6. In the channelled pathway the free-intermediate concentration decreased with the increase in the enzyme concentrations, whereas in the same pathway lacking the channel it remained constant (Fig. 8, left panel). Moreover, the concentration of all species in the bulk phase, including the enzymes, also decreased (Fig. 8, left panel).

This demonstration was not for constant total flux. However, in all cases the total flux can be maintained constant by simultaneous equal modulation of all rate constants additional to the modulation of total protein concentration. Indeed, such modulation leaves all the pathway concentrations unchanged, affecting only the pathway fluxes [41,59]. Consequently our results are also relevant for the constant-flux condition. Fig. 8 (right panel) confirms this by plotting the bulk-phase pool versus the total flux through either pathway. The inset shows how the pool size depends on the fraction of flux flowing through the channel. We also note that at constant total flux there are ways of driving more flux through the channel branch that leave the concentration of the free intermediate unaltered, decrease it or increase it.

We conclude that channelling may cause either a decrease or an increase in pool size when compared with an analogous pathway lacking a channel. The behaviour of the bulk-phase intermediate when the enzymes become more concentrated greatly depends on the absolute values of the rate constants (i.e. on the activation barriers) of elemental steps located upstream and downstream from the branch points rather than on the standard Gibbs energy differences across these steps. We have shown that a channelling pathway and an identical pathway lacking a channel may pass the same flux (although the enzyme concentrations in the pathways differ), whereas pool size and the concentration of all species are smaller in the case of channelling. Specifically, when the elemental step supplying the bulk-phase intermediate (X) is sufficiently fast and the concentration of a dynamic enzyme–enzyme complex is much smaller than that of monomeric enzyme forms, X falls as the proteins become more concentrated. Consequently, at least for some kinetic conditions, channelling does provide a mechanism for decreasing pool size. Such a mechanism may have some advantages for organisms which are subjected to transient changes in the cytoplasmic water content due to changes in environmental conditions.

Fig. 7   Variation with protein concentration of the extent to which the enzymes control the bulk-phase intermediate X

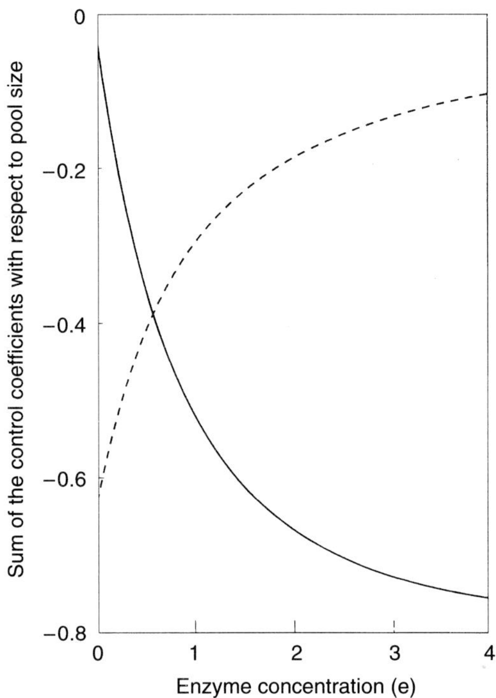

For the pathway of Fig. 1 the dependencies are shown of the sum $(C_{e_1}^{X} + C_{e_2}^{X})$ of the enzyme control coefficients (solid line) and of the sum $(C_2^{X} + C_3^{X})$ of the elemental control coefficients of steps 2 and 3 (broken line) on the total concentration (e) of either enzyme (these equal concentrations, $e_1 = e_2 = e$, are shown in dimensionless units). The parameter values were (dimensionless units): $S = 1$, $P = 0.1$, $k_1^{+} = 1$, $k_1^{-} = 0.5$, $k_2^{+} = 10$, $k_2^{-} = 0.05$, $k_3^{+} = 0.01$, $k_3^{-} = 0.5$, $k_4^{+} = 50$, $k_4^{-} = 1$, $k_5^{+} = 20$, $k_5^{-} = 250$, $k_6^{+} = 50$, $k_6^{-} = 1$.

Conclusions

In this chapter we have reviewed attempts to develop a quantitative theory for the control of metabolite channelling. We have shown that, although earlier analyses were able to deal with certain types of channelling, notably static channelling, the more subtle dynamic channelling could not be described quantitatively. Static enzyme–enzyme complexes are likely to be more stable upon isolation and seem to be less suitable for allowing enzymes to deliver metabolites to more than one target. In addition, it is the reversible, probably dynamic, type of channelling that is likely to be induced by the phenomenon of macromolecular crowding that increases the apparent

Fig. 8   **Comparison of the behaviour of the bulk-phase intermediate in a dynamic channel with that in an ideal pathway**

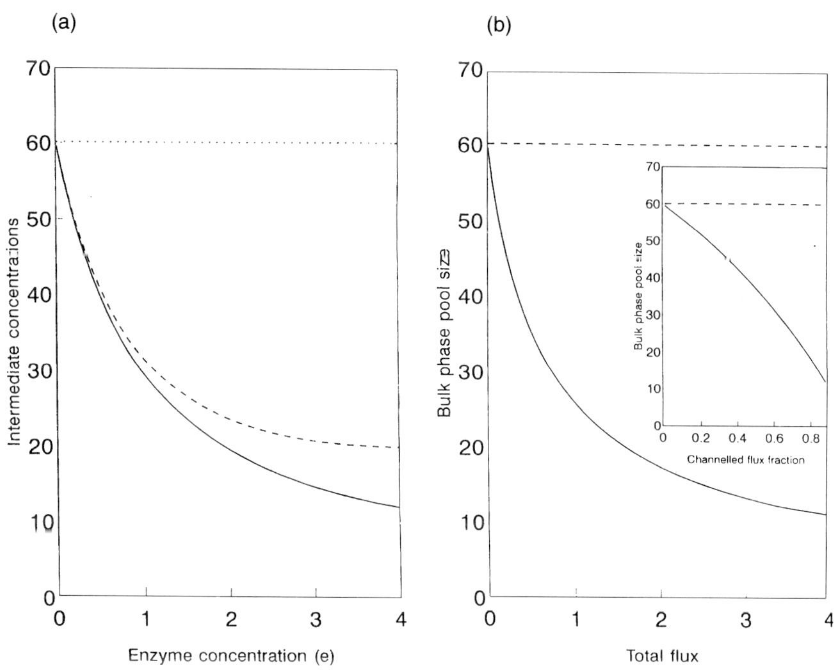

A dynamic channel and an ideal pathway are shown in Figs. 1 and 4 respectively. Left panel: dependence of the concentration of the intermediate X on the total concentration (e) of either enzyme for a dynamic channel (solid line) and an ideal pathway (dotted line), and the analogous dependence of the concentration of all substances in the bulk phase for a dynamic channel (broken line). Right panel: concentration of the bulk-phase intermediate (X) versus the total pathway flux (J) for a dynamic channel (solid line) and for an ideal pathway (dotted line). Inset: X for either pathway versus the flux fraction through the channel (J$_{chan}$/J). The parameter values are indicated in the legend to Fig. 7.

effective concentration of enzymes much more than that of the low-molecular-mass metabolites, in some cases to dramatic extents ([70,71]; see also Chapter 3 in the current volume).

Very recent work, however, can deal with both dynamic and static channelling. The breakthrough has been to regress to the description of the channelled pathway in terms of all its elemental steps and then to define control coefficients with respect to those steps. The control coefficients of the steps can then be understood in terms of the enzyme kinetic properties. In addition, the control coefficients of the enzymes can be expressed in terms of the control exerted by sets of elemental steps, and can hence also be expressed in terms of the kinetic properties of the pathway enzymes. The pay-off, of course, is that the enzyme control coefficients become mechanism-dependent, and there are few cases where the elemental control coefficients can be measured directly. However, this is how complex reality is, and reality should not be ducked. In channelled metabolism the sum of the control coefficients of the enzymes need no longer equal 1, but is likely to be within 1 and 2 ([59,72]; see, however, [41,52,57]). Surprisingly, in channelled metabolic pathways the enzymes do not control the flux in a single mode; they control it by their concentration, but also through all the elemental processes in which an enzyme is involved, i.e. by their impact [29,41].

The extent to which directing the flux of a pathway through the channelling branch can decrease the concentration of the free metabolite has been analysed both numerically and analytically. It turns out that the concentration of the free metabolite can either increase or decrease as the fraction of flux flowing through the channel increases. In terms of evolution, this means that if a decrease in the concentration of a free metabolite exerted positive selection pressure, this may have led to the selection of such changes in metabolism. Increased channelling could have been a side effect. However, it should be pointed out that there are other ways of decreasing the concentrations of free metabolite, i.e. without increasing the extent of channelling.

We thank D.B. Kell, P. Mendes and G.R. Welch for reading the manuscript and for making valuable suggestions as to its improvement. This work was supported by CIRIT de la Generalitat de Catalunya, by DGICYT (grant PB92–0852) and by the Netherlands Organization for Scientific Research (NWO).

References

1. De Vries, H. (1871) Arch. Neerl. Sci. **6**, 117
2. Ling, G.N. (1984) Search of the Physical Basis of Life, Plenum Press, New York
3. Clegg, J.S. (1986) in The Organization of Cell Metabolism (Welch, G.R. and Clegg, J.S., eds.), pp. 41–56, Plenum Press, New York

4. Srere, P.A. (1987) Annu. Rev. Biochem. **56**, 89–124
5. Welch, G.R. (1977) Prog. Biophys. Mol. Biol. **32**, 103–191
6. Keleti, T., Ovàdi, J. and Batke, J. (1989) Prog. Biophys. Mol. Biol. **53**, 105–152
7. Mendes, P., Kell, D.B. and Welch, G.R. (1995) Adv. Mol. Cell. Biol. **11**, 1–19
8. Yanofsky, C. (1989) Biochim. Biophys. Acta **1000**, 133–137
9. Hyde, C.C., Ahmed, S.A., Padlan, E.A., Miles, E.W. and Davies, D.R. (1988) J. Biol. Chem. **263**, 17857–17871
10. Lamb, H.K., van den Hombergh, J.P.T.W., Newton, G.H., Moore, J.D., Roberts, C.F. and Hawkins, A.R. (1992) Biochem. J. **284**, 181–187
11. Welch, G.R. and Gaertner, F.H. (1980) Curr. Top. Cell. Regul. **16**, 113–162
12. Postma, P.W., Lengeler, J.W. and Jacobson, G.R. (1993) Microbiol. Rev. **57**, 543–594
13. Ovádi, J. (1991) J. Theor. Biol. **152**, 1–22
14. Brindle, K., Fulton, S., Sheldon, J. and Williams, S. (1995) Biochem. Soc. Trans. **23**, 376–381
15. Hess, B. and Mikhailov, A. (1994) Ber. Bunsen-Ges. Phys. Chem. **98**, 1198–1201
16. Westerhoff, H.V. and Welch, G.R. (1992) Curr. Top. Cell. Regul. **33**, 361–390
17. Westerhoff, H.V., Kell, D.B., Kamp, F. and Van Dam, K. (1988) in Microcompartmentation (Jones, D.P., ed.), pp. 114–154, CRC Press, Boca Raton, FL
18. Prigogine, I. (1980) From Being to Becoming: Time and Complexity in the Physical Sciences, Freeman, San Franscisco
19. Higgins, J.J. (1965) in Control of Energy Metabolism (Chance, B., Estabrook, R.W. and Williamson, J.R., eds.), pp. 13–46, Academic Press, New York
20. Kacser, H. and Burns, J.A. (1973) in Rate Control of Biological Processes (Davies, D.D., ed.), pp. 65–104, Cambridge University Press, London
21. Heinrich, R. and Rapoport, T.A. (1974) Eur. J. Biochem. **42**, 89–95
22. Kacser, H. and Burns, J.A. (1979) Biochem. Soc. Trans. **7**, 1149–1160
23. Savageau, M.A. (1972) Curr. Top. Cell. Regul. **6**, 63–130
24. Flint, H.J., Tateson, R.W., Barthelmess, I.B., Porteous, D.J., Donachie, W.D. and Kacser, H. (1981) Biochem. J. **200**, 231–246
25. Groen, A.K., Wanders, R.J.A., Westerhoff, H.V., Van der Meer, R. and Tager, J.M. (1982) J. Biol. Chem. **257**, 2754–2757
26. Jensen, P.R., Westerhoff, H.V. and Michelsen, O. (1993) Eur. J. Biochem. **211**, 181–191
27. Westerhoff, H.V. (1995) Trends Biotechnol. **13**, 242–244
28. Easterby, J.S. (1990) in Control of Metabolic Processes (Cornish-Bowden, A. and Cárdenas, M.L., eds.), pp. 281–290, Plenum Press, New York
29. Kholodenko, B.N. and Westerhoff, H.V. (1995) Trends Biochem. Sci. **20**, 52–54
30. Kacser, H., Sauro, H.M. and Acerenza, L. (1990) Eur. J. Biochem. **187**, 481–491
31. Reder, C. (1988) J. Theor. Biol. **135**, 175–201
32. Kholodenko, B.N. (1988) Mol. Biol. (USSR) **22**, 1238–1256 [English translation (1989) **22**, 990–1005]
33. Schuster, S. and Heinrich, R. (1992) BioSystems **27**, 1–15
34. Kholodenko, B.N. and Westerhoff, H.V. (1994) in Modern Trends in BioThermoKinetics. (Schuster, S., Rigoulet, M., Ouhabi, R. and Mazateds, J.P., eds.), pp. 205–210, Plenum Press, New York and London
35. Fell, D.A. and Sauro, H.M. (1990) Eur. J. Biochem. **192**, 183–187
36. Kholodenko, B.N., Lyubarev, A.E. and Kurganov, B.I. (1992) Eur. J. Biochem. **210**, 147–153
37. Kholodenko, B.N. (1993) Biokhimiya (Moscow) **58**, 424–437 (English translation **58**, 325–337)
38. Kholodenko, B.N. and Westerhoff, H.V. (1995) Biochim. Biophys. Acta **1229**, 275–289
39. Kholodenko, B.N., Molenaar, D., Schuster, S., Heinrich, R. and Westerhoff, H.V. (1995) Biophys. Chem. **56**, 215–226
40. Giersch, C. (1988) Eur. J. Biochem. **174**, 509–513
41. Kholodenko, B.N. and Westerhoff, H.V. (1993) FEBS Lett. **320**, 71–74
42. Welch, G.R. and Easterby, J.S. (1994) Trends Biochem. Sci. **19**, 193–197
43. Srivastava, D.K. and Bernard, S.A. (1987) Annu. Rev. Biophys. Biophys. Chem. **16**, 175–204

44. Ushiroyama, T., Fukushima, T., Styre, J.D. and Spivey, H.O. (1992) Curr. Top. Cell. Regul. **33**, 291–307
45. Cori, C.F., Velick, S.F. and Cori, G.T. (1950) Biochim. Biophys. Acta **4**, 160–169
46. Friedrich, P. (1974) Acta Biochim. Biophys. Acad. Sci. Hung. **9**, 159–173
47. Srivastava, D.K. and Bernhard, S.A. (1984) Biochemistry **23**, 4538–4545
48. Smolen, P. and Keizer, J. (1990) Biophys. Chem. **38**, 241–263
49. Kell, D.B. and Westerhoff, H.V. (1990) in Structural and Organizational Aspects of Metabolic Regulation (Srere, P.A., Jones, M.E. and Mathews, C.K., eds.), pp. 273–289, Wiley–Liss, New York
50. Welch, G.R., Keleti, T. and Vertessy, B.J. (1988) Theor. Biol. **130**, 407–422
51. Sorribas, A. and Savageau, M.A. (1989) Math. Biosci. **94**, 161–193
52. Sauro, H.M. and Kacser, H. (1990) Eur. J.Biochem. **187**, 493–500
53. Kell, D.B. and Westerhoff, H.V. (1985) in Organized Multienzyme Systems (Welch, G.R., ed.), pp. 63–138, Academic Press, New York
54. Brindle, K.M. (1988) Biochemistry **27**, 6187–6196
55. Kholodenko, B.N., Cascante, M. and Westerhoff, H.V. (1993) FEBS Lett. **336**, 381–384
56. Kholodenko, B.N. and Westerhoff, H.V. (1995) Biochim. Biophys. Acta **1229**, 256–274
57. Kholodenko, B.N., Westerhoff, H.V., Puigjaner, J. and Cascante, M. (1995) Biophys. Chem. **53**, 247–258
58. Kholodenko, B.N., Demin, O.V. and Westerhoff, H.V. (1993) FEBS Lett. **320**, 75–78
59. Van Dam, K., Van der Vlag, J., Kholodenko, B.N. and Westerhoff, H.V. (1993) Eur. J. Biochem. **212**, 791–799
60. Kholodenko, B.N., Sauro, H.M. and Westerhoff, H.V. (1994) Eur. J. Biochem. **225**, 179–186
61. Kholodenko, B.N., Cascante, M., Molenaar, D., Demin, O.V., van der Gugten, A.A. and Westerhoff, H.V. (1995) J. Biol. Syst. **3**, 145–154
62. Cornish-Bowden, A. (1991) Eur. J. Biochem. **195**, 103–108
63. Mendes, P., Kell, D.B. and Westerhoff, H.V. (1992) Eur. J. Biochem. **204**, 257–266
64. Cornish-Bowden, A. and Cárdenas, M.L. (1993) Eur. J. Biochem. **213**, 87–92
65. Mendes, P., Kell, D.B. and Westerhoff, H.V. (1996) Biochim. Biophys. Acta **1289**, 175–186
66. Kholodenko, B.N., Cascante, M. and Westerhoff, H.V. (1995) Mol. Cell. Biochem. **143**, 151–168
67. Sauro, H.M. (1994) BioSystems **33**, 55–67
68. Kholodenko, B.N. and Westerhoff, H.V. (1994) Biochim. Biophys. Acta **1208**, 294–305
69. Fell, D.A. and Sauro, H.M. (1985) Eur. J. Biochem. **148**, 555–561
70. Garner, M.M. and Burg, M.B. (1994) Am. J. Physiol. **266**, C877–C892
71. Walter, H. and Brooks, D.E. (1995) FEBS Lett. **361**, 135–139
72. Brand, M.D., Vallis, B.P.S. and Kesseler, A. (1994) Eur. J. Biochem. **226**, 819–829

7

Multifunctional 2-oxoacid dehydrogenase complexes

Thomas E. Roche* and David J. Cox†

*Department of Biochemistry, Kansas State University, Manhattan, KS 66506, U.S.A., and †School of Arts and Sciences, Indiana University-Purdue University, Fort Wayne, IN 46805, U.S.A.

Introduction

Enzymes that catalyse successive steps in a metabolic sequence are sometimes discovered bound to one another in stable multienzyme complexes. There has been continuous speculation as to the functional usefulness of multienzyme complexes since they were first noticed [1,2] more than 30 years ago. Increased catalytic efficiency, channelling of intermediates and protection of unstable metabolites have been suggested as hypothetical advantages of multienzyme complexes over independently soluble enzymes (e.g. [1–7]). Over the same period, information has gradually accumulated on the structure and behaviour of some complexes that has begun to place speculation on a concrete experimental basis.

The 2-oxoacid dehydrogenases have been particularly rewarding subjects of both speculation and experiment. All of the members of this family are responsible for the oxidative decarboxylation of 2-oxoacids and are large, symmetrical multienzyme complexes (for reviews see [8–11], and all chapters in [12]). These complexes are found in nearly all organisms, and they function at strategic points in sugar metabolism [pyruvate dehydrogenase complexes (PDHCs)], in the Krebs cycle [2-oxoglutarate dehydrogenase complexes (OGDHCs)] and in amino acid catabolism [branched-chain 2-oxoacid dehydrogenase complexes (BCODHCs)]. PDHC and OGDHC are specific for pyruvate and 2-oxoglutarate respectively, whereas one BCODHC oxidatively decarboxylates all three short branched-chain 2-oxoacids produced by the transamination of isoleucine, leucine and valine. The complexes differ among themselves in important details, but they have a number of features in common. Each of them comprises multiple copies of three catalytically active components, which are listed for each complex in Fig. 1, along with a general reaction scheme. E1, containing bound thiamin pyrophosphate (TPP), first decarboxylates the appropriate 2-oxoacid and in a second step generates electrons and the acyl group, which are transferred to a lipoyl prosthetic group that is covalently bound to a lysine of E2. E1 is specific, not only for a particular 2-oxoacid, but also for the lipoate-bearing

Fig. 1 **Reaction sequence and components of 2-oxoacid dehydrogenase complexes**

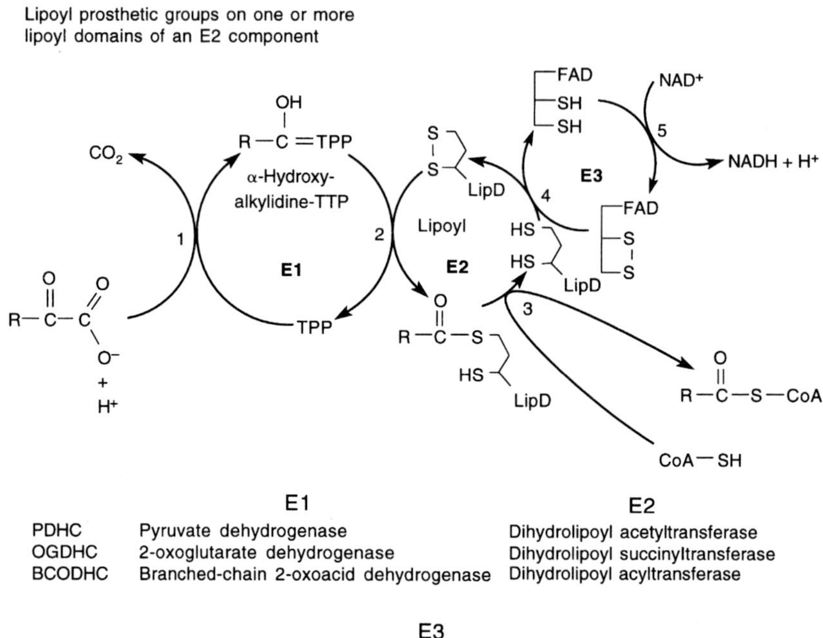

	E1	E2
PDHC	Pyruvate dehydrogenase	Dihydrolipoyl acetyltransferase
OGDHC	2-oxoglutarate dehydrogenase	Dihydrolipoyl succinyltransferase
BCODHC	Branched-chain 2-oxoacid dehydrogenase	Dihydrolipoyl acyltransferase

E3
Dihydrolipoyl dehydrogenase (common to all three complexes)

R = − CH₃ (pyruvate), − CH₂COOH (2-oxoglutarate) or side chains of the amino acids leucine, isoleucine or valine. TPP is bound to E1 components. A lipoyl moiety is covalently attached to each lipoyl domain (LipD) of the E2 (or E3BP) components. The names of E1 and E2 components for PDHC, OGDHC and BCODHC are listed, as well as that of their shared E3 component.

domain of E2 from the same complex and the same organism. Free lipoamide, lipoyl peptides and non-cognate lipoyl domains are poor substrates [11,13]. E2 transfers the acyl group from bound lipoate to CoA. It also serves a structural role, self-associating to form the symmetrical core of the complex and providing attachment sites for the other components. E3 uses a reducible disulphide–FAD system to reoxidize the dihydrolipoyl group, transferring reducing equivalents to NAD$^+$.

Transacylase cores

The unique structures of the E2 components are of central importance to the organization and function of these complexes. E2 components from all sources consist of several independently folded domains set off from each other by mobile linker regions 18–35 amino acids long [9–11]. These domains are of three different types. The largest domain is the C-terminus of the molecule. A trimer of C-terminal domains is the structural and catalytic unit of E2. The trimers assemble themselves as a structural core in two different ways. They occupy the eight corners of a cube in OGDHCs and 'pure' BCODHCs from all sources and in PDHCs from Gram-negative bacteria. In PDHCs from Gram-positive bacteria and from eukaryote sources, the C-domain trimers lie at the 20 vertices of a dodecahedron.

The next E2 domain, attached to the core by a flexible chain segment, is usually a subunit-binding domain that serves to bind either the E3 component only (in PDHCs and OGDHCs from Gram-negative bacteria [11,14]), the E1 component only (in mammalian and yeast PDHCs [15–17]) or both the E1 and E3 components (in PDHCs from Gram-positive bacteria and in mammalian BCODHCs [11,18,19]). The three-dimensional structure of the subunit-binding domain of *Bacillus stearothermophilus* PDHC E2 was determined by NMR [20], and a single domain of this small independently folded structure (35 amino acids) was shown to bind either one E3 dimer [21] or one E1 tetramer [22]. Nakano et al. [23] have demonstrated that the mammalian OGDHC lacks this binding domain in E2; instead an E3-binding domain is apparently attached to its E1 component [24].

The N-terminal segment of E2 consists of one to three lipoyl domains connected to each other and to the subunit-binding domain by mobile links [9–11]. The functional significance of the mobility of these tethered lipoyl domains will be a major theme of this chapter. NMR spectroscopy was used to determine the three-dimensional structure of the lipoyl domain of *B. stearothermophilus* PDHC E2 [25] and a lipoyl domain of *Escherichia coli* PDHC [26]. Both 80-amino-acid structures are composed of two four-stranded β sheets with the lipoate attached to a lysine at the tip of a tight β turn. The lipoyl-bearing H-protein of the glycine cleavage system [27] has the same fold despite a very low level of sequence identity. Moreover, the amino acid sequences of biotinyl-lysine domains of ATP-dependent carboxylases are similar enough to those of lipoyl domains that the same folding pattern has been proposed [28].

Organization

The attachment of the other components to the E2 framework differs among the various complexes. The organization of mammalian PDHC in particular is shown in Fig. 2 [15,16,29–36]. In this complex, E1, an $\alpha_2\beta_2$ tetramer, binds to the B domain of E2 through its β subunit [15,16]. Each tetramer probably binds to the B domains of two E2 chains unless E1 is in excess. Mammalian PDHC is controlled by a phosphorylation/dephosphorylation cycle; the relevant kinase and phosphatase are bound to the innermost of the two lipoyl domains of mammalian E2 ([16,33–36]; L. Wang, S. Liu and T.E. Roche, unpublished work). In eukaryotic complexes E3 is not bound directly to E2;

instead, it is secured through an additional component, the E3-binding protein (E3BP) [30–32]. The domain structure of E3BP (Fig. 2) resembles that of E2: a C-terminal domain that binds very strongly to the E2 core, a binding domain specific for E3, and a single lipoyl domain that can undergo reduction and acetylation during the catalytic cycle [32,37–39]. Recent studies indicate that the inner domains of 12 E3BP subunits bind to the inside of the porous dodecahedral core of E2 and that each B domain binds one E3 dimer [40].

The ratios of E1 and E3 to E2 are uncertain in most cases and may not, in fact, be precisely defined. The composition of a given complex

Fig. 2   Domain structure of E2 and E3 of mammalian PDHC and domain interactions with other components

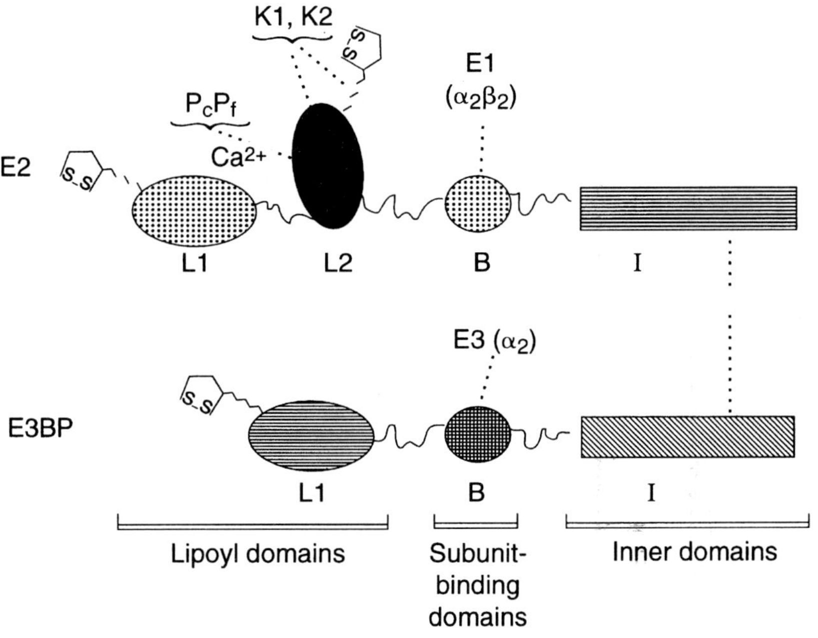

The globular domains of the E2 and E3BP components [9–11] are shown with their connecting linker regions (wiggly lines). The related lipoyl domains, designated L1 and L2 in E2 and L in E3BP, are shown with a representation of attached lipoyl groups. The interactions between components and specific domains of E2 and E3BP are indicated with dotted lines. For the components required for the PDHC reaction, associations are shown between the inner domain, I, of E2 and E3BP [29], between the β subunit of E1 and the component-binding domain, B, of E2 [15,16], and between E3 and E3BP [15,30,31] by the B domain of E3BP [32]. As detailed in this chapter, the regulatory E1a kinase (K1 and K2 isoforms) binds to the lipoyl domain region of E2 by an interaction with the L2 domain that also requires the lipoyl prosthetic group [16,33–35]; the E1b phosphatase (P$_c$ and P$_f$ subunits) also interacts with the L2 domain of E2 ([36]; L. Wang, S. Liu and T.E. Roche, unpublished work).

appears to vary somewhat from one preparation to another. PDHC from bovine heart consistently contains about 30 E1 tetramers, while the same complex isolated from kidney has only about 20 [8]; E1, E2 and E3 polypeptides are identical in the two tissues. PDHC isolated from *E. coli* is heterogeneous in sedimentation coefficient, and presumably in mass, since sedimenting boundaries spread more rapidly than can be accounted for by diffusion [41]. Isolated complexes can often bind additional E1 (e.g. [42,42a]). All of this could, of course, be accounted for by progressive loss of E1 and E3 in the course of isolation, even though the components are quite tightly bound in the isolated complexes. It may be, however, that the number of components and their distribution on the surface of the complex really is heterogeneous *in vivo*. With large numbers of each active site collected into one particle, synthesis of the various peptide chains would not need to be precisely co-ordinated to provide reaction partners for all of the available components.

It has been suggested in some studies that the 2-oxoacid dehydrogenase complexes associate with organelle membranes [43,44]. In higher organisms, all three complexes are located in mitochondria; a distinct form of PDHC is located in plant chloroplasts [45]. Procedures that physically disrupt the enclosing membranes and release 'soluble' components liberate a portion of these complexes. However, there is considerable variation in the ease and extent of release. PDHC is solubilized more completely from mitochondria prepared in a swollen, somewhat damaged, form and is then much more readily released from liver and kidney mitochondria (a major portion by freezing and thawing) than from heart or brain mitochondria, which require a disruption step such as sonication, implosion or repeated freeze–thawing [46–48]. There is also some evidence for specific associations of PDHC and OGDHC with components of the tricarboxylic acid cycle and with the electron transport system [43,49–51]. One might speculate that such interactions could serve to channel metabolites into and out of the complexes. However, the evidence is sparse and, beyond one finding mentioned below, these observations will not be addressed in the present chapter.

Catalytic transfers

The complete complexes are enormous, with molecular masses ranging upward to 9×10^6 Da. Moreover, the effective volumes of the complexes are very much larger than would be predicted for compact structures; that is, they occlude a great deal of solvent. Even the rigid cubic or dodecahedral cores assembled from the C-terminal domains of E2 are porous structures, enclosing a body of solvent accessible through the core faces. A three-dimensional structure is available for the cubic core of the *Azotobacter vinelandii* PDHC E2 [52]. The trimeric catalytic units at the corners of the cube each contain three equivalent active sites. Two subunits line a channel into which a lipoyl lysine reaches from outside the core, and the equally long CoA molecule penetrates from the inside [52–54]. CoA can approach the active site only by entering the interior of the core through the faces of the cube. CoA-SH can reach far enough into the channel to accept an acetyl group from 8-acetyl-lipoate, but not from a disulphide with the free 6-thiol.

The temptation is irresistible to extrapolate from the *Azotobacter* structure to comment on some recent observations on complexes for which structural information is less complete. Sumegi et al. [49] observed that citrate synthase was precipitated at low poly(ethylene glycol) levels in the presence of mammalian PDHC. Preliminary studies (S. Ravindran and T.E. Roche, unpublished work) indicate that an E2–E3BP subcomplex is more effective than an E2 oligomer produced by recombinant techniques in precipitating citrate synthase. This observation suggests that citrate synthase associates with E3BP. Studies are under way to test the hypothesis that it is the inner domain of E3BP, which is located inside the dodecahedral inner core of E2, that is responsible for the binding. If so, acetyl-CoA produced inside the inner core could be immediately used by citrate synthase. This speculative idea is consistent with earlier evidence for a select pool of acetyl-CoA in mitochondria that is produced by PDHC and preferentially used by citrate synthase [55,56].

The three-dimensional structures of E3 components have also been determined [57,58]. The active site of the E3 homodimer, like that of the E2 trimer, lies between the subunits, with the lipoate being inserted into this interface. This insertion places the reactive thiols next to a disulphide–FAD, and reducing equivalents are passed through the FAD to the pyridine ring of NAD^+ held in position by a typical NAD^+-binding domain. For identical subunits (E2 and E3), to have their activity constituted in channels between subunits would seem to require an evolutionary background in which formation of the aggregated state precedes the development of a specific catalytic role. In this respect, it may be significant that E3 is homologous to glutathione reductase [59] and E2 is homologous to chloramphenicol acetyltransferase [60].

Evidence is accumulating that the active sites of E1 components are similarly distributed between subunits, at least in the $\alpha_2\beta_2$ tetramers found in Gram-positive and eukaryotic PDHCs and BCODHCs [61–67]. The E1s of Gram-negative PDHCs and of all OGDHCs are homodimers; since the subunits have masses greater than 90 kDa, they are very probably folded into multiple domains that could, perhaps, be functionally equivalent to separate α and β subunits. In mammalian PDHC E1, both the α and the β chains contribute significant groups to the active site [62–65]; TPP contacts both subunits [61,64]. It seems likely these subunits form a channel that the lipoyl group enters upon specific binding of the lipoyl domain at the entrance in an interaction that involves both chains.

Both E1 and E3 catalyse Ping Pong reactions [68,69], in which intermediates are first made and then used in very different reaction steps. In the case of E3, the FAD bridges two sides in the active site, capturing reducing equivalents on one side and passing them to the other side. In E1, the 'active aldehyde'–TPP arising from decarboxylation of a 2-oxoacid is anchored by a flexible pyrophosphate–Mg^{2+} tether. It could easily move within the interlobular channel and allow additional residues of E1 to catalyse reductive acylation of a lipoate. The movement could be driven by decarboxylation itself, which converts a zwitterionic 2-hydroxyacid–TPP intermediate into a neutral, relatively non-polar α-hydroxyalkylidene–TPP. Mammalian E1 also exhibits a Flip-Flop mechanism, in which the two active sites must operate alternately [70,71]. Phosphorylation of one α subunit of the tetramer inactivates both sites [72]. These facts, along with major spectral changes that occur during the reaction [65,71], suggest that relative motion of the subunits forming the active site may be involved in the catalytic mechanism.

This common mechanistic feature of moving a lipoate into a channel formed between subunits or domains, suggested for E1 and established for E2 and E3, may be exploited in a variety of ways. The reactions could be controlled by gated interactions of tethered mobile proteinaceous lobes at the entrance to the active sites. Binding a lipoyl domain at the channel entrance should contribute to the specificity of catalysis and might also force the lipoyl lysine prosthetic group into an energetically unfavourable interaction with the active site or protect reactive intermediates. The role of the lipoyl domain in contributing to specificity is best documented in the case of E1, but even in the case of E3, we (J.C. Baker and T.E. Roche, unpublished work) have found a much lower K_m and higher V_{max} for a lipoyl domain of human E2 versus free lipoamide. Furthermore, the trimer units of *Azotobacter* PDHC E2 appear to have pockets that may accommodate the lipoyl domain, suggesting favourable interactions between the catalytic and lipoyl domains of E2 (J. Hendle and W.G.J. Hol, personal communication).

Surface dynamics

The rest of this chapter will focus on the outer layer of mammalian PDHC and, in particular, on the mobility of the tails that dangle from the vertices of the core, which has important consequences for catalysis and for regulation. This layer is sparsely occupied by up to 30 E1 tetramers and by one or two E1α kinase dimers bound to the N-terminal tails of 60 E2 subunits, each folded into two lipoyl domains and one binding domain, along with about 12 E3 dimers bound to the tails of E3BP subunits. Most of the surface layer, however, is occupied by solvent. Very early sedimentation velocity measurements gave remarkably high frictional ratios for intact complexes and for E2 cores with tails intact [73,73a,74], despite the symmetrical appearance of these objects under the electron microscope [75,76]. When subcomplexes of E2 undersaturated with E1 or E3 are examined by cryoelectron microscopy, which does not shrink the particles by drying, gaps as large as 4–6 nm are regularly seen between the bound components and the inner core [77,78]. Kidney PDHC includes about 20 E1 tetramers; the heart complex contains about 30, and so has a mass larger by 1.5×10^6 Da. Nevertheless, the effective sizes of the two complexes are the same, as measured by quasielastic light scattering [79]. Images of intact mammalian complexes have a diameter of about 50 nm [78], in agreement with light scattering measurements. The diameter of the dodecahedral inner core, viewed along a 5-fold axis, is about 22.5 nm, so that the volume of the surface layer is about 6×10^4 nm^3. Of this volume only about 9×10^3 nm^3, or 15%, is accounted for by the protein components of the heart complex, assuming a partial specific volume of 1.21×10^{-3} nm^3/Da (0.73 cm^3/g). A similar crude calculation indicates that the dodecahedral core, whose rigidity is suggested by well-resolved electron microscopic images, is an open framework containing twice as much solvent as protein.

The fact that the E2 tails have room to move would not necessarily mean that they do move. Nevertheless, there is direct evidence that the tails are in fact mobile. They are not easily visible in electron micrographs [76–78], and they are efficiently cleaved from the core by proteases [80–82]. The most persuasive evidence for movement of the N-terminal half of E2 chains comes from proton NMR spectra. Perham and his associates have found in *E. coli* complexes a group of resonances whose narrow line-widths show that the rotational movement of the amino acid residues responsible for them must be much more rapid than that of the complexes as a whole [11,83–85]. They have traced the signals to the interdomain linkers of E2 by comparing the NMR spectra of the normal complex and of genetically engineered complexes having the linkers truncated, deleted or modified. The catalytic activities of a series of modified complexes also documented the functional significance of movement in the E2 tails. As the linker between the binding domain and the innermost lipoyl domain was progressively shortened, the rate of the reaction catalysed by the complex decreased [86]. Activity did not disappear when this one linker was completely eliminated; presumably the chains remained flexible around the linkers between the lipoyl domains.

In contrast to the globular domains, the various linker peptides show no common pattern in their amino acid sequences, but there are some general similarities in their composition. They are high in Ala and Pro residues, contain little His or Met and no aromatic amino acids and, in most cases, are surprisingly low in Gly. Both charged and uncharged hydrophilic residues are fairly common. NMR studies have shown that synthetic peptides that mimic sequences of linkers from *E. coli* PDHC are not completely disordered [87,88]; these model regions contain several Ala-Pro sequences and the peptide group in each is detected exclusively in the *trans* conformation. This suggestion of conformational constraint has been generalized to imply a certain stiffness in the linkers that would tend to hold the E2 domains apart along the chain axis. The domains themselves carry net negative charges, which might disperse them laterally in the surface layer.

The flexible E2 tails carrying lipoyl domains closely resemble the 'swinging arm' model suggested many years ago by Reed [89] to account for the integrated activity of the complexes, during which the dithiol of lipoate must cycle through the active sites of E1, E2 and E3. Mounting the prosthetic group on a mobile protein arm increases the potential range of movement beyond the length of an extended lipoyl-lysine chain (≤ 3 nm). Energy-transfer studies by Hammes and associates [90–92] indicated that active sites are indeed separated by some 4.5 nm. Movement of the E2 tails can also bring the lipoyl domains of different chains into contact with each other and provide a way of moving acyl groups and electrons from one lipoyl group to another [89]. Acetyl groups and reducing equivalents certainly do spread around the surface of isolated PDHC [93,94]. There is, however, reason to doubt that such transfers are obligatory steps in the catalytic sequence. Decarboxylation catalysed by E1 appears rate-limiting [95,96]; that is, all downstream reactions are faster than this first step [10,11]. It is difficult to evaluate whether mechanisms may exist to facilitate transfers between lipoyl groups within a complex. Active-site coupling probably involves several lipoyl groups servicing an active site. Certainly uncatalysed transacylation [97,98] and electron transfer by disulphide interchange [99] are slow. Furthermore, any calculated rate of interdomain transfer in a complex would rest on a speculative estimate of the effective concentration of tethered lipoyl domains in the surface layer. The highly mobile but apparently stiff interdomain linkers might bend in preferred directions, making transfer more efficient. For the moment, the functional significance of acyl or electron exchange between lipoates remains an open question.

The apparent redundancy of lipoyl domains is a puzzling feature of many PDHCs. *E. coli* PDHC, for example, has three such domains in each E2 tail; mammalian E2 chains have two, and there is an additional lipoyl domain in each E3BP subunit [9–12]. In a given complex, the amino acid sequences of the lipoyl domains differ but are related and probably fold similarly. Under normal conditions, all of the domains are lipoylated and all of the lipoyl groups can be reduced and acylated during the catalytic cycle. It might be reasonable to suppose that each lipoyl domain plays some essential, specialized role, but, at least where catalysis is concerned, the evidence is against this notion. OGDHCs and BCODHCs have only one lipoyl domain per E2 chain, as do PDHCs from many organisms; all of these complexes operate efficiently. Removal of half of the lipoates from mammalian or *E. coli* PDHC E2 has very little effect on the rate of the overall reaction catalysed by the complex [16,100]. The most persuasive evidence that the number of lipoyl domains exceeds what is required for catalysis is provided by genetically modified *E. coli* complexes in which lipoyl domains are deleted, spliced together, or crippled by replacing the lysine to which lipoate is attached [86,101,102]. As long as at least one lipoyl domain per chain is present and functional, the engineered complexes are fully active.

The single lipoyl domain of E3BP in yeast and mammalian PDHCs may be an exception to the functional interchangeability of lipoyl domains. Complete removal of E3BP decreases the activity of the mammalian complex by 96% ([30]; D. Yang, J. Song, T. Wagenknecht and T.E. Roche, unpublished work) and inactivates the yeast complex almost entirely [103]. By itself, this result is not surprising; although unbound E3 readily uses free forms of E2 lipoyl domains as substrates, anchoring E3 to the E2 core ought to enhance the reaction rate. However, removal of the E3BP lipoyl domain alone, leaving the binding domain that secures E3, causes the loss of $\sim 40\%$ of the activity of the complex ([103]; S.L. Powers-Greenwood and T.E. Roche, unpublished work; a lesser effect was noted in [104]). This effect is greatly disproportionate, since E3BP accounts for only 12 of more than 120 lipoyl domains in the mammalian PDHC; in contrast, removal of half of the E2 lipoyl domains of the complex has little effect on activity [16]. This observation suggests that the E3BP lipoyl domain may be particularly efficient in funnelling reducing equivalents to E3 [105]. Since removing this domain decreases but does not eliminate activity, it seems that a path for electrons through E3BP is preferred but not required.

Regulation

Mobility of components in the surface layer is certainly involved in regulation of the mammalian PDHC. The complex controls the irreversible commitment of carbohydrate to aerobic energy production [106]. In general, it is physiologically desirable to conserve carbohydrate when energy is available from fatty acids or ketone bodies. Energy sufficiency is signalled by increases in the intramitochondrial $NADH/NAD^+$ and acetyl-CoA/CoA ratios. When these ratios increase, a dedicated kinase is activated and transfers phosphate from ATP to an α chain of the rate-limiting E1, shutting down the activity of the complex [36,107]. When the metabolite ratios fall, signalling the need for energy from carbohydrate, the kinase activity is decreased, phosphate is removed from E1 by a competing complex-specific phosphatase, and the complex is turned on.

E1a kinases appear to be a series of species: in rat tissues, two PDHC-specific kinase chains are known (K1 and K2) and have 70% identical sequences [108,109]. A third kind of kinase polypeptide is associated with rat BCODHC which is uniquely regulated [110,111] and has about 30% of its sequence in common with PDH kinase isoenzymes. When E1a kinase, separated from the PDHC, is subjected to native-gel electrophoresis, a pattern consistent with all three possible dimers is observed (K1$_2$, K1K2, and K2$_2$) (J.C. Baker and T.E Roche, unpublished work). Although E1a kinases phosphorylate serine hydroxy groups, their amino acid sequences [108–111] are not detectably similar to any of the serine-, threonine- or tyrosine-specific kinases of mammalian cells. Instead, they resemble distantly the bacterial histidine kinases which are involved in detecting extracellular signals [112,113]. The latter role has recently been observed in eukaryotic cells (e.g. [114,115]).

Recent studies have addressed two issues that relate the down-regulation of PDHC by E1a kinase to the organization and movement of components of the complex. First, how can a limited number of strongly bound kinase dimers efficiently modify a much larger number of E1 tetramers distributed around the surface of the complex? Secondly, how is the metabolic signal represented by NADH/NAD$^+$ and acetyl-CoA/CoA ratios transmitted to the kinase?

Dissection of the E2 tail of mammalian PDHC by limited proteolysis and by genetic constructs has shown that E1 associates with the binding domain [15,16], the module closest to the core. The kinase is bound to the inner lipoyl domain (L2, numbered from the N terminus) [35]; binding is greatly weakened if the lipoyl prosthetic group is removed [35,116]. Both components are very tightly bound [34,42a,117,118]. The kinase does not dissociate detectably; very slow dissociation of E1 can be observed at extreme dilution of the complex [42a,118]. However, bound E1 is preferentially phosphorylated by the kinase; initially free E1s are phosphorylated at a rate that corresponds to the rate of reassociation [120]. Dissociation and reassociation of E1 and the kinase are far too slow to account for the rapid phosphorylation of all the E1 of a complex by one or two bound kinase dimers. Therefore E1 and the kinase can find each other only if one or both partners move across the surface of the complex without dissociating.

Although the kinase does not dissociate from the complex, it can be passed directly from one L2 domain to another. For example, L2 domains, fused to glutathione S-transferase and anchored in a glutathione–Sepharose column, rapidly strip kinase from E2 passed through the column [35]. A model for kinase movement has been proposed based on this observation [34,35]. A kinase dimer, normally bound to the L2 domains of two E2 tails, dissociates briefly from one of them. Since the tails are mobile, the momentarily free end of the kinase may find a new partner as it reassociates. By repeatedly dissociating and rebinding one end at a time, a kinase dimer can patrol the surface of the complex 'hand over hand', finding and phosphorylating all of the bound E1 without losing its grip on the complex.

We now turn to the mechanism by which the activity of the kinase responds appropriately to the NADH/NAD$^+$ and acetyl-CoA/CoA ratios, throttling down the complex when a rise in the ratios signals energy sufficiency. Kinase and E1 can be isolated from the complex. When ATP is added to a mixture of these components, free in solution, E1 is phosphorylated; that is, the reaction does not absolutely require that either the kinase or its substrate be bound to E2. However, the reaction rate is increased, at physiological ionic strength, when E2 is added to the assay mixture. If the lipoyl residues of the added E2 are in the oxidized form, the rate increase is about 4-fold [34,121]. This augmented rate increases by 80% when the lipoyl residues are reduced and triples when they are reduced and acetylated [99,122–125].

Two factors are presumably at work. Binding of the kinase and its protein substrate to adjacent domains should increase the efficiency of the reaction whatever the state of the lipoyl residues. In addition, acetyl-lipoate specifically and directly stimulates the activity of the kinase. This latter stimulation can be distinguished from the juxtaposition effect by experiments in which intact E2 is replaced by isolated L2 domains [125]. Reduction and acetylation of the isolated domains increases the rate of the kinase reaction. Stimulation also occurs when a peptide substrate is substituted for E1. The mechanism of kinase stimulation by acetyl-L2 is uncertain. The rate of the kinase reaction is limited by dissociation of the product ADP from the active site. Pyruvate, which directly inhibits the kinase, does so by slowing release of ADP [126]. Ravindran et al. [125] have suggested that acetyl-L2 may act, conversely, by accelerating ADP dissociation.

In the intact complex, the lipoyl groups of E2 can be reduced and acetylated either by oxidative decarboxylation of pyruvate through E1 or by electrons and acetyl groups backing up from NADH and acetyl-CoA through E3 and the E2 active site. Under most conditions, the faster downstream reactions should govern the reduction/acetylation state of the lipoyl residues [96,125]. As a result, the degree of reduction and acetylation of the lipoyl prosthetic groups reflects directly the $NADH/NAD^+$ and acetyl-CoA/CoA ratios. The state of the lipoates in turn governs the kinase activity and so modulates the activity of the complex.

This enhancement of kinase inactivation of mammalian PDHC is remarkably sensitive to the level of acetylation of sites in the complex. Half-maximal stimulation of the kinase occurs with only 6% of the lipoates of the complex reduced and acetylated; 15% acetylation gives near-maximal stimulation [123–125]. The 15% level of acetylation is reached when the $NADH/NAD^+$ and acetyl-CoA/CoA ratios are around 0.1, far too low to give significant direct product inhibition of the PDHC reaction [48,125]. The response of the kinase to very low levels of acetylation cannot be accounted for by preferential acetylation of the L2 domains where the kinase is bound. The acetyl groups are distributed over lipoyl residues in E3BP and E2 [37]; there is no evidence that L2 is disproportionately acetylated (M. Rahmatullah and T.E. Roche, unpublished work). Moreover, isolated L2 domains, included in assay mixtures at a concentration 60-fold below their calculated concentration at the surface of the core, stimulate the kinase half-maximally when only 20% of the free domains are acetylated [125].

The exaggerated effect of low levels of acetylation is very probably due to tighter binding of the kinase to whatever L2 domains happen to be reduced and acetylated [36,125]. As a kinase dimer moves around the surface of the complex, it would spend a disproportionate part of the time bound to, and stimulated by, acetylated sites. Binding must not be so tight as to fix the kinase at one site and to prevent its moving on to phosphorylate E1 over the entire surface. However, some degree of localization need not be a problem. Since the E2 tails are mobile, a kinase dimer pausing at an acetylated L2 domain should be within reach of several E1s, and phosphorylation of a single α subunit of an E1 tetramer is sufficient to inactivate it. This line of reasoning suggests that the organization and mobility of the surface of the complex serve to amplify the metabolic signal.

The phosphatase that re-activates the complex slowly removes phosphate from E1b when the enzyme and substrate are free of the complex. Catalytic activity increases 10-fold when both are bound to E2 [127]. The phosphatase associates with the L2 domain of E2 (L.Wang, S. Liu and T.E. Roche, unpublished work); association and consequent increases in catalytic rate require micromolar Ca^{2+}. The phosphatase is less strongly bound than the kinase, and so unassisted dissociation and reassociation are probably sufficiently rapid to account for the efficient dephosphorylation of all the E1b bound to an E2 core by one phosphatase molecule [128,129]. The catalytic subunit of the phosphatase has a sequence that places it in the protein phosphatase 2C family [130]. A major advance in understanding phosphatase function is anticipated following the recent finding that the 90 kDa FAD-containing regulatory subunit (P_f) has 35% sequence identity with the mitochondrial matrix enzyme dimethylglycine dehydrogenase [131]. Specific roles of the phosphatase subunits in its control by effectors have not yet been determined. The activity of the phosphatase is not affected by the reduction/acetylation state of recombinant L2, although there is a modest inhibition by NADH, the mechanism of which has not been established. The phosphatase does, however, respond directly to intramitochondrial Ca^{2+} [132,133] and indirectly to insulin [134,135].

Intramitochondrial Ca^{2+} rises when Ca^{2+} enters the cytoplasm from intracellular or extracellular pools in response to hormonal signals or during muscle contraction. The mitochondrion responds to elevated Ca^{2+} by accelerated production of NADH, which enhances the rate of oxidative phosphorylation [133,136]. PDHC is one of the three intramitochondrial sites at which production of NADH is increased [133]; the effect of Ca^{2+} is to activate the phosphatase by binding it to the complex close to its substrate E1b [127–129]. In addition, Ca^{2+} causes a large decrease in the K_m of the OGDHC for 2-oxoglutarate [137,138] and greatly decreases inhibition by NADH of that enzyme [139,140]. Ca^{2+} also increases NADH production by activating isocitrate dehydrogenase [141].

In addition to its activation by Ca^{2+}, the phosphatase responds to a quite different metabolic signal: its activity is increased by insulin in white and brown adipose tissue and in lactating mammary gland, tissues in which the synthesis of fatty acids from carbohydrate is important [135]. The activity of the phosphatase is Mg^{2+}-dependent; at saturating Mg^{2+}, the maximal turnover rate of the phosphatase exceeds that of E1a kinase [130,131]. However, the concentration of Mg^{2+} required for near-maximal activity in the absence of insulin is well above that normally found in mitochondria. When an appropriate target tissue is treated with insulin, the K_m of the phosphatase for Mg^{2+} drops into the physiological range, and the activity of the phosphatase increases markedly, switching E1 to its active form [134]. The heightened response to Mg^{2+} persists in mitochondria isolated intact from insulin-treated adipose tissue but is lost when the mitochondria are disrupted [134,135]. Evidently, the stimulation of the phosphatase by insulin is mediated by an intramitochondrial second messenger, possibly an inositol phosphate glycan [142]. Its effect is mimicked by spermine or spermidine [143], but only at concentrations higher than those found in mitochondria. Moreover, polyamine concentrations have not been shown to vary in response to insulin [135].

Thus carbohydrate reserves are maintained in mammals by a set of very sensitive signal translation mechanisms that control PDHC activity. Flow through the complex responds to product/substrate ratios, to Ca^{2+} and to insulin in 'rational' ways that are closely connected with the organization of the complex. There is limited knowledge as to the way this general control scheme for PDHC is adjusted or augmented to serve the divergent physiological functions of specific organs. The pattern of E1a kinase isoenzymes appears to vary from one tissue to another and these enzymes have quantitatively different responses to kinase effectors [111]. Under starvation and in the diabetic state, the kinase isoenzyme pattern shifts in a tissue-dependent way, the total amount of kinase increases, and PDHC activity is decreased to a very low level to conserve carbohydrate [106,111,144,145]. PDHC and its relatives will clearly reward continuing study.

We wish to acknowledge support from National Institutes of Health Grant DK18320, from the Kansas Affiliate of the American Heart Association, and from the Kansas State Agricultural Experiment Station (contribution 96–33-B). We thank Jason Baker and Amy Paulin for help in preparation of the figures, and Connie Schmidt and Marci Irey for help in manuscript preparation.

References

1. Reed, L.J. and Cox, D.J. (1966) Annu. Rev. Biochem. **35**, 57–84
2. Lynen, F. (1964) in New Perspectives in Biology (Sela, M., ed.), pp. 132–146, American Elsevier, New York
3. Reed, L.J. and Cox, D.J. (1970) Enzymes 3rd Edn. **1**, 213–240
4. Ginsburg, A. and Stadtman, E.R. (1970) Annu. Rev. Biochem. **39**, 429–472
5. Welch, G.R. (1977) Prog. Biophys. Mol. Biol. **32**, 103–191
6. Welch, G.R., ed. (1985) Organized Multienzyme Systems: Catalytic Properties, pp. 1–458, Academic Press, New York

7. Srere, P.A. (1987) Annu. Rev. Biochem. **56**, 89–124
8. Reed, L.J. (1974) Acc. Chem. Res. **7**, 40–46
9. Reed, L.J. and Hackert, M.L. (1990) J. Biol. Chem. **265**, 8971–8974
10. Patel, M.S. and Roche, T.E. (1990) FASEB J. **4**, 3224–3233
11. Perham, R.N. (1991) Biochemistry **30**, 8501–8517
12. Roche, T.E. and Patel, M.S., eds. (1989) Ann. N.Y. Acad. Sci. **573**, 1–462
13. Graham, L.D., Packman, L.C. and Perham, R.N. (1989) Biochemistry **28**, 1574–1581
14. Packman, L.C. and Perham, R.N. (1986) FEBS Lett. **206**, 193–198
15. Rahmatullah, M., Gopalakrishnan, S., Andrews, P.C., Chang, C.L., Radke, G.A. and Roche, T.E. (1989) J. Biol. Chem. **264**, 2221–2227
16. Rahmatullah, M., Radke, G.A., Andrews, P.C. and Roche, T.E. (1990) J. Biol. Chem. **265**, 14512–14517
17. Lawson, J.E., Niu, X.D. and Reed, L.J. (1991) Biochemistry **30**, 11249–11254
18. Packman, L.C., Borges, A. and Perham, R.N. (1988) Biochem. J. **252**, 79–86
19. Wynn, R.M., Chuang, J.L., Davie, J.R., Fisher, C.W., Hale, M.A., Cox, R.P. and Chuang, D.T. (1992) J. Biol. Chem. **267**, 1881–1887
20. Kalia, Y.N., Brocklehurst, S.M., Hipps, D.S., Appella, E., Sakaguchi, K. and Perham, R.N. (1993) J. Mol. Biol. **230**, 323–341
21. Hipps, D.S., Packman, L.C., Allen, M.D., Fuller, C., Sakaguchi, K., Apella, E. and Perham, R.N. (1994) Biochem. J. **297**, 137–143
22. Lessard, I.A.D. and Perham, R.N. (1995) Biochem. J. **306**, 727–733
23. Nakano, K., Matuda, S., Yamanaka, T., Tsubouchi, H., Nakagawa, S., Titani, K., Ohta, S. and Miyata, T. (1991) J. Biol. Chem. **266**, 19013–19017
24. Rice, J.E., Dunbar, B. and Lindsay, J.G. (1992) EMBO J. **11**, 3229–3235
25. Dardel, F., Davis, A.L., Laue, E.D. and Perham, R.N. (1993) J. Mol. Biol. **229**, 1037–1048
26. Green, J.D.F., Laue, E.D., Perham, R.N., Ali, S.T. and Guest, J.R. (1995) J. Mol. Biol. **248**, 328–343
27. Pares, S., Cohen-Addad, C., Sieker, L., Neuburger, M. and Douce, R.(1994) Proc. Natl. Acad. Sci. U.S.A. **94**, 4850–4853
28. Brocklehurst, S.M. and Perham, R.N. (1993) Protein Sci. **2**, 626–639
29. Rahmatullah, M., Gopalakrishnan, S., Radke, G.A. and Roche, T.E. (1989) J. Biol. Chem. **264**, 1245–1251
30. Powers-Greenwood, S.L., Rahmatullah, M., Radke, G.A. and Roche, T.E. (1989) J. Biol. Chem. **264**, 3655–3657
31. Gopalakrishnan, S., Rahmatullah, M., Radke, G.A., Powers-Greenwood, S.L. and Roche, T.E. (1989) Biochem. Biophys. Res. Commun. **160**, 715–721
32. Lawson, J.E., Behal, R.H. and Reed, L.J. (1991) Biochemistry **30**, 2834–2839
33. Li, L., Radke, G.A., Ono, K. and Roche, T.E. (1992) Arch. Biochem. Biophys. **296**, 497–504
34. Ono, K., Radke, G.A., Roche, T.E. and Rahmatullah, M. (1993) J. Biol. Chem. **268**, 26135–26143
35. Liu, S., Baker, J.C. and Roche, T.E. (1995) J. Biol. Chem. **270**, 793–800
36. Roche, T.E., Liu, S., Ravindran, S., Baker, J.C. and Wang, L. (1996) in α-Keto Acid Dehydrogenase Complexes (Patel, M.S., Roche, T.E. and Harris, R.A., eds.), pp. 33–52, Birkhäuser Verlag, Basel
37. Jilka, J.M., Rahmatullah, M., Kazemi, M. and Roche, T.E. (1986) J. Biol. Chem. **261**, 1858–1867
38. Behal, R.H., Browning, K.S., Hall, T.B. and Reed, L.J. (1989) Proc. Natl. Acad. Sci. U.S.A. **86**, 8732–8736
39. Rahmatullah, M. and Roche, T.E. (1987) J. Biol. Chem. **262**, 10265–10271
40. Maeng, C.-Y., Yazdi, M.A., Niu, X.-D., Lee, H.Y. and Reed, L.J. (1994) Biochemistry **33**, 13801–13807
41. Gilbert, G.A. and Gilbert, L.M. (1980) J. Mol. Biol. **144**, 405–408
42. Reed, L.J., Pettit, F.H., Eley, M.H., Hamilton, L., Collins, J.H. and Oliver, R.M. (1975) Proc. Natl. Acad. Sci. U.S.A. **72**, 3068–3072
42a. Wu, T.-L. and Reed, L.J. (1984) Biochemistry **23**, 221–226
43. Sumegi, B. and Srere, P.A. (1984) J. Biol. Chem. **259**, 15040–15045
44. Sumegi, B., Zsolt, L., Lindsey, I., Paull, W.K. and Srere, P.A. (1987) Eur. J. Biochem. **169**, 223–230

45. Williams, M. and Randall, D.D. (1979) Plant Physiol. **64**, 1099–1103
46. Linn, T.C., Pelley, J.W., Pettit, F.H., Hucho, F., Randall, D.D. and Reed, L.J. (1972) Arch. Biochem. Biophys. **148**, 327–342
47. Cooper, R.H., Randle, P.J. and Denton, R.M. (1974) Biochem, J. **143**, 625–641
48. Roche, T.E. and Cate, R.L. (1977) Arch. Biochem. Biophys. **183**, 664–677
49. Sumegi, B., Gyocsi, L. and Alkonyi, I. (1983) Biochim. Biophys. Acta **749**, 163–171
50. Porpazy, Z., Sumegi, B. and Alkonyi, I. (1986) J. Biol. Chem. **262**, 9509–9514
51. Fahren, L.A., MacDonald, M.J., Teller, J.K., Fibich, B. and Fahien, C.M. (1989) J. Biol. Chem. **264**, 12303–12312
52. Mattevi, A., Obmolova, G., Schulze, E., Kalk, K.H., Westphal, A., de Kok, A. and Hol, W.G.J. (1992) Science **255**, 1544–1550
53. Mattevi, A., Obmolova, G., Kalk, K.H., Westphal, A.H., de Kok, A. and Hol, W.G.J. (1993) J. Mol. Biol. **230**, 1183–1199
54. Mattevi, A., Obmolova, G., Kalk, K.H., Teplyakov, A. and Hol, W.G.J. (1993) Biochemistry **32**, 3887–3901
55. Delisle, G. and Fritz, I.B. (1967) Proc. Natl. Acad. Sci. U.S.A. **58**, 790–797
56. Glutz, U.G. and Walter, P. (1975) Eur. J. Biochem. **66**, 147–152
57. Schierbeek, A.J., Swarte, M.B.A., Dijkstra, B.W., Vriend, G., Read, R.J., Hol, W.G.J., Drenth, J. and Betzel, C. (1989) J. Mol. Biol. **206**, 365–379
58. Mattevi, A., Obmolova, G., Sokatch, J.R., Betzel, C. and Hol, W.G.J. (1992) Protein J. **13**, 336–351
59. Williams, C.H., Arscott, L.D. and Schulz, G.F. (1981) Proc. Natl. Acad. Sci. U.S.A. **79**, 2199–2201
60. Guest, J.R., Angier, S.J. and Russell, G.C. (1989) Ann. N.Y. Acad. Sci. **573**, 76–99
61. Hawkins, C.F., Borges, A. and Perham, R.N. (1990) Eur. J. Biochem. **191**, 337–346
62. Zhao, Y., Kuntz, M.J., Harris, R.A. and Crabb, D.W. (1992) Biochim. Biophys. Acta **1132**, 207–210
63. Robinson, B.H. and Chun, K. (1993) FEBS Lett. **328**, 99–102
64. Ali, M.S., Roche, T.E. and Patel, M.S. (1993) J. Biol. Chem. **268**, 22353–22356
65. Ali, M.S., Shenoy, B.C., Eswaran, D., Andersson, L.A., Roche, T.E. and Patel, M.S. (1995) J. Biol. Chem. **270**, 4570–4574
66. Davie, J.R., Wynn, R.M., Cox, R.P. and Chuang, D.T. (1992) J. Biol. Chem. **267**, 16601–16606
67. Korotchkina, L.G., Tucker, M.M., Tekkumkara, T.J., Madhusudhan, K.T., Pons, G., Kim, H. and Patel, M.S. (1995) Protein Expression Purif. **6**, 79–90
68. Reed, J.K. (1970) J. Biol. Chem. **248**, 4834–4839
69. Roche, T.E. and Liu, S. (1994) FASEB J. **8**, A1350
70. Khailova, L.S. and Korochkina, L.G. (1985) Biochem. Int. **11**, 509–516
71. Kharlova, L.S., Korochkina, L.G. and Severin, S.E. (1989) Ann. N.Y. Acad. Sci. **573**, 36–54
72. Yeaman, S.J., Hutcheson, E.T., Roche, T.E., Pettit, F.H., Brown, J.R., Reed, L.J., Watson, D.C. and Dixon, G.H. (1978) Biochemistry **17**, 2364–2370
73. Koike, M., Reed, L.J. and Carroll, W.R. (1960) J. Biol. Chem. **235**, 1924–1930
73a. Fernandez-Moran, H., Reed, L.J., Koike, M. and Williams, C.R. (1964) Science **145**, 930–932
74. Danson, M.J., Hile, G., Johnson, P. and Perham, R.H. (1979) J. Mol. Biol. **129**, 603–617
75. Reed, L.J. and Oliver, R.M. (1968) Brookhaven Symp. Biol. **21**, 397–412
76. Oliver, R.M. and Reed, L.J. (1982) in Electron Microscopy of Proteins (Harris, R., ed.), vol. 2, pp. 1–48, Academic Press, London
77. Wagenknecht, T., Grassucci, R. and Frank, J. (1988) J. Mol. Biol. **199**, 137–147
78. Wagenknecht, T., Grassucci, R., Radke, G.A. and Roche, T.E. (1991) J. Biol. Chem. **266**, 24650–24656
79. Roche, T.E., Powers-Greenwood, S.L., Shi, W., Zhang, W., Ren, S.Z., Roche, E.D., Cox, D.J. and Sorensen, C.M. (1993) Biochemistry **32**, 5629–5637
80. Bliele, D.M., Munk, P., Oliver, R.M. and Reed, L.J. (1979) Proc. Natl. Acad. Sci. U.S.A. **76**, 4385–4389
81. Kresge, B.B. and Ronft, H. (1980) Eur. J. Biochem. **112**, 589–599
82. Bliele, D.M., Hackert, M.L., Pettit, F.H. and Reed, L.J. (1981) J. Biol. Chem. **256**, 514–519

83. Perham, R.N., Duckworth, H.W. and Roberts, G.C.K. (1981) Nature (London) **297**, 474–477
84. Radford, S.E., Laue, E.D., Perham, R.N., Miles, J.S. and Guest, J.R. (1987) Biochem. J. **247**, 641–649
85. Texter, F.L., Radford, S.E., Laue, E.D., Perham, R.N., Miles, J.S. and Guest, J.R. (1988) Biochemistry **27**, 289–296
86. Miles, J.S., Guest, J.R., Radford, S.E. and Perham, R.N. (1988) J. Mol. Biol. **202**, 97–106
87. Radford, S.E., Laue, E.D., Perham, R.N., Martin, S.R. and Appella, E. (1989) J. Biol. Chem. **264**, 767–775
88. Green, D.F., Perham, R.N., Ulrich, S.J. and Appella, E. (1992) J. Biol. Chem. **267**, 23484–23488
89. Reed, L.J. (1962) Vitam. Horm. **20**, 1–38
90. Papadakis, N. and Hammes, G.G. (1977) Biochemistry **16**, 1890–1896
91. Shepherd, G.B. and Hammes, G.G. (1977) Biochemistry **16**, 5234–5241
92. Hammes, G.G. (1981) Biochem. Soc. Symp. **46**, 73–90
93. Bates, D.L., Danson, M.J., Hale, G., Hopper, E.A. and Perham, R.N. (1977) Nature (London) **268**, 313–316
94. Collins, J.H. and Reed, L.J. (1977) Proc. Natl. Acad. Sci. U.S.A. **74**, 4223–4227
95. Danson, M.J., Fersht, A.R. and Perham, R.N. (1978) Proc. Natl. Acad. Sci. U.S.A. **75**, 5386–5390
96. Cate, R.L., Roche, T.E. and Davis, L.C. (1980) J. Biol. Chem. **255**, 7556–7562
97. O'Connor, T.P., Roche, T.E. and Paukstellis, J.V. (1982) J. Biol. Chem. **257**, 3110–3112
98. Yang, V.-S. and Frey, P.A. (1986) Biochemistry **25**, 8173–8178
99. Roche, T.E. and Cate, R.L. (1976) Biochem. Biophys. Res. Commun. **72**, 1375–1383
100. Stepp, L.R., Bleile, D.M., McRorie, D.K., Pettit, F.H. and Reed, L.J. (1981) Biochemistry **20**, 4555–4560
101. Guest, J.R., Lewis, H.M., Graham, L.D., Packman, P.C. and Perham, R.N. (1985) J. Mol. Biol. **185**, 743–754
102. Allen, A.G., Perham, R.N., Allison, N., Miles, J.S. and Guest, J.R. (1989) J. Mol. Biol. **208**, 623–633
103. Lawson, J.E., Behal, R.H. and Reed, L.J. (1991) Biochemistry **30**, 2834–2839
104. Neagle, J.C. and Lindsay, J.G. (1991) Biochem. J. **278**, 423–427
105. Roche, T.E., Rahmatullah, M., Chang, C.L., Radke, G.A., Powers-Greenwood, S.L., Gopalakrishnan, S. and Li, L. (1991) in Biochemistry and Physiology of Thiamine Diphosphate Enzymes (Bisswanger, H. and Ulrich, H., eds.), pp. 164–169, VCH Publishers, Weinheim
106. Randle, P.J. (1986) Biochem. Soc. Trans. **14**, 799–806
107. Pettit, F.H., Pelley, J.W. and Reed, L.J. (1975) Biochem. Biophys. Res. Commun. **65**, 575–582
108. Popov, K.M., Kedishvili, N.Y., Zhao, Y., Shimomura, Y., Crabb, D.W. and Harris, R.A. (1993) J. Biol. Chem. **268**, 26602–26606
109. Popov, K.M., Kedishvili, N.Y., Zhao, Y., Guidi, R. and Harris, R.A. (1994) J. Biol. Chem. **269**, 29720–29724
110. Popov, K.M., Zhao, Y., Shimomura, Y., Kuntz, M.J. and Harris, R.A. (1992) J. Biol. Chem. **267**, 13127–13130
111. Harris, R.A. and Popov, K.M. (1996) in α-Keto Acid Dehydrogenase Complexes (Patel, M.S., Roche, T.E. and Harris, R.A., eds.), pp. 139–149, Birkhäuser Verlag, Basel
112. Bourret, R.B., Borkovich, K.A. and Simon, M.I. (1991) Annu. Rev. Biochem. **60**, 401–441
113. Stock, J.B., Ninfa, A.J. and Stock, A.M. (1989) Microbiol. Rev. **53**, 450–490
114. Chang, C., Kwok, S.F., Bleecker, A.B. and Meyerowitz, E.M. (1993) Science **262**, 539–511
115. Ota, I.M. and Alexander, A. (1993) Science **262**, 566–569
116. Radke, G.A., Ono, K., Ravindran, S. and Roche, T.E. (1993) Biochem. Biophys. Res. Commun. **190**, 982–991
117. Linn, T.C., Pelley, J.W., Pettit, F.H., Hucho, F., Randall, D.D. and Reed, L.J. (1972) Arch. Biochem. Biophys. **148**, 327–342

118. Brandt, D.R., Roche, T.E. and Pratt, M.L. (1983) Biochemistry **22**, 2958–2966
119. Reference deleted
120. Brandt, D.R. and Roche, T.E. (1983) Biochemistry **22**, 2966–2971
121. Hucho, F., Randall, D.D., Roche, T.E., Burgett, M.W., Pelley, J.W. and Reed, L.J. (1972) Arch. Biochem. Biophys. **151**, 328–340
122. Cate, R.L. and Roche, T.E. (1978) J. Biol. Chem. **253**, 496–503
123. Cate, R.L. and Roche, T.E. (1979) J. Biol. Chem. **254**, 1659–1665
124. Rahmatullah, M. and Roche, T.E. (1985) J. Biol. Chem. **260**, 10146–10152
125. Ravindran, S., Radke, G.A. and Roche, T.E. (1996) J. Biol. Chem. **271**, 653–662
126. Pratt, M.L. and Roche, T.E. (1979) J. Biol. Chem. **254**, 7191–7196
127. Pettit, F.H., Roche, T.E. and Reed, L.J. (1972) Biochem. Biophys. Res. Commun. **49**, 563–571
128. Teague, W.M., Pettit, F.H., Wu, T.-L., Silberman, S.R. and Reed, L.J. (1982) Biochemistry **21**, 5585–5592
129. Pratt, M.L., Maher, J.F. and Roche, T.E. (1982) Eur. J. Biochem. **125**, 349–355
130. Lawson, J.E., Niu, X.-D., Browning, K.S., Trong, H.L., Yan, J. and Reed, L.J. (1993) Biochemistry **32**, 8987–8993
131. Reed, L.J., Lawson, J.E., Niu, X.-D. and Yan, J. (1996) in α-Keto Acid Dehydrogenase Complexes (Patel, M.S., Roche, T.E. and Harris, R.A., eds.), pp. 131–138, Birkhäuser Verlag, Basel
132. Denton, R.M., Randle, P.J. and Martin, B.R. (1972) Biochem. J. **128**, 161–163
133. Denton, R.M. and McCormack, J.G. (1990) Annu. Rev. Physiol. **52**, 451–466
134. Thomas, A.P. and Denton, R.M. (1986) Biochem. J. **238**, 93–101
135. Denton, R.M., Midgley, P.J.W., Rutter, G.A., Thomas, A.P. and McCormack, J.G. (1989) Ann. N.Y. Acad. Sci. **573**, 285–296
136. Hansford, R.G. (1991) J. Bioenerg. Biomembr. **23**, 823–854
137. McCormack, J.G. and Denton, R.M. (1979) Biochem. J. **180**, 533–544
138. Lawlis, V.B. and Roche, T.E. (1981) Biochemistry **20**, 2512–2518
139. Lawlis, V.B. and Roche, T.E. (1981) Biochemistry **20**, 2519–2524
140. Roche, T.E. and Lawlis, V.B. (1981) Ann. N.Y. Acad. Sci. **378**, 236–249
141. Denton, R.M., Richards, D.A. and Chen, J.G. (1978) Biochem. J. **176**, 899–906
142. Larner, J., Huang, L.C., Suzuki, S., Tang, G., Zhang, C., Schwartz, C.F.W., Romero, G., Luttrell, L. and Kennington, A.S. (1989) Ann. N.Y. Acad. Sci. **573**, 297–305
143. Demuni, Z., Humphreys, J.S. and Reed, L.J. (1984) Biochem. Biophys. Res. Commun. **124**, 95–99
144. Kerbey, A.L. and Randle, P.J. (1982) Biochem. J. **206**, 103–111
145. Preistman, D.A., Mistry, S.C., Halsall, A. and Randle, P.J. (1994) Biochem. J. **300**, 659–664

8

Covalent mechanisms in multifunctional and monofunctional polypeptides: eukaryotic and prokaryotic fatty acid synthases

Stuart Smith

Children's Hospital, Oakland Research Institute, 747 Fifty-second Street, Oakland, CA 94609, U.S.A.

The reaction sequence

Fatty acids are essential components of all biological membranes and represent an important form of energy storage in plants and animals, so their biosynthesis occurs ubiquitously in living organisms. Although the enzymes involved in this pathway exist in nature in complexes of different architectural design, and the details of the substrate trafficking events differ somewhat in different types of organism, some of the characteristics of the pathway are universally conserved in all living organisms [1–4]. The key feature of the *de novo* pathway is the sequential extension of an alkanoic chain, two carbon atoms at a time, by a series of Claisen condensation reactions. The 'primer' substrate, usually an acetyl moiety, is first translocated to the active-site cysteine residue of the condensing enzyme, 3-oxoacyl synthase (EC 2.3.1.41). The two-carbon extender unit is supplied as a thioester of malonic acid, linked to the 4′-phosphopantetheine of a small acyl carrier protein (ACP) component of the fatty acid synthase (FAS) systems, so that formation of a new C–C bond is coupled with an energetically favourable decarboxylation reaction. Each condensation reaction generates a 3-oxoacyl moiety which undergoes the same three-step β-carbon reduction, catalysed by the sequential action of 3-oxoacyl reductase (EC 1.1.1.100), 3-hydroxyacyl dehydratase (EC 4.2.1.61) and enoyl reductase (EC 1.3.1.10), to give a fully saturated acyl moiety two carbon atoms longer than in the previous cycle. The newly formed saturated acyl moiety is then translocated back to the active-site cysteine of the 3-oxoacyl synthase in preparation for the next round of condensation and β-carbon processing reactions. Thus, after completion of seven cycles of elongation and reduction, the product is a saturated C_{16} acyl moiety (Fig. 1). The major differences in the

Fig. I   **Universal reaction sequence for the biosynthesis of fatty acids *de novo***

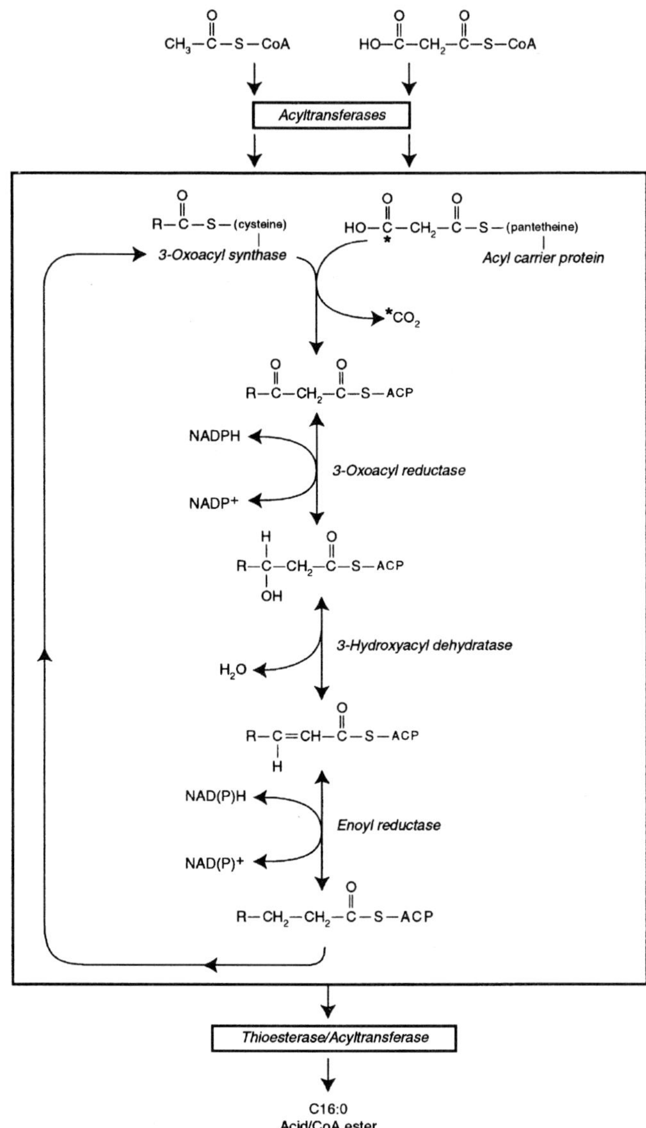

Details of the substrate-loading and product-release reactions differ in different FAS systems and are discussed separately in the text. The enoyl reductases of micro-organisms contain a bound flavin and utilize the pro-4S H of NADH [5,6], whereas those of the animal FASs lack a bound flavin and utilize the pro-4R H of NADPH [7]. An asterisk identifies the carbon atom lost as CO_2 in the condensation reaction. β-Ketoacyl ≡ 3-oxoacyl; dehydrase ≡ dehydratase.

catalytic mechanisms of the various architectural forms of FAS are in the processes utilized to direct substrates to the proper location for catalysis of the condensation reaction and in the type of chain-termination reaction employed. A detailed account of the substrate translocation events involved in the different forms of FAS is presented later in this chapter.

Depending on whether the particular type of FAS utilizes a thioesterase or acyltransferase as the chain-terminating enzyme, the palmitoyl moiety is released either as the free acid or CoA thioester and the overall reaction sequence can be summarized as shown in Scheme 1. In some prokaryotes the palmitoyl-ACP may be used directly as an acyl donor in complex lipid synthesis.

Scheme 1   **Overall reaction of fatty acid biosynthesis**

$$\text{Acetyl-CoA} + 7\text{malonyl-CoA} + 14\text{NAD(P)H} + 14\text{H}^+ \rightarrow$$
$$\text{palmitic acid} + 7\text{CO}_2 + 8\text{CoA} + 14\text{NAD(P)}^+ + 6\text{H}_2\text{O}$$
$$\text{or}$$
$$\text{palmitoyl-CoA} + 7\text{CO}_2 + 7\text{CoA} + 14\text{NAD(P)}^+ + 7\text{H}_2\text{O}$$

Subunit architecture in different forms of FAS

In most prokaryotes and in plants, the enzymes catalysing the *de novo* biosynthesis of fatty acids from malonyl-CoA exist as discrete monofunctional proteins that can be readily purified from one another; in cyanobacteria [8], phytoflagellates [9], algae [10] and plants [11] these enzymes are located in the chloroplast. However, in more advanced prokaryotes [12], fungi [13], heterotrophic dinoflagellates [14], etiolated phytoflagellates [15] and animals [2], the enzymes are integrated into multifunctional proteins that are located in the soluble cytoplasm. Two distinct architectural forms of multifunctional FASs appear to have evolved that differ both in the ordering of the catalytic domains on their constituent polypeptides and in their subunit organization (Fig. 2).

The animal FAS is a dimer of identical subunits each containing (from N- to C-terminus) a 3-oxoacyl synthase, malonyl/acetyltransferase, 3-hydroxyacyl dehydratase, enoyl reductase, 3-oxoacyl reductase, ACP and thioesterase [4]. In these FASs chain termination is catalysed by a thioesterase and results in the formation of free palmitic acid as the major product [4]. In some advanced prokaryotes, e.g. the brevibacteria, mycobacteria and corynebacteria, the FAS is a hexamer of identical subunits, each containing an acetyltransferase, enoyl reductase, 3-hydroxyacyl dehydratase,

Fig. 2   Domain organization in multifunctional FASs

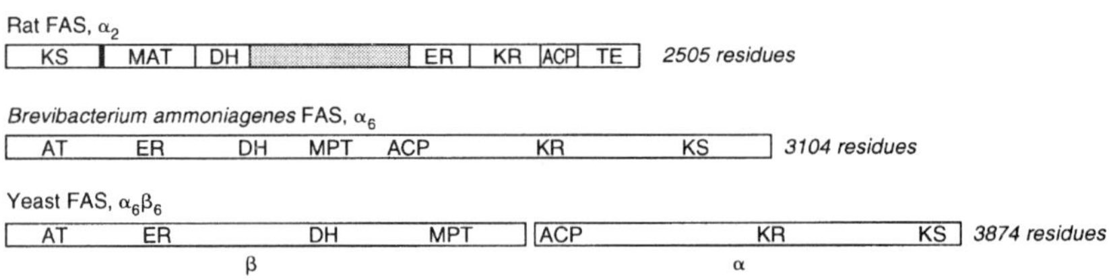

The rat FAS, which is probably typical of all animal FASs, is a homodimer of 0.54×10^6 Da [16–18]. The FAS of Brevibacterium ammoniagenes, *which is probably typical of the prokaryotic multifunctional FASs, is a homohexamer of 1.96×10^6 Da [19]. The FAS of* Saccharomyces cerevisiae, *a typical fungal FAS, contains six copies each of two non-identical subunits ($\alpha_6\beta_6$) and has a molecular mass of 2.57×10^6 Da [20,21]. The locations of interdomain boundaries and regions thought to play structural rather than catalytic roles are shown as shaded areas in the rat FAS [22]; the location of structural domains and interdomain boundaries in the hexameric FASs is uncertain. The amino acid sequences of the $\alpha_6\beta_6$ and α_6 forms of FAS are 30% identical but exhibit no statistically significant similarity with the α_2 form. Abbreviations: KS, 3-oxoacyl (ketoacyl) synthase; MAT, malonyl/acetyltransferase; DH, 3-hydroxyacyl dehydratase; ER, enoyl reductase; KR, 3-oxoacyl (ketoacyl) reductase; TE, thioesterase; AT, acetyltransferase; MPT, malonyl/palmitoyltransferase.*

malonyl/palmitoyltransferase, ACP, 3-oxoacyl reductase and 3-oxoacyl synthase [19,23]. In fungal FASs the ordering of functional domains is identical to that found in the prokaryotic multifunctional FASs except that the first four and the last three components are encoded by two separate genes: these FASs then are composed of six copies of each of the two non-identical subunits. In both the $\alpha_6\beta_6$ and α_6 forms of FAS, chain termination is catalysed by a palmitoyltransferase and the major product is therefore palmitoyl-CoA. Similarity in yeast and bacterial multifunctional FASs is also evident at the level of the amino acid sequences of the individual domains, suggesting that one type has evolved from the other by either a gene fusion or gene splitting event [19].

The multifunctional dimeric FASs

The animal FASs consist of two identical polypeptides of molecular mass 270 kDa [16]. Electron microscopic and small-angle neutron scattering studies indicate that the dimer is an ellipsoid structure containing two 'holes', one at each end of the molecule (Fig. 3A). Electron micrographic images of FAS labelled with Fab fragments derived from antibodies raised against the C-terminal thioesterase domain show two anti-thioesterase Fab fragments bound at opposite ends of the major axis of the dimers. This observation is consistent with the finding that the two subunits of the animal FAS can be cross-linked by dibromopropanone via the active-site cysteine of one subunit and the 4'-phosphopantetheine of the companion subunit [24]. Thus the two subunits of the animal FAS are oriented in an antiparallel arrangement. The stoichiometry of acyl-chain assembly has been measured directly using an enzyme preparation from which the chain-terminating enzyme has been removed by limited proteolysis. These modified FASs synthesize two long-chain-length fatty-acyl moieties per truncated dimer. Based on this evidence, the established ordering of the constituent domains in the polypeptide and

---

Fig. 3 **Organization of domains within the α_2 protomer of the animal FAS**

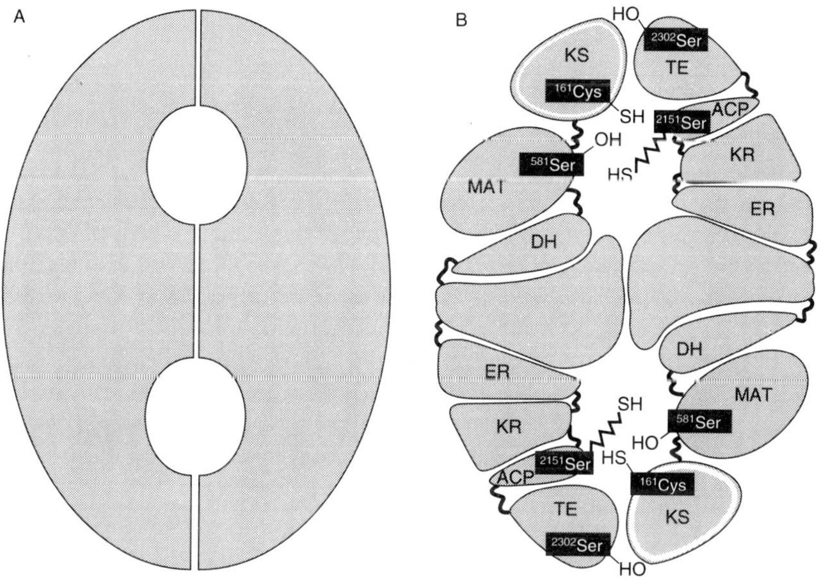

(A) Overall shape of the protein as revealed by electron micrographic evidence [25,26]. The molecule consists of two identical subunits arranged in an antiparallel configuration. Estimated dimensions are 216 Å long, 144 Å wide and 72 Å deep; the two 'holes' are approximately 40 Å in diameter. (B) Domain map based primarily on amino acid sequence data and limited proteolytic dissection experiments [4]. The N-terminal domain is identified by highlighting. Individual catalytic domains are linked covalently by loops which are exposed at the protein surface, some in the dimer, others only in the monomers, and are therefore susceptible to proteolysis [22,27]. The central core regions have no known catalytic activity and may play a structural role in stabilization of the dimer [22,25,27]. The sites of covalent attachment of the substrates and intermediates are shown: the 4'-phosphopantetheine thiol (represented by a jagged line) attached to serine-2151 in the ACP domain, the active-site serine-581 of the malonyl/acetyltransferase, the active-site cysteine-161 of the 3-oxoacyl synthase and the active-site serine-2302 of the chain-terminating thioesterase domain. A key feature of this model is that two centres for acyl chain assembly and release are formed by co-operation of three catalytic domains (KS/MAT/DH) of one subunit with four catalytic domains (ER/KR/ACP/TE) of the adjacent subunit. Abbreviations: KS, 3-oxoacyl (ketoacyl) synthase; MAT, malonyl/acetyltransferase; DH, 3-hydroxyacyl dehydratase; ER, enoyl reductase; KR, 3-oxoacyl (ketoacyl) reductase; TE, thioesterase.

the observation that only the dimer can catalyse the overall reaction of fatty acid synthesis, a model for the animal FAS has been proposed (Fig. 3B). In this model each of the two centres for acyl-chain assembly are formed by the co-operation of the 3-oxoacyl synthase, malonyl/acetyltransferase and 3-hydroxyacyl dehydratase of one subunit with the enoyl reductase, oxoacyl reductase, ACP and thioesterase of the other subunit [4].

The multifunctional hexameric FASs

The best characterized of this type of multifunctional FAS is the yeast $\alpha_6\beta_6$ complex. This FAS is composed of six copies of α and β subunits having molecular masses of 208 kDa and 220 kDa respectively [28,29]. Electron micrographic evidence suggests a somewhat baroque, barrel-like structure consisting of six disc-like α subunits arranged in a central hexagonal ring from which radiate six arch-like β subunits (Fig. 4). Although individual functional domains cannot be identified from these images, discrete globular regions can be distinguished within the β subunits. The number of discernible globular regions appears higher than the number of catalytic units present, suggesting that some of these domains may play a structural role, perhaps in stabilizing subunit interactions in the oligomer. Consistent with this idea is the observation that the polypeptides of the hexameric FASs are considerably longer than their counterparts in the α_2 FASs and contain long stretches of amino acids to which no catalytic function can be readily assigned [19]. Analysis of the electron micrographic images is hampered by the fragility of the molecules during preparation, and the tendency of molecules to 'flatten' has been attributed to the very open and flexible nature of the protein; possibly this high flexibility may be essential for proper functioning of the FAS, allowing domains of the β chains to access substrates bound to the thiol sites on the α chains.

The model for the yeast FAS derived from these studies consists of three $\alpha_2\beta_2$ protomers such that within each protomeric unit the ends of the pair of β arches interact with opposite sides of the pair of α discs. Chemical modification studies indicate that the bifunctional reagent dibromopropanone is able to cross-link the active-site cysteine of the 3-oxoacyl synthase on one α subunit with the 4'-phosphopantetheine of an adjacent α subunit, suggesting that, as in the animal α_2 FAS, adjacent head-to-tail-oriented α subunits within the protomer co-operate to form a site for the condensation reaction [32]. Since the yeast FAS terminates the chain elongation process by an acyltransferase reaction, exclusion of CoA from the assay blocks release of the product, allowing direct measurement of the number of palmitoyl moieties formed on the FAS. Results of these experiments indicate a stoichiometry of six functional centres per $\alpha_6\beta_6$ oligomer and suggest that each centre is composed of two complementary 'half α' subunits and one β subunit [33]. Thus the minimum functional unit, consisting of two α subunits and two β subunits, contains two centres for fatty acid synthesis and is consistent with the proposed $\alpha_2\beta_2$ protomeric structure of the complex. Based on these considerations and the established order of the various enzymes within the α and β subunits, a map showing the relative locations of the functional domains within the $\alpha_2\beta_2$ protomer can be constructed (Fig. 5). In this model a centre for acyl-chain synthesis is composed of the acetyltransferase, enoyl reductase, 3-hydroxyacyl dehydratase and malonyl/acetyl/palmitoyltransferase of a β subunit in co-operation with the 3-oxoacyl synthase of one α subunit and the ACP and oxoacyl reductase domains of the adjacent α subunit. The prokaryotic α_6 and eukaryotic $\alpha_6\beta_6$ FASs display similar electron micrographic images and share identical ordering of the domains in the constituent polypeptides, so it seems likely that juxtaposition of functional domains in the two oligomeric forms of FAS is essentially the same (Figs. 5B and 5C). Nevertheless, the bacterial multifunctional FASs differ from their eukaryotic counterparts in that they

---

Fig. 4   Model for the yeast FAS

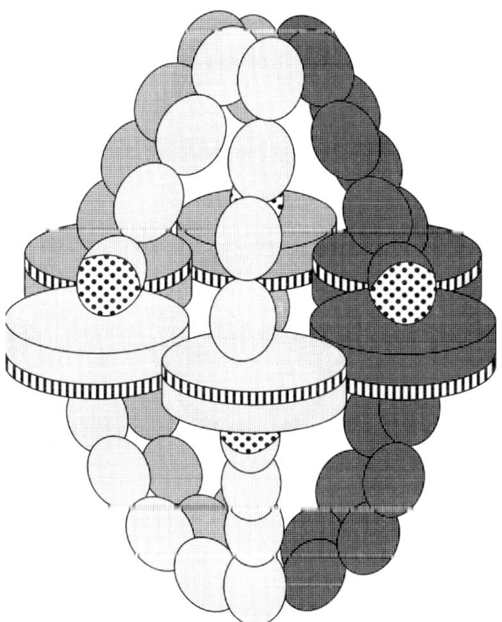

The model, based on electron microscopic evidence [30,31], is shown in side view tilted to reveal the spatial relationship between the α and β subunits. The α subunits appear as discs arranged in a central hexagonal wall such that adjacent α subunits are related by a 180° rotation about an axis normal to the ring and are connected by pairs of β subunits that form arch-like structures, one above and one below the plane of the α subunits. The diameter of the ring of α subunits is estimated to be approx. 218 Å and the overall length of the molecule approx. 247 Å. The structure exhibits threefold symmetry, i.e. $(\alpha_2\beta_2)_3$. The three $\alpha_2\beta_2$ protomers are distinguished by differential shading, the antiparallel arrangement of α subunits is indicated by striping and the orientation of the β subunits is indicated by stippling at the N-terminal end of the polypeptides. Adapted from [30,31].

are able to synthesize unsaturated as well as saturated fatty acids. This unique property of the α_6 form of FAS has been attributed to its ability to perform β,γ-dehydration of a 3-hydroxyacyl thioester intermediate and to elongate the β,γ-enoate without reduction of the double bond [34]. In this regard the bacterial multifunctional α_6 form of FAS resembles the bacterial monofunctional FAS systems which also use the same enzymes for the synthesis of saturated and unsaturated fatty acids, retaining the double bond formed at the C_{10} dehydration step by an α,β to β,γ isomerization [35]. This isomerase activity appears to be an integral part of the α_6 multifunctional FAS.

Fig. 5   **Organization of domains within the $\alpha_2\beta_2$ protomer of the yeast $\alpha_6\beta_6$ FAS and the α_2 protomer of the prokaryotic α_6 multifunctional FAS**

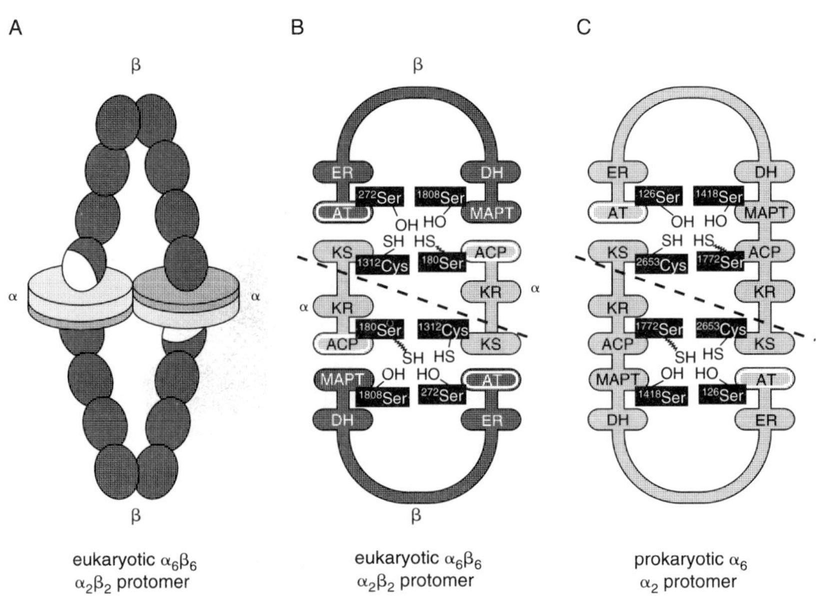

(A) Model of the yeast $\alpha_2\beta_2$ protomer based on electron micrographic evidence [30,31]. The antiparallel orientation of α subunits and the orientation of β subunits is indicated by highlighting at the N-terminal ends of the polypeptides. (B) Domain map of the yeast $\alpha_2\beta_2$ protomer based on the order of the functional elements within the α and β subunits, as determined by mutational analysis and amino acid sequencing [20,21,36]. The sites of covalent attachment of the substrates and intermediates, one 4'-phosphopantetheine thiol (represented as a jagged line), one cysteine thiol and two serine hydroxy groups are indicated. Some minor differences in the sequences determined in the Schweizer and Wakil laboratories affect the numbering of the residues, as discussed by Mohamed et al. [37]. The broken line marks the functional division of the protomer into two catalytic centres for fatty acid synthesis. (C) Domain map of the α_2 protomer of the prokaryotic FAS, based on analogy with the eukaryotic $\alpha_2\beta_2$ protomeric form [19]. Abbreviations: AT, acetyltransferase; ER, enoyl reductase; DH, 3-hydroxyacyl dehydratase; MAPT, malonyl/acetyl/palmitoyltransferase; KR, 3-oxoacyl (ketoacyl) reductase; KS, 3-oxoacyl (ketoacyl) synthase.

However, it is unclear whether a single 3-hydroxyacyl dehydratase domain is responsible for catalysis of all dehydration reactions as well as the isomerization reaction or whether a separate 3-hydroxyacyl dehydratase, in an as yet unidentified location, is responsible for catalysing the dehydration and isomerization reactions that lead to retention of the double bond.

The monofunctional FASs

Unlike the enzymes associated with multifunctional polypeptides, which make contacts only with heterologous domains, many of the individual enzymes that comprise the monofunctional FAS systems are themselves oligomers (Table 1). In general the monofunctional enzymes found in bacteria share similar structural and functional characteristics with their plant counterparts. However, the bacterial and plant systems differ in two significant aspects. First, only the bacterial systems possess the unique 3-hydroxydecanoyl dehydratase/isomerase enzyme that is utilized for the retention of the double bond introduced during *de novo* fatty acid synthesis. Secondly, whereas thioesterases clearly play an important role as chain-terminating enzymes in plants [38], their role in bacterial systems is at present unclear. Two thioesterase enzymes, termed thioesterases I and II, have been characterized in *Escherichia coli* and are included in Table 1 for the sake of completeness. However, strains containing double null mutations in the structural genes for the two thioesterases exhibit unaltered fatty acid composition and growth characteristics; additionally, unlike other lipogenic enzymes in *E. coli*, thioesterase I is located in the periplasm. It is quite possible, then, that these enzymes do not participate directly in fatty acid synthesis and their true physiological substrates remain in question. One possibility is that the enzymes are involved in the transport and metabolism of exogenously supplied fatty acids that are initially activated to CoA thioesters [39]. In this eventuality the true substrates would be acyl-CoA rather than acyl-ACP thioesters [40], and indeed both thioesterases I and II are active towards acyl-CoA thioesters *in vitro* [41,42]. In any event, the prokaryotic monofunctional FAS systems appear to differ from the monofunctional plant FASs and multifunctional animal FASs, which utilize thioesterases as chain-terminating enzymes, and from the hexameric FASs of fungi and prokaryotes, which use acyltransferases. In the prokaryotic monofunctional FAS systems the acyl-ACP species can be used directly as acyl donors for complex-lipid synthesis [43,44].

The three-dimensional structure of the *E. coli* ACP has been determined in solution from NMR measurements [60]. The principal structural feature appears to be a hydrophobic cavity formed by the juxtaposition of three long helices. The vacant 4′-phosphopantetheine prosthetic group is extended away from the protein into the solvent in a flexible conformation. However, it seems probable that a fatty-acyl chain attached to the 4′-phosphopantetheine thiol would be accommodated in the hydrophobic cavity formed by the three helices [60]. The ACP component of the multi-

Table 1   **Subunit structure of monofunctional FAS enzymes**

Enzyme	Source	Structure	Reference
ACP	E. coli	Monomer, 8.8 kDa	45
ACP	Spinach*	Monomer, 9.3 kDa	46
Acetyl-CoA:ACP transacylase	Avocado	Monomer, 18 kDa	47
Malonyl-CoA:ACP transacylase	E. coli	Monomer, 32 kDa	48
Malonyl-CoA:ACP transacylase	Spinach	Monomer, 31 kDa	49
3-Oxoacyl synthase I	E. coli	α_2, $\alpha = 39$ kDa	50
3-Oxoacyl synthase I	Barley	α_2, $\alpha = 45$ kDa	51
3-Oxoacyl synthase II	E. coli	α_2, $\alpha = 44$ kDa	50
3-Oxoacyl synthase III	Avocado	α_2, $\alpha = 37$ kDa	47
3-Oxoacyl synthase III	E. coli	Monomer†, 35 kDa	52
3-Oxoacyl reductase	Spinach	α_4, $\alpha = 24$ kDa	53
3-Oxoacyl reductase	E. coli	?, $\alpha = 25$ kDa	54
3-Hydroxyacyl dehydratase	Spinach	α_4, $\alpha = 19$ kDa	53
3-Hydroxydecanoyl dehydratase/isomerase	E. coli	α_2, $\alpha = 18.8$ kDa	55
Enoyl reductase	Spinach	α_4, $\alpha = 32$ kDa	53
Thioesterase II, medium-chain-length‡	E. coli	α_4, $\alpha = 32$ kDa	56
Thioesterase I, long-chain-length‡	E. coli	Monomer, 20 kDa	57
Thioesterase, medium-chain-length	Bay	Monomer, 34 kDa	38
Thioesterase, long-chain-length	Rapeseed	Monomer, 38 kDa	58

*Plants express different isoforms of ACP, often in a tissue-specific manner. The different isoforms, when present in the same tissue, appear to be utilized indiscriminately [59].

†J.E. Cronan, Jr., personal communication.

‡The role of the E. coli thioesterases as chain-terminating enzymes in fatty acid synthesis is in doubt (see text).

functional animal FAS is predicted to have similar secondary structure to that of the *E. coli* system and it is likely that the two types of ACP bind the various fatty-acyl intermediates in a similar manner.

Recently the three-dimensional structure of the malonyl-CoA:ACP transacylase of *E. coli* has been solved at 1.5 Å resolution [61]. The protein has an α/β type architecture, but its fold is unique. The active-site serine (residue 92) is hydrogen-bonded to a histidine (residue 201) in a fashion similar to that in the serine hydrolases. However, the oxyanion hole appears displaced such that a water molecule cannot be suitably oriented for activation and hydrolysis of the acyl-enzyme intermediate, whereas the sulphur atom of a thiol co-substrate might be expected to be ideally positioned to act as an acceptor. The malonyl transacylase of *E. coli* exhibits significant sequence similarity with the malonyl/acetyltransferase of the animal multifunctional FASs; both the serine and histidine residues implicated in the catalytic mechanism for the *E. coli* enzyme are positionally conserved in the animal FASs and have been shown to be essential for catalytic activity by site-directed mutagenesis (V.S. Rangan and S. Smith, unpublished work). Both the *E. coli* and animal enzymes are excellent transferases but poor hydrolases, and it seems likely that they employ similar mechanisms. Nevertheless the enzymes are distinguished by their substrate specificities; the animal enzyme is able to shuttle either acetyl or malonyl groups equally well but the *E. coli* enzyme is limited to malonyl transfer. Unfortunately the crystal structure does not offer an immediate explanation for the restricted specificity of the *E. coli* enzyme [60].

At this point in time no complexes between heterologous components of a monofunctional FAS system have been isolated or reconstituted and so nothing is known as to the likely molecular architecture of such complexes. Nevertheless an argument can be made, based on circumstantial evidence, that heterologous complexes may be formed in the course of the fatty acid biosynthetic reactions, and this issue is addressed later in the chapter.

Translocation of substrates and intermediates between active sites

Three types of covalent acyl-enzyme intermediates are formed during fatty-acyl chain assembly by both the monofunctional and multifunctional forms of FAS, involving the active-site serine hydroxy group of the malonyl- and/or acetyltransferase, the 4'-phosphopantetheine of the ACP and the active-site cysteine of the 3-oxoacyl synthase [2]. Some of these sites fulfil multiple roles and are used to transport the primer substrate, the chain extender substrate and the growing intermediate-chain-length acyl moieties. For these systems to function effectively it is important that the FASs are able to avoid saturating the various binding sites with substrate combinations incompatible with a successful condensation reaction. This problem has been solved in different ways in the animal α_2 and yeast $(\alpha_6\beta_6)$ multifunctional FASs and in the monofunctional FASs of plants and prokaryotes.

The multifunctional dimeric FASs

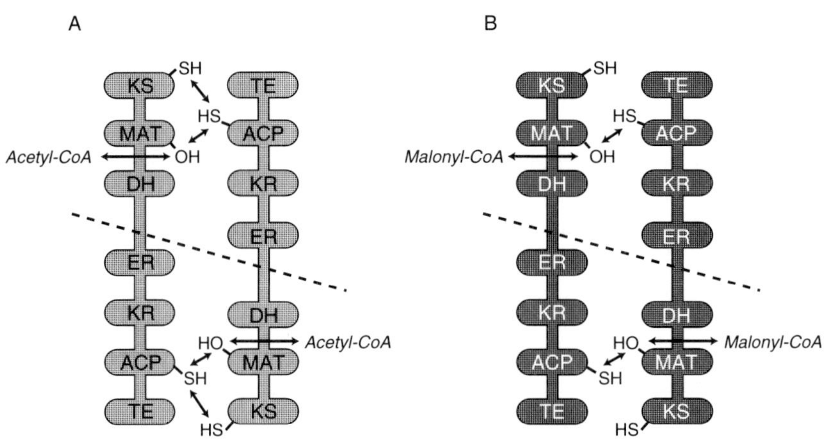

The model shows two sites for acyl-chain initiation and growth separated by the broken line. In the rat FAS the active-site serine of the malonyl/acetyltransferase is residue 581, the 4'-phosphopantetheine of the ACP domain is covalently linked to serine-2151 and the active-site cysteine of the 3-oxoacyl synthase is residue 161. (A) Loading of acetyl moieties; (B) loading of malonyl moieties. The malonyl/acetyltransferase does not discriminate between acetyl- and malonyl-CoA, and sorting for the correct pair of substrates compatible with condensation is a random process. Abbreviations: KS, 3-oxoacyl (ketoacyl) synthase; MAT, malonyl/acetyltransferase; DH, 3-hydroxyacyl dehydratase; ER, enoyl reductase; KR, 3-oxoacyl (ketoacyl) reductase; TE, thioesterase.

In this form of multifunctional FAS (Fig. 6), both acetyl and malonyl moieties initially form covalent acyl-enzyme intermediates at the same active-site serine residue (serine-581 in the rat FAS) before being transferred to the same 4'-phosphopantetheine residue (located at serine-2151 of the second subunit); the acetyl moiety alone subsequently can be transferred to the active-site cysteine residue of the 3-oxoacyl synthase (residue 161 of the first subunit) [62]. Only when an acetyl moiety has been positioned on the active-site cysteine residue and a malonyl moiety on the 4'-phosphopantetheine can the first condensation event occur. The use of common loading sites for the two substrates results in each substrate being a competitive inhibitor for the other, so that high concentrations of either malonyl-CoA or acetyl-CoA inhibit fatty acid formation [62]. Furthermore, the loading of substrates is random in the sense that either acetyl or malonyl moieties may be loaded on to the active-site serine of the FAS with the result that unproductive enzyme–substrate complexes can be formed. Thus the resting enzyme can load up to 4.4 acetyl moieties per dimer (in the absence of malonyl-CoA and NADPH) or 3.7 malonyl moieties per dimer (in the absence of acetyl-CoA and NADPH) [63]. Even when the enzyme is incubated with saturating concentrations of acetyl-CoA, all six sites per dimer are not occupied. Analysis of the location of the substrate moieties in these experiments indicates that, whereas the serine loading site and 4′-phosphopantetheine site can be almost fully occupied with either acetyl or malonyl moieties, the cysteine active site cannot approach full occupancy by acetyl moieties even when concentrations of acetyl-CoA are used that result in maximum loading of the enzyme. These results have been interpreted to indicate that the equilibrium constant for translocation of acetyl and malonyl moieties between the serine loading site and the 4′-phosphopantetheine site is close to unity and that both of these sites potentially can be saturated by either of the two substrates. Only the cysteine active site cannot be saturated, since acetyl translocation between the two thiol sites greatly favours formation of the 4′-phosphopantetheine thioester [63,64].

For acyl-chain initiation to occur, the enzyme–substrate complex malonyl-O-transferase–acetyl-S-4′-phosphopantetheine must first be formed. Only with this combination of substrates bound specifically at these sites can the subsequent translocations of the acetyl moiety to the 3-oxoacyl synthase active site and the malonyl moiety to the 4′-phosphopante-theine site occur, allowing the first condensation step to take place (see Fig. 1). For chain initiation to proceed efficiently, all potentially unproduc-tive enzyme–substrate complexes (malonyl-O-transferase–malonyl-S-4′-phosphopantetheine; acetyl-O-transferase–acetyl-S-4′-phosphopantetheine; acetyl-O-transferase–malonyl-S-4′-phosphopantetheine) must be rapidly dissociated by transfer of the acetyl or malonyl moiety back to its CoA thioester form. Since the loading reaction catalysed by the malonyl/ acetyltransferase is readily reversible, a 'self-editing' role can be assumed for this enzyme provided that free CoA is available as acceptor [65]. Paradoxic-ally then, although CoA appears in the overall equation for fatty acid synthesis on the product side (Scheme 1), it must be continually available for synthesis to proceed. This requirement for free CoA in the FAS reaction can be readily demonstrated by scavenging the CoA formed by the loading of acetyl or malonyl moieties on to the enzyme, for example using ATP:citrate lyase or phosphotransacetylase; when the scavenging system is activated, no fatty acids are formed [66]. The self-editing process occurs extremely rapidly, with catalytic-centre activities greater than 100 s^{-1}, and does not limit the rate of acyl-chain assembly provided that an appropriate concentration of free CoA is available. If the free CoA concentration becomes too high, however, the equilibrium in the translocation of substrates between CoA and enzyme-bound forms is shifted towards CoA-ester, i.e. to substrate *unloading*; under these conditions the FAS is effectively starved of substrates and fatty acid synthesis is impeded [65]. Thus CoA functions both as an activator, at low concentrations, and as an inhibitor, at high concentrations, of the overall FAS reaction.

Implicit in the proposed model for the animal α_2 FAS is the concept that the two centres for acyl-chain assembly are formed at the interface of two antiparallel arranged subunits (Figs. 3 and 6). Thus several of the substrate-transfer reactions are intersubunit events. The transfer of acetyl and malonyl moieties from the serine hydroxy group loading site to the 4′-phosphopantetheine thiol site occurs across the subunit interface. Similarly, the transfer of the acetyl moiety and all of the intermediate-chain-length saturated acyl moieties from the 4′-phosphopantetheine thiol site to the active-site cysteine of the 3-oxoacyl synthase, in preparation for the condensation reaction, are also intersubunit events. Additionally the model predicts that although reduction of the 3-oxoacyl and enoyl moieties attached to the 4′-phosphopantetheine thiol involves interaction of the ACP, 3-oxoacyl reductase and enoyl reductase domains of the same subunit, dehydration of the 3-hydroxyacyl intermediates involves co-operation between the 3-hydroxyacyl dehydratase and ACP domains of adjacent subunits. The final step in the pathway is the release of the palmitoyl moiety formed on the 4′-phosphopantetheine thiol in a reaction catalysed by the adjacent thioesterase domain on the same subunit. Although this model is entirely consistent with the earlier finding that only the dimer can catalyse the overall reaction of fatty acid synthesis, some of the evidence supporting details of the model is at present circumstantial [4]. A rigorous testing of the model is presently under way in our laboratory.

The 4′-phosphopantetheine 'swinging arm' of the multifunctional FAS has long been accepted as a key component in coupling the various partial reactions required for fatty acid synthesis. Nevertheless, data that have emerged in recent years indicate that the simple swinging-arm hypothesis alone does not adequately account for the functioning of the complex. Although the length of the phosphopantetheine arm is only 20 Å, distances between the active sites have been estimated by fluorescence energy transfer experiments to be considerably greater [67,68]; e.g. more than 40 Å between the phosphopantetheine and the active sites of the oxoacyl reductase, enoyl reductase and thioesterase domains on the same subunit. These observations indicate that a degree of domain mobility is required to accomplish coupling of the partial reactions. Each of the two 'holes' in the molecule identified in electron micrographic images may represent an open region in which occur dynamic interactions between domains that co-operate in catalysis of the overall reaction sequence. We have suggested that mobility of the catalytic domains may be facilitated, at least in part, by the presence of flexible interdomain linkers [69]. Growing evidence indicates this to be the case in other multidomain proteins, notably the pyruvate dehydrogenase complex, where some degree of conformational flexibility in the interdomain segments of the E2 polypeptide chains permits these domains to link to the different, widely separated, active sites [70]. The putative interdomain linker sequences are poorly conserved in the animal FASs [22] so it is highly unlikely that specific residues within the linker play direct roles in communicating with adjacent domains, as they do for example in tryptophan synthase [71]. The only obvious common feature is that they tend to be rich in alanine, proline and charged residues, and they are predicted to be random-coil, hydrophilic, surface loops, a conclusion supported by the observation that they are the primary targets for proteolytic attack in the folded protein [22]. Interestingly, the linkers in the E2 subunit of dihydrolipoamide acetyltransferase are also rich in alanine and proline residues, and there is strong evidence indicating that these sequences offer flexibility while retaining a degree of rigidity that may minimize the adoption of collapsed conformations by the linker, ensuring that the connected domains are held for the most part at the distance most suited for functional interaction [72].

The multifunctional hexameric FASs

Although most biochemical studies on the hexameric FASs have been performed with the yeast complex, the structural similarities between the yeast $\alpha_6\beta_6$ and prokaryotic α_6 FASs suggest that these two types of FAS employ the same catalytic mechanisms. As in the case of the animal α_2 FAS, several of the substrate-translocation events take place across the subunit interfaces (Fig. 7). There are no reports in the literature indicating that the hexameric multifunctional FASs require the presence of free CoA for the efficient initiation of acyl-chain growth, and it is unlikely that these enzyme systems employ the self-editing mechanism to facilitate loading of the correct combination of substrates at the appropriate sites [33]. Nevertheless free CoA is required as a co-substrate since the chain-terminating reaction is catalysed by a transferase rather than a thioesterase enzyme, with CoA playing the role of acceptor for the palmitoyl moiety [1]. The hexameric FASs appear to have solved the substrate-translocation problem by an entirely different strategy. First of all, these complexes utilize different transferases for loading the acetate and malonate substrates [73,74], although the on-loading of malonyl moieties and the off-loading of palmitoyl moieties are catalysed by the same enzyme [75,76]. Recent studies [77] with various active-site mutants of the yeast FAS have revealed that whereas the specificity of the acetyltransferase is limited to loading of the primer substrate, the specificity of the malonyltransferase is less restricted and this loading site can be used for the on-loading of both malonate and acetate as well as the off-loading of palmitate (Fig. 7).

A second unique feature of the yeast FAS is that, even under saturating conditions, the extent by which the complex can be either acetylated or malonated is extremely limited. Thus a maximum of 2–3 mol of malonate rather than the theoretical maximum of 12, or 6–7 mol of acetate rather than the theoretical maximum of 24, can be loaded per hexamer. Schweizer and his co-workers have termed this phenomenon a negative co-operativity and suggest that this mechanism ensures that the FAS does not become overloaded with substrate combinations that will impede the condensation process [77].

The monofunctional FASs

Although the monofunctional FAS systems found in plants and micro-organisms exhibit many similarities, they differ in that the bacterial FAS

Fig. 7   **Substrate-translocation events in the initiation of acyl-chain growth on the fungal $\alpha_6\beta_6$ FAS**

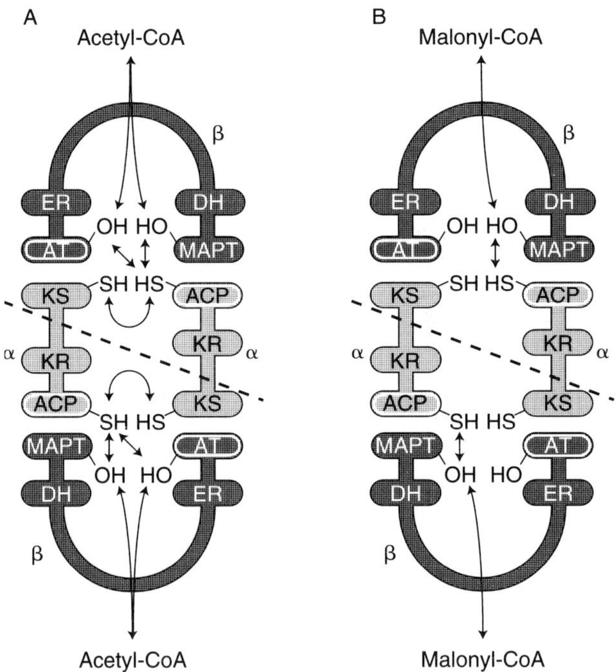

The model shows two sites for acyl-chain initiation and growth, each formed by two 'half α' subunits and two β subunits, separated by the broken line. In the yeast FAS the active-site serines of the acetyltransferase and the malonyl/acetyl/palmitoyltransferase are located at residues 272 and 1808 respectively of the β subunit; the 4'-phosphopantetheine of the ACP domain and the active-site cysteine of the 3-oxoacyl synthase domain are located at residues 180 and 1312 respectively of the α subunit [20,21,36,37]. Acetyl moieties can be loaded either via the specific acetyltransferase domain or via the domain previously named a malonyl/palmitoyltransferase. (A) Loading of acetyl moieties; (B) loading of malonyl moieties. Abbreviations: AT, acetyltransferase; ER, enoyl reductase; DH, 3-hydroxyacyl dehydratase; MAPT, malonyl/acetyl/palmitoyltransferase; KR, 3-oxoacyl (ketoacyl) reductase; KS, 3-oxoacyl (ketoacyl) synthase.

---

system serves to produce both saturated and unsaturated fatty acids [35], whereas plants have more in common with higher organisms in that they employ separate enzymes dedicated to desaturation pathways [11]. Because the bacterial FAS enzymes play this dual role, discussion of the system necessarily includes reference to the synthesis of both saturated and unsaturated fatty acids.

Based on a combination of genetic evidence, enzyme purification and inhibitor studies, it has recently been established that the monofunctional FASs of prokaryotes and plants utilize three distinct 3-oxoacyl synthases in the conversion of malonyl-CoA into long-chain-length fatty acids. One of these enzymes, 3-oxoacyl synthase I, is able to catalyse all of the condensation reactions necessary for palmitate synthesis [50]. On the other hand 3-oxoacyl synthase III, an enzyme that uniquely uses a CoA thioester (i.e. acetyl-CoA) rather than an ACP thioester as primer, appears capable of catalysing only the early condensation steps of the pathway [78] and 3-oxoacyl synthase II is most active in the final condensation reactions [50]. The 3-oxoacyl synthase III enzyme also exhibits acetyl-CoA:ACP transacylase activity and possibly could generate acetyl-ACP for use as a primer by 3-oxoacyl synthase I. However, since 3-oxoacyl synthase III can itself perform the entire first condensation step from acetyl-CoA, the significance of this transacylase activity may be of minor importance in the chain-initiation process. Reports in the earlier literature of the isolation of discrete acetyl-CoA:ACP transacylase enzymes [79,80] have recently been reinterpreted and the activity ascribed to 3-oxoacyl synthase III enzymes [81]. Nevertheless a recent publication has described the chromatographic separation of discrete 3-oxoacyl synthase III and acetyl-CoA:ACP transacylase activities, so this controversy is not yet resolved [47]. Although both 3-oxoacyl synthases I and II can also catalyse condensation reactions necessary for the biosynthesis of unsaturated fatty acids in *E. coli* [12:1(5) → 14:1(7) → 16:1(9)], it seems likely that only 3-oxoacyl synthase I is able to catalyse the first committed step, from 10:1(3) to 12:1(5), and only 3-oxoacyl synthase II is able to catalyse the final step from palmitoleoyl-ACP to *cis*-vaccenyl-ACP [16:1(9) → 18:1(11)] [82,83]. Clearly, although the three 3-oxoacyl synthases exhibit different substrate preferences, there is also some overlap in their specificities and it is not possible to implicate exclusively one enzyme for each of the condensation reactions. A scheme identifying the roles of the three 3-oxoacyl synthases in the biosynthesis of saturated and unsaturated fatty acids by *E. coli* is shown in Fig. 8.

Fatty acid synthesis in *E. coli* is directly coupled to the synthesis of phospholipids and lipopolysaccharides, so the long-chain acyl-ACPs produced by the FAS enzymes are utilized directly as substrates for the appropriate acyltransferases. Thus the non-esterified fatty acid pool in *E. coli* is normally very small and thioesterases do not appear to be obligatory enzymes in the biosynthetic pathway [84]. Two thioesterases active towards

Fig. 8 **Role of *E. coli* 3-oxoacyl synthases I, II and III in fatty acid synthesis**

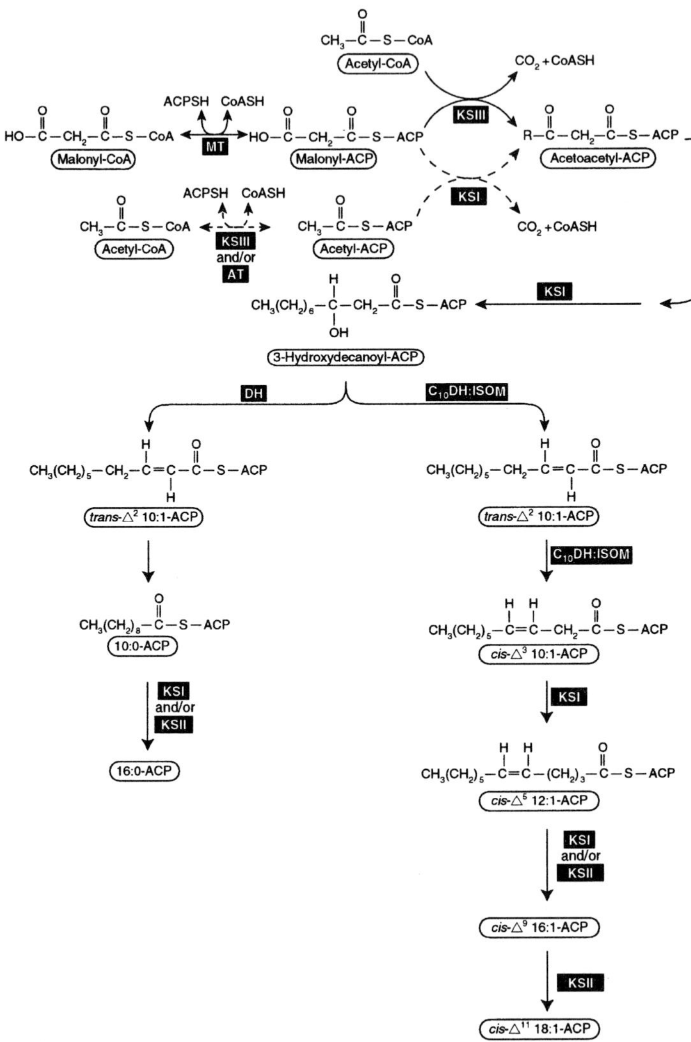

All *β-carbon atom processing reactions are catalysed by the same oxoacyl reductase, 3-hydroxyacyl dehydratase and enoyl reductase, with the exception of those at the C_{10} stage. At this branch point in the pathway the dehydration reaction can be catalysed either by the same 3-hydroxyacyl dehydratase, thus continuing down the pathway towards long-chain saturated fatty acids, or by a chain-length-specific 3-hydroxydecanoyl dehydratase/isomerase that retains the double bond, thus leading down the pathway to long-chain monounsaturated fatty acids. Subsequent β-carbon atom processing reactions are catalysed by the same enzymes in both pathways. Reactions of questionable significance are presented as broken lines (see the text for details). Abbreviations: KSI, II and III, 3-oxoacyl (ketoacyl) synthases I, II and III respectively; MT, malonyltransferase; DH, 3-hydroxyacyl dehydratase (broad chain-length specificity); $C_{10}DH$:ISOM, 3-hydroxydecanoyl-ACP dehydratase and Δ^2-trans-Δ^3-cis-isomerase.*

acyl-ACPs have been described in *E. coli* but their exact role in the pathway remains unclear [56,57]. There is strong evidence indicating that when phospholipid synthesis slows upon cessation of cell growth, long-chain acyl-ACPs accumulate, exerting a feedback inhibition on fatty acid synthesis [57,84]. This inhibition can be relieved either by overexpression of the endogenous *E. coli* thioesterases [84] or by heterologous expression of a plant acyl-ACP thioesterase [85]. These enzymes all reduce the size of the fatty-acyl-ACP pool, and it is possible that the thioesterases play a role in the regulation of lipogenesis through modulation of the fatty-acyl-ACP concentrations.

The possibility of overloading the FAS enzymes with substrate combinations incompatible with catalysis of the condensation reactions and the mechanisms devised to counter this problem was discussed earlier in the case of both the α_2 and $\alpha_6\beta_6$ multifunctional FASs. This potential difficulty is completely circumvented in the monofunctional FASs since the primer and chain-extender substrates are loaded by completely independent mechanisms involving different covalent acyl-protein species. Thus the primer acetyl moiety is loaded directly from a CoA ester to the condensation site, on the active-site cysteine of 3-oxoacyl synthase III, in a reaction catalysed by 3-oxoacyl synthase III itself, whereas the chain-extender malonyl moiety is loaded on to its condensation site on ACP via a malonyl-specific transferase.

Kinetics

The multifunctional dimeric FASs

Analysis in Hammes' laboratory of the reaction intermediates bound to the animal FAS revealed that at all stages of chain elongation the 3-oxo intermediates predominate, suggesting that the 3-oxoacyl reductase reaction is the slowest step in the overall reaction sequence [62]. This conclusion is supported by measurements of the catalytic-centre activities for the individual steps using fast reaction techniques, again in Hammes' laboratory [62]. Whereas the 3-oxoacyl synthase, 3-hydroxyacyl dehydratase and enoyl reductase have similar activities in the range 30–40 s^{-1}, the value for the 3-oxoacyl reductase is somewhat lower, approx. 17 s^{-1}. Although for technical reasons it is not possible to measure directly the catalytic-centre activity for the thioesterase (data in Table 2 were obtained using palmitoyl-CoA as a model substrate), clearly this reaction is not rate-limiting overall, since very little palmitate accumulates as an intermediate on the FAS. In fact the predominant intermediates are of short chain length, mainly as the 3-oxo and, to a lesser extent, the saturated forms, indicating that the early oxoreduction and condensation steps are slower than those for the longer-chain-length intermediates. The measured overall steady-state catalytic-centre activity for palmitate synthesis (measured as C_{16} moieties) is approx. 2 s^{-1} at 37 °C, in good agreement with the value computed from the activities of the

Table 2   Catalytic-centre activities for animal FAS enzymes

Enzyme	Catalytic-centre activity (s^{-1})
Transferase	
Acetyl-CoA → acetylserine	~ 150
Acetylserine → acetylpantetheine	< 110
Acetylpantetheine → acetylcysteine	< 43
3-Oxoacyl synthase	~ 31
3-Oxoacyl reductase	17
3-Hydroxyacyl dehydratase	> 37
Enoyl reductase	~ 37
Thioesterase	~ 35

For comparative purposes, all catalytic-centre activities are presented in terms of C_2 moieties. The value for the thioesterase is approximated using palmitoyl-CoA as a model substrate and multiplying the value by 7 to allow for the seven C_2 moieties added to the primer C_2 during biosynthesis. The kinetics of malonylation have not been examined in detail. Original data taken from Chang and Hammes [62].

individual reactions [62]. By examining the distribution of chain lengths covalently bound to the FAS during catalysis, Hammes and colleagues have assessed the possible influence of acyl chain length on the activities of the individual enzymes. The data fitted best to a kinetic model in which the rate constants for the 3-oxoacyl synthase and 3-oxoacyl reductase reactions increase by a factor of two for every two-carbon unit added to the acyl chain [62]. Several factors are collectively responsible for the overall product specificity of the pathway. First, since the condensation rates for intermediate-chain-length acyl moieties are faster than those for the early condensation steps, once chain elongation has been initiated it proceeds rapidly to long chain lengths. On the other hand, acyl moieties with 16 or more carbon atoms cannot readily be elongated, as revealed by studies with FAS from which the chain-terminating thioesterase has been removed [62,86]. Whereas saturated intermediates containing fewer than 16 carbon atoms partition predominantly to the active-site cysteine of the 3-oxoacyl synthase, those containing more than 16 carbon atoms partition predominantly to the 4′-phosphopantetheine thiol, suggesting that steric hindrance offered by these long acyl chains restricts translocation from the 4′-phosphopantetheine to the site of condensation, the active-site cysteine residue of the 3-oxoacyl synthase [62]. So, whereas intermediate-chain-length acyl moieties do not accumulate on the FAS and have little opportunity to be hydrolysed by the resident thioesterase enzyme, palmitoyl moieties once formed are not readily elongated further and therefore are more likely to dwell on the 4′-phosphopantetheine moiety where they are potential targets for the resident chain-terminating thioesterase enzyme. Finally, the thioesterase enzyme itself has a marked specificity for long-chain substrates, exhibiting a

10-fold preference for C_{16} over C_{14} straight-chain thioester substrates [87]. These various features of the FAS ensure that palmitate is normally the major product.

The multifunctional hexameric FASs

The measured overall steady-state catalytic-centre activity for fatty acid synthesis by the yeast enzyme at 25 °C is approx. 1.8 s^{-1} for each of the six catalytic centres, very similar to the value obtained for the animal α_2 complex [88]. Detailed kinetic analysis of the individual reaction steps has not been performed.

The monofunctional FASs

To date no prokaryotic or plant FAS system has been reconstituted from its purified individual monofunctional protein components. Attempts to isolate such complexes, for example by gentle gel filtration of crude extracts, have always resulted in fractionation of the FAS into discrete proteins catalysing individual reactions in the pathway; no aggregates with molecular masses greater than those of the individual oligomeric FAS enzymes have been detected [89]. Thus assessment of the overall FAS activity of these systems has not been made directly with purified enzymes, as can be done readily with the multifunctional FASs.

Unfortunately, reported measurements of the overall rate of fatty acid synthesis in *E. coli* cells *in vivo* vary considerably, possibly because of the large and variable isotope dilution effects produced by endogenous substrates. Similarly, published estimates of the rate of fatty acid biosynthesis in crude soluble extracts of *E. coli* vary widely and do not provide a reliable estimate of the catalytic potential of the *E. coli* lipogenic system. Therefore a minimum estimate of the capacity of the lipogenic system can probably best be made based on the known fatty acid content of an *E. coli* cell by assuming that these fatty acids are completely duplicated during a single generation. The calculation is as follows. On the basis of the following data: (1) a single *E. coli* cell contains 2×10^7 molecules of phospholipid (4×10^7 molecules of fatty acid) and 2×10^6 molecules of lipopolysaccharide (12×10^6 molecules of fatty acid), i.e. 5.2×10^7 molecules of total fatty acid; (2) a single *E. coli* cell contains 0.5 pg of protein; and (3) the doubling time for an *E. coli* cell is 30 min, one can calculate: rate of fatty acid synthesis $= 5.2 \times 10^7/6 \times 10^{23}$ mol of fatty acid/30 min per 0.5 pg of total protein, i.e. $(5.2 \times 10^7 \times 10^9 \times 10^9)/(6 \times 10^{23} \times 30 \times 0.5)$ nmol of fatty acid/min per mg of total protein, i.e. 5 nmol/min per mg. Thus using this approach the lipogenic capacity of *E. coli* is estimated to be approx. 5 nmol of fatty acid synthesized/min per mg of total protein.

According to the scheme in Fig. 8, of the seven condensation reactions required to form a 16-carbon fatty acid, only one is catalysed by 3-oxoacyl synthase III and at least five are catalysed by oxoacyl synthase I. Thus the calculated rate of fatty acid synthesis would require oxoacyl synthase III and oxoacyl synthase I activities of at least 5 and 25 nmol of malonate condensed/min per mg of total protein respectively. The activities of 3-oxoacyl synthases III and I in crude extracts of *E. coli* are estimated to be 8 and 58 nmol of malonate condensed/min per mg of total protein respectively, using acetyl-CoA as substrate for 3-oxoacyl synthase III and 12:0-ACP as substrate for 3-oxoacyl synthase I [50]. Thus these values appear adequate to support the calculated rate of fatty acid synthesis *in vivo*. Furthermore the apparent K_m value of 3-oxoacyl synthase III for acetyl-CoA has been estimated to be approx. 150 μM, well within the physiological concentration of $\sim$ 300 μM in *E. coli* cells. Analysis of the relative pool sizes of ACP thioester intermediates in *E. coli in vivo* indicates that during exponential growth the total ACP concentration is $\sim$ 50 μM, most of which is accounted for by approximately equal concentrations of free ACP, acetyl-ACP and malonyl-ACP [78]. Longer-chain-length acyl-ACPs are barely detectable, suggesting that the first condensation reaction is probably the rate-limiting step in the conversion of malonyl-CoA into fatty acid [78]. However, the kinetic data obtained from experiments with purified 3-oxoacyl synthase I give K_m values of the order of 20–100 μM for the substrates 12:0- and 14:0-ACP thioesters [and with purified oxoacyl synthase II, values in the range 20–220 μM for the substrates 14:0-, 12:1(5)-, 14:1(7)- and 16:1(9)-ACP] [50]. Clearly, if these kinetic parameters were operative *in vivo*, the concentrations of intermediate-chain-length saturated acyl-ACP thioesters (probably submicromolar) are not adequate to allow 3-oxoacyl synthases I and II to operate at a rate that could support the calculated rate of fatty acid synthesis. It would seem, therefore, that the conditions used *in vitro* to study the kinetic properties of 3-oxoacyl synthases, and perhaps other FAS enzymes, may not properly reflect the conditions existing *in vivo*. In particular, the enzyme concentrations employed for *in vitro* assays typically are several orders of magnitude lower than those that exist *in vivo*. For example the concentration of 3-oxoacyl synthase I used for a typical *in vitro* assay is $\sim$ 60 nM whereas the actual concentration *in vivo* is $\sim$ 50 μM. A possible explanation, then, is that *in vivo* the FAS enzymes form a 'loose' multienzyme complex that permits efficient channelling of the acyl-ACP intermediates between the various catalytic centres without mixing in the bulk cytoplasm. Since the concentration of FAS proteins in the *E. coli* cell is quite high, e.g. 50–60 μM for 3-oxoacyl synthase and ACP (J.E. Cronan, Jr., personal communication), the association constants for complex-formation need not be particularly high: low enough, perhaps, to make detection of the complex *in vitro* a difficult task.

In 1970 Van den Bosch et al. [90] grew cells of a *panD E. coli* strain in a medium containing β-[^{3}H]alanine, a precursor of the pantetheine moiety of CoA and the ACP, and by analysing the distribution of radioactivity in electron microscope autoradiographs concluded that the ACP is localized at, or just inside, the plasma membrane. This finding stimulated speculation that *in vivo* the FAS enzymes might be compartmentalized and that the cell membrane might provide an organizational matrix. Subsequently, however, the work of Jackowski et al. [91] showed that in the earlier study the apparent association of ACP with the cell membrane was probably an artifact. Employing affinity-purified rabbit anti-(*E. coli* ACP) IgG and goat anti-(rabbit IgG) antibodies conjugated to colloidal gold, these workers found that in carefully fixed cells the immunogold particles were distributed throughout the cytoplasm and were not associated with the cell membrane. Meanwhile no new experimental evidence for the existence of a compartmentalized or associated cluster of FAS enzymes in simple prokaryotes has been forthcoming. The situation is no clearer for plant FAS systems. The rate of fatty acid synthesis in isolated spinach leaf chloroplasts is estimated to be about 4.5 nmol of acetate incorporated/min per mg of stromal protein, equivalent to about 1.8 nmol/mg of total soluble cell protein, and is thought to closely approximate the rate *in vivo* [92]. Based on the assay of the individual FAS activities in extracts of various plants it would appear that the limiting enzymes in the conversion of malonyl-CoA into fatty acid are most likely the 3-oxoacyl synthases (Table 3).

Although the activities of several of the individual enzymes measured in extracts of spinach leaves appear adequate to account for the rate of fatty acid synthesis observed in intact chloroplasts, those of others, notably the oxoacyl synthases and possibly the dehydratase, are not. Examination of the *in vivo* pools of free and acylated ACP in both seed and leaves of the spinach plant revealed that approx. 55–60% of the ACP was present in the free, non-acylated form, with malonyl-ACP and acetyl-ACP each representing $\sim$ 10%, and 4:0-ACP and 6:0-ACP each $\sim$ 3% [59]. The remaining $\sim$ 25% of the ACP was fairly evenly distributed over all of the medium- and long-chain saturated intermediates 8:0–18:0, with the 16:0 and 18:0 thioesters predominating slightly. This finding contrasts with the observations that in *E. coli* cells none of the intermediates accumulates significantly [78] and suggests that in plants all of the condensation steps proceed at similar rates [59]. Since the total ACP concentration in chloroplasts is $\sim$ 4 μM [11] (the original published value of 8 μM was based on an estimated stromal volume of 36 μl/mg of chlorophyll, whereas the correct value is 66 μl/mg [94]), the steady-state levels of the intermediates 4:0–14:0 must each be no more than $\sim$ 0.1 μM. The K_m values of plant 3-oxoacyl synthases I and II for 2:0–16:0 acyl-ACPs are all in the range 5–10 μM [95], suggesting that were these kinetic parameters to hold *in vivo*, then both enzymes should be operating well below their respective V_{max}. Thus the available kinetic data for the component enzymes of both the plant and *E. coli* FAS systems cannot account for the overall rate of fatty acid synthesis estimated to occur *in vivo* unless the intermediates are restrained from diffusing away from the individual enzymes. The direct channelling of intermediates from one active centre to another would probably necessitate intimate physical association between the component FAS enzymes. The absence of any evidence for the formation of physical complexes between the ACP and the component enzymes of the

Table 3   **Enzyme activities of the FAS systems in crude extracts from plant tissues**

Enzyme	Activity (nmol/min per mg of protein)				
	Cuphea lutea	Safflower seeds	Rape seeds	Pea leaves	Spinach leaves
Malonyl-CoA:ACP transacylase	9.8	24	24	8.8	12
3-Oxoacyl-ACP synthase I	0.6	0.05	0.1	0.05	0.02
3-Oxoacyl-ACP synthase II	0.1	0.04	0.1	0.04	0.15
3-Oxoacyl-ACP synthase III*	–	–	–	–	< 2
3-Oxoacyl-ACP reductase	17	19	37	13	19
3-Hydroxyacyl-ACP dehydratase†	8.3	13	15	7.3	6.7
Enoyl-ACP reductase	37	33	42	31	32

Data are from Shimakata and Stumpf [80] except for the β-oxoacyl-ACP synthase III measurement which was reported by Clough et al. [93]. The 3-oxoacyl-ACP synthase I and II activities were assayed using as substrates decanoyl-ACP and palmitoyl-ACP respectively.
*Clough et al. [93] assayed 3-oxoacyl-ACP synthase III activity using acetyl-CoA and malonyl-ACP as substrates only after the first step in purification, so that their value probably overestimates the specific activity in the crude extract.
†Activities were measured for the back reaction; for the spinach enzyme the forward, dehydration, reaction is 5.7-fold slower [53].

monofunctional FAS systems of plants and prokaryotes, then, is perplexing, particularly in view of the finding that even in the case of the multifunctional FAS systems there exist demonstrable non-covalent interactions between component domains [27]. It is possible, perhaps, that the formation of a loosely associated FAS multienzyme complex in the bacterial cytosol or in the plant chloroplast requires the presence of an essential scaffolding component that is destroyed on disruption of the cell. Alternatively, the interaction between components of the monofunctional FAS systems may be a dynamic process in the sense that the individual enzymes are accommodated in the complex only transiently during the catalytic process. A precedent for such a mechanism has been described for the multifunctional animal FAS which can interact with a unique chain-terminating enzyme, thioesterase II from lactating mammary gland, resulting in the release of medium-chain-length fatty acids from the FAS [86,96]. Although clearly the thioesterase II enzyme must form an enzyme–substrate complex with the acyl-FAS, all attempts to isolate a physical complex between the two proteins have failed [97]. Remarkably, these target substrates of thioesterase II are the very intermediates that do not accumulate on the FAS under steady-state conditions, yet they are efficiently released from the multifunctional enzyme through the action of this transiently associated enzyme.

Concluding remarks

The multifunctional polypeptide form of molecular architecture is commonly assumed to offer unique advantages for efficient compartmentalization of complex metabolic pathways, and it has been argued that the multifunctional FAS is particularly well adapted to ensure the efficient synthesis of palmitic acid without significant accumulation and leakage of intermediates. This assumption is supported by the calculations of the overall fatty acid synthetic capacity of both the animal FAS (12 μmol of malonate condensed/min per mg of 3-oxoacyl synthase domain, calculated from the observed specific activity of purified rat FAS) and the *E. coli* FAS (1.2 μmol of malonate condensed/min per mg of 3-oxoacyl synthase I, calculated as described earlier, assuming that 3-oxoacyl synthase I constitutes 2% of the soluble protein in *E. coli*) as well as by the catalytic-centre activities for the 3-oxoacyl synthases (31 s^{-1} for the animal 3-oxoacyl synthase and 3.3 s^{-1} for *E. coli* 3-oxoacyl synthase I).

Maintenance of covalent connections between the catalytic domains of the multifunctional FASs is essential for efficient coupling of the sequential reactions since, for example, when the thioesterase domain of the animal FAS is removed by limited proteolysis its ability to catalyse the chain-terminating reaction is reduced by at least two orders of magnitude, even though the integrity of its catalytic centre is preserved [87,98]. Nevertheless it would be incorrect to conclude that a conjugated multienzyme complex is necessarily always the only way of efficiently organizing a metabolic pathway. The mammary gland thioesterase II enzyme referred to earlier is a case in point. This 29 kDa monofunctional protein, which is not an integral component of the animal FAS, can perform the chain-terminating reaction equally as well as the thioesterase resident in the conjugated multienzyme complex. Presumably the mammary gland thioesterase II exploits specific non-covalent interactions with the FAS that are unnecessary for the normal functioning of the resident chain-terminating thioesterase. Once the covalent attachment between the resident thioesterase and the FAS core is broken, this enzyme is ill-equipped to function as the chain-terminating enzyme when relying on non-covalent association with the complex. Thus the multifunctional animal FAS, together with the thioesterase II enzyme, provide examples of metabolic organization based both on structural association of components and on functional complementarity of non-conjugated components. Clearly further investigation is required to determine whether organization of the monofunctional FAS systems is purely functional, in that the kinetic properties of the component enzymes mesh suitably with those of other enzymes in the reaction sequence, or whether it has a structural component.

Finally, in considering the merits of the multifunctional polypeptide design, one should not overlook possible benefits to the host organism other than in improved catalytic efficiency. Since only one copy of each catalytic component is required for each centre of fatty acid synthesis, this design feature simplifies regulation of expression of the enzymes in the pathway, and all components are formed synchronously in the correct stoichiometry through the expression of either a single gene, as in the animal α_2 and bacterial α_6 FASs, or two genes, as in the fungal $\alpha_6\beta_6$ FAS.

I thank Drs. Charles O. Rock, Grattan Roughan, John E. Cronan Jr., James K. Stoops and Antoni R. Slabas for their helpful discussions, and Drs. Andrzej Witkowski and Raymond R. Dils for their careful reading of the manuscript. The author is supported by grant DK 16073 from the National Institutes of Health.

References

1. Lynen, F. (1980) Eur. J. Biochem. **112**, 431–442
2. Wakil, S.J. (1989) Biochemistry **28**, 4523–4530
3. Magnuson, K., Jackowski, S., Rock, C.O. and Cronan, J.E., Jr. (1993) Microbiol. Rev. **57**, 522–542
4. Smith, S. (1994) FASEB J. **8**, 1248–1259
5. Sedgwick, B. and Morris, C. (1980) J. Chem. Soc. Chem. Commun. 96–97
6. Seyama, Y., Kawaguchi, A., Okuda, S. and Yamakawa, T. (1980) J. Sci. Ind. Res. **39**, 802–808
7. Anderson, V.E. and Hammes, G.G. (1984) Biochemistry **23**, 2088–2094
8. Stapleton, S.R. and Jaworski, J.G. (1984) Biochim. Biophys. Acta **794**, 249–255

9. Worsham, L.M.S., Tucker, M.M. and Ernst-Fonberg, M.L. (1988) Biochim. Biophys. Acta **963**, 423–428

10. Hwang, S.-R. and Tabita, R.F. (1991) J. Biol. Chem. **266**, 13492–13494

11. Ohlrogge, J.B., Kuhn, D.N. and Stumpf, P.K. (1979) Proc. Natl. Acad. Sci. U.S.A. **76**, 1194–1198

12. Brindley, D.N., Matsumura, S. and Bloch, K. (1969) Nature (London) **224**, 666–669

13. Schwietz, H., Dietlein, G., Schiltz, E. and Schweizer, E. (1976) Biochim. Biophys. Acta **453**, 453–458

14. Sonnenborn, U. and Kunau, W. (1982) Biochim. Biophys. Acta **712**, 523–534

15. Siebenlist, U., Wohlgemuth, S., Finger, K. and Schweizer, E. (1991) Eur. J. Biochem. **202**, 515–519

16. Amy, C., Witkowski, A., Naggert, J., Williams, B., Randhawa, Z. and Smith, S. (1989) Proc. Natl. Acad. Sci. U.S.A. **86**, 3114–3118

17. Schweizer, M., Takabayashi, K., Laux, T., Beck, K.-F. and Schreglmann, R. (1989) Nucleic Acids Res. **17**, 567–587

18. Holzer, K.P., Liu, W. and Hammes, G.G. (1989) Proc. Natl. Acad. Sci. U.S.A. **86**, 4387–4391

19. Meurer, G., Biermann, G., Schütz, A., Harth, S. and Schweizer, E. (1992) Mol. Gen. Genet. **232**, 106–116

20. Schweizer, M., Roberts, L.M., Holtke, J., Takabayashi, K., Hollerer, E., Hoffmann, B., Muller, G., Kottig, H. and Schweizer, E. (1986) Mol. Gen. Genet. **203**, 479–486

21. Schweizer, E., Müller, G., Roberts, L.M., Schweizer, M., Rosch, J., Wiesner, P., Beck, J., Stratmann, D. and Zauner, I. (1987) Fat Sci. Technol. **89**, 570–577

22. Witkowski, A., Rangan, V.S., Randhawa, Z.I., Amy, C.M. and Smith, S. (1991) Eur. J. Biochem. **198**, 571–579

23. Seyama, Y. and Kawaguchi, A. (1987) in Pyridine Nucleotide Coenzymes: Chemical, Biochemical and Medical Aspects (Dolphin, D. and Poulson, R., eds.), pp. 381–431, Wiley, New York

24. Stoops, J.K. and Wakil, S.J. (1981) J. Biol. Chem. **256**, 5128–5133

25. Kitamoto, T., Nishigai, M., Sasaki, T. and Ikai, A. (1988) J. Mol. Biol. **203**, 183–195

26. Stoops, J.K., Wakil, S.J., Uberbacher, E.C. and Bunick, G.J. (1987) J. Biol. Chem. **262**, 10246–10251

27. Rangan, V.S., Witkowski, A. and Smith, S. (1991) J. Biol. Chem. **266**, 19180–19185

28. Schweizer, E., Werkmeister, K. and Jain, M.K. (1978) Mol. Cell. Biochem. **21**, 95–106

29. Wakil, S.J., Stoops, J.K. and Joshi, V.C. (1983) Annu. Rev. Biochem. **52**, 537–579

30. Hackenjos, W.-A. and Schramm, H.J. (1987) Biol. Chem. Hoppe-Seyler **368**, 19–36

31. Stoops, J.K., Kolodziej, S.L., Schroeter, J.P., Bretaudiere, J. and Wakil, S.J. (1992) Proc. Natl. Acad. Sci. U.S.A. **89**, 6585–6589

32. Stoops, J.K. and Wakil, S.J. (1981) J. Biol. Chem. **256**, 8364–8370

33. Singh, N., Wakil, S.J. and Stoops, J.K. (1985) Biochemistry **24**, 6598–6602

34. Kawaguchi, A. and Okuda, S. (1977) Proc. Natl. Acad. Sci. U.S.A. **74**, 3180–3183

35. Bloch, K. (1971) Enzymes 3rd Edn. **5**, 441–464

36. Chirala, S.S., Kuziora, M.A., Spector, D.M. and Wakil, S.J. (1987) J. Biol. Chem. **262**, 4231–4240

37. Mohamed, A.H., Chirala, S.S., Mody, N.H., Huang, W.-Y. and Wakil, S.J. (1988) J. Biol. Chem. **263**, 12315–12325

38. Voelker, T.A., Worrell, A.C., Anderson, L., Bleibaum, J., Fan, C., Hawkins, D.J., Radke, S.E. and Davies, H.M. (1992) Science **257**, 72–74

39. Klein, K., Steinberg, R., Frithen, B. and Overath, P. (1971) Eur. J. Biochem. **19**, 442–450

40. Ray, T.K. and Cronan, J.E., Jr. (1976) Proc. Natl. Acad. Sci. U.S.A. **73**, 4374–4378

41. Barnes, E.M., Jr., Swindell, A.C. and Wakil, S.J. (1970) J. Biol. Chem. **245**, 3122–3128

42. Barnes, E.M., Jr. and Wakil, S.J. (1968) J. Biol. Chem. **243**, 2955–2962

43. Ailhaud, G.P. and Vagelos, P.R. (1966) J. Biol. Chem. **241**, 3866–3868

44. Raetz, C.R.H. (1993) J. Bacteriol. **175**, 5745–5753

45. Vanaman, T.C., Wakil, S.J. and Hill, R.L. (1968) J. Biol. Chem. **243**, 6420–6431

46. Kuo, T.M. and Ohlrogge, J.B. (1984) Arch. Biochem. Biophys. **234**, 290–296

47. Gulliver, B.S. and Slabas, A.R. (1994) Plant Mol. Biol. **25**, 179–191

48. Ruch, F.E. and Vagelos, P.R. (1973) J. Biol. Chem. **248**, 8086–8094

49. Stapleton, S.R. and Jaworski, J.G. (1984) Biochim. Biophys. Acta **794**, 240–248

50. Garwin, J.L., Klages, A.L. and Cronan, J.E., Jr. (1980) J. Biol. Chem. **255**, 11949–11956
51. Siggaard-Andersen, M., Kauppinen, S. and Wettstein-Knowles, P.V. (1991) Proc. Natl. Acad. Sci. U.S.A. **88**, 4114–4118
52. Tsay, J.-T., Oh, W., Larson, T.J., Jackowski, S. and Rock, C.O. (1992) J. Biol. Chem. **267**, 6807–6814
53. Shimakata, T. and Stumpf, P.K. (1982) Arch. Biochem. Biophys. **218**, 77–91
54. Rawlings, M. and Cronan, J.E., Jr (1992) J. Biol. Chem. **267**, 5751–5754
55. Helmkamp, G.M., Jr. and Bloch, K. (1969) J. Biol. Chem. **243**, 6014–6022
56. Naggert, J., Narasimhan, M.L., Veaux, L.D., Cho, H., Randhawa, Z.I., Cronan, J.E., Jr., Green, B.N. and Smith, S. (1991) J. Biol. Chem. **266**, 11044–11050
57. Cho, H. and Cronan, J.E. (1993) J. Biol. Chem. **268**, 9238–9245
58. Loader, N.M., Woolner, E.M., Hellyer, A., Slabas, A.R. and Safford, R. (1993) Plant Mol. Biol. **23**, 769–778
59. Post-Beittenmiller, D., Jaworski, J.G. and Ohlrogge, J.B. (1991) J. Biol. Chem. **266**, 1858–1865
60. Holak, T.A., Nilges, M., Prestegard, J.H., Gronenborn, A.M. and Clore, G.M. (1988) Eur. J. Biochem. **175**, 9–15
61. Serre, L., Verbree, E.C., Dauter, Z., Stuitje, A.R. and Derewenda, Z.S. (1995) J. Biol. Chem. **270**, 12961–12964
62. Chang, S.I. and Hammes, G.G. (1990) Acc. Chem. Res **23**, 363–369
63. Mikkelsen, J., Smith, S., Stern, A. and Knudsen, J. (1985) Biochem. J. **230**, 435–440
64. Cognet, J.A.H. and Hammes, G.G. (1983) Biochemistry **22**, 3002–3007
65. Stern, A., Sedgwick, B. and Smith, S. (1982) J. Biol. Chem. **257**, 799–803
66. Linn, T.C., Stark, M.J. and Srere, P.A. (1980) J. Biol. Chem. **255**, 1388–1392
67. Foster, R.J., Poulose, A.J., Bonsall, R.F. and Kolattukudy, P.E. (1985) J. Biol. Chem. **260**, 2826–2831
68. Yuan, Z. and Hammes, G.G. (1986) J. Biol. Chem. **261**, 13643–13651
69. Joshi, A.K. and Smith, S. (1993) J. Biol. Chem. **268**, 22508–22513
70. Perham, R.N. (1991) Biochemistry **30**, 8501–8512
71. Yang, X.-J. and Miles, E.W. (1992) J. Biol. Chem. **267**, 7520–7528
72. Turner, S.L., Russell, G.C., Williamson, M.P. and Guest, J.R. (1992) Protein Eng. **6**, 101–108
73. Ziegenhorn, J., Niedermeier, R., Nüssler, C. and Lynen, F. (1972) Eur. J. Biochem. **30**, 285–300
74. Schweizer, E., Piccinini, F., Duba, C., Günther, S., Ritter, E. and Lynen, F. (1970) Eur. J. Biochem. **15**, 483–499
75. Ayling, J., Pirson, R. and Lynen, F. (1972) Biochemistry **11**, 526–532
76. Knobling, A., Schiffmann, D., Sickinger, H.-D. and Schweizer, E. (1975) Eur. J. Biochem. **56**, 359–367
77. Schuster, H., Rautenstrauss, B., Mittag, M., Stratmann, D. and Schweizer, E. (1995) Eur. J. Biochem. **228**, 417–424
78. Jackowski, S. and Rock, C.O. (1987) J. Biol. Chem. **262**, 7927–7931
79. Alberts, A.W., Majerus, P.W., Talamo, B. and Vagelos, P.R. (1964) Biochemistry **3**, 1563–1571
80. Shimakata, T. and Stumpf, P.K. (1983) J. Biol. Chem. **258**, 3592–3598
81. Jackowski, S., Murphy, C.M., Cronan, J.E., Jr. and Rock, C.O. (1989) J. Biol. Chem. **264**, 7624–7629
82. Cronan, J.E.J. and Rock, C. (1987) in *Escherichia coli* and *Salmonella typhimurium*: Cellular and Molecular Biology (Neidhardt, F.C., ed.), pp. 474–497, American Society for Microbiology, Washington, DC
83. Boom, T.V. and Cronan, J.E., Jr. (1989) Annu. Rev. Microbiol. **43**, 317–343
84. Jiang, P. and Cronan, J.E., Jr. (1994) J. Bacteriol. **176**, 2814–2821
85. Ohlrogge, J., Savage, L., Jaworski, J., Voelker, T. and Post-Beittenmiller, D. (1995) Arch. Biochem. Biophys. **317**, 185–190
86. Libertini, L.J. and Smith, S. (1979) Arch. Biochem. Biophys. **192**, 47–60
87. Lin, C.Y. and Smith, S. (1978) J. Biol. Chem. **253**, 1954–1963
88. Singh, N., Wakil, S.J. and Stoops, J.K. (1985) Biochem. Biophys. Res. Commun. **131**, 786–792
89. Shimakata, T. and Stumpf, P.K. (1982) Plant Physiol. **69**, 1257–1262

90. Van Den Bosch, H., Williamson, J.P. and Vagelos, P.R. (1970) Nature (London) **228**, 338–341
91. Jackowski, S., Edwards, H.H., Davis, D. and Rock, C.O. (1985) J. Bacteriol. **162**, 5–8
92. Soll, J. and Roughan, G. (1982) FEBS Lett. **146**, 189–192
93. Clough, R.C., Matthis, A.L., Barnum, S.R. and Jaworski, J.G. (1992) J. Biol. Chem. **267**, 20992–20998
94. Winter, H., Robinson, D.G. and Heldt, H.W. (1994) Planta **193**, 530–535
95. Shimakata, T. and Stumpf, P.K. (1982) Proc. Natl. Acad. Sci. U.S.A. **79**, 5808–5812
96. Libertini, L.J. and Smith, S. (1978) J. Biol. Chem. **253**, 1393–1401
97. Mikkelsen, J., Witkowski, A. and Smith, S. (1987) J. Biol. Chem. **262**, 1570–1574
98. Naggert, J., Witkowski, A., Wessa, B. and Smith, S. (1991) Biochem. J. **273**, 787–790

9

Control of metabolic flux within and between the quinate and pre-chorismate (shikimate) pathways in filamentous fungi

Heather K. Lamb, Kerry A. Wheeler and Alastair R. Hawkins*

Department of Biochemistry and Genetics, New Medical School, Catherine Cookson Building, Framlington Place, University of Newcastle upon Tyne, Newcastle upon Tyne NE2 4HH, U.K.

Introduction

The quinate utilization (*qut*) pathway in *Aspergillus nidulans* and other micro-bial eukaryotes is a dispensable alternative carbon utilization pathway that exploits quinate, which constitutes around 10% of the abundant biomass provided by leaf litter [1]. Production of the three enzymes necessary to convert quinate into protocatechuate (Table 1 and Fig. 1) is induced by the presence of quinate; however, this induction is itself subject to carbon catabolite repression [2]. Two of the intermediates in the catabolism of quinate, namely dehydroquinate (DHQ) and dehydroshikimate (DHS), are also metabolites in the pre-chorismate section of the shikimate pathway (see Fig. 1), where they are interconverted by a separate isoenzyme. In the shiki-mate pathway, DHQ and DHS are interconverted by the complex pentafunc-tional AROM enzyme which is produced constitutively at a low level [3]. The shikimate pathway is of great industrial importance as it leads to the production not only of the aromatic amino acids and *p*-aminobenzoic acid, but also of a diverse array of compounds including vitamins E and K, folic acid, ubiquinone and plastoquinone, and certain metal chelators such as enterochelin [4]. Other branches of the shikimate pathway provide inter-mediates for the synthesis of the ansamycins, which have a long aliphatic bridge of polyketide origin and a diverse array of biological properties such as antibiotic, antiviral and anticancer effects [4].

**To whom correspondence should be addressed.*

Table 1   **Genes involved in quinate catabolism and its regulation**

Locus	Mutant phenotype	Function	Size of encoded protein		Comments
			Amino acids	Mass (kDa)	
qutA	Recessive loss of induction of all three enzymes	Activator	825	90.432	QUTA protein has a zinc binuclear cluster and is related to the two N-terminal domains of the AROM protein
qutR	Recessive constitutive production of all three enzymes; dominant or semi-dominant loss of induction for all three enzymes	Repressor	929	103.601	QUTR protein sequence is related to the three C-terminal domains of the AROM protein
qutB	Recessive loss of quinate dehydrogenase	Codes for quinate dehydrogenase	329	36.093	
qutC	Recessive loss of DHS dehydratase	Codes for DHS dehydratase	348	39.096	
qutD	Recessive loss of induction of all three enzymes	Codes for quinate permease	533	59.484	Protein has several membrane-spanning hydrophobic motifs; mutant phenotype is pH-reparable; gene has two putative introns
qutE	Recessive loss of 3-dehydroquinase	Codes for 3-dehydroquinase	153	16.519	
qutG	Not determined	Unknown, possibly a phosphatase	330	36.796	Protein sequence highly similar to bovine *myo*-inositol monophosphatase; gene has four putative introns
qutH	Not determined	Unknown, possibly a DNA-binding protein	378	41.109	Protein sequence has a zinc binuclear cluster motif; gene has one putative intron

Fig. 1 Genes, enzymes and metabolites comprising the quinate and pre-chorismate (shikimate) pathways in *A. nidulans*

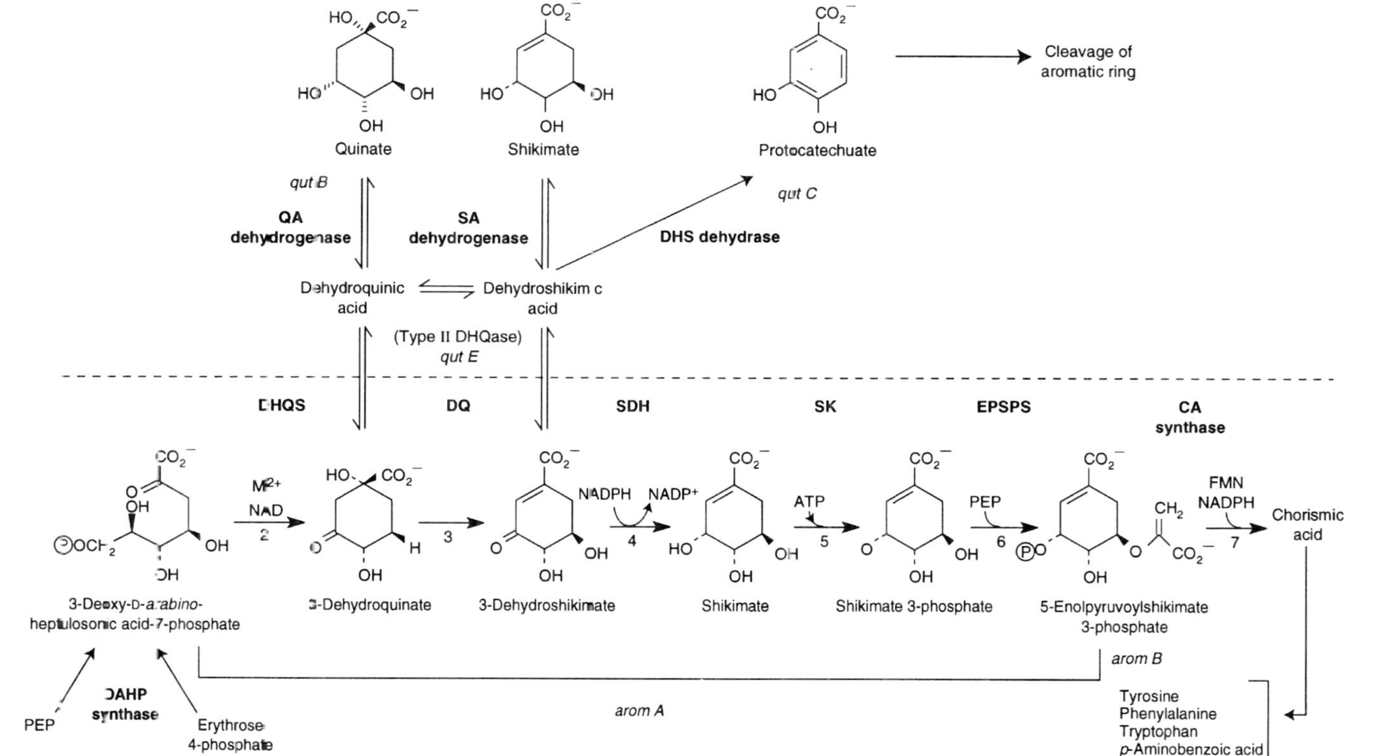

The AROM protein catalyses steps 2–6 in the pre-chorismate section of the shikimate pathway, converting 3-deoxy-D-arabino-heptulosonate 7-phosphate into 5-enolpyruvylshikimate 3-phosphate. The individual enzymes are: DHQ synthase (EC 4.6.1.3), 3-dehydroquinase (EC 4.2.1.10; DHQase), shikimate dehydrogenase (EC 1.1.1.25), shikimate kinase (EC 2.7.1.71; SA kinase) and 5-enolpyruvylshikimate-3-phosphate synthase (EC 2.5.1.19; EPSP synthase). The initial step in the shikimate pathway is catalysed by 3-deoxy-D-arabino-heptulosonate-7-phosphate synthase (EC 4.1.2.15; DAHP synthase); the final step in the pre-chorismate section is catalysed by chorismate synthase (EC 4.6.1.4; CA synthase). Abbreviations used: DHQS, DHQ synthase; DQ, type-1 DHQase; SDH, shikimate dehydrogenase; SK, SA kinase; EPSPS, EPSP synthase; PEP, phosphoenopyruvate. Reprinted with permission from [31].

Genetical and biochemical historical overview

The original dissection of the *qut* and shikimate pathways was pioneered by Case and Giles [5], starting in the 1960s, using *Neurospora crassa*. Initial genetic evidence identified four linked genes, one for each of the three *qut* pathway enzymes (designated *qa* in *N. crassa*) and one interpreted to encode a control protein that could be split into two distinct regulatory domains [6]. Not surprisingly, these early genetic data were interpreted within a framework provided by prokaryotic operon model systems, an interpretation strengthened by parallel studies on the pre-chorismate section of the shikimate pathway [7]. Mutants singly lacking the enzymes necessary for the synthesis of chorismate from 3-deoxy-D-*arabino*-heptulosonic acid 7-phosphate were identified; however, this analysis showed that one class, that lacking the ability to convert DHQ into DHS, was missing [8–10]. This missing class (lacking dehydroquinase) was interpreted in terms of the equivalent *qut* pathway isoenzyme being able to substitute in the shikimate pathway, causing the corresponding shikimate pathway mutants to elude the mutant screening procedure [11,12]. This interpretation was borne out when the missing shikimate pathway mutant (lacking dehydroquinase) was isolated in a mutant strain unable to synthesize all three quinate pathway enzymes.

When the mutation causing the loss of the shikimate pathway dehydroquinase was placed in a genetic background that was wild type with respect to the quinate pathway, it proved to have interesting properties. Such strains, in addition to being auxotrophic for the aromatic amino acids, also produced the quinate pathway enzymes constitutively, even in the absence of exogenously supplied quinate [13]. This constitutive production of the quinate pathway enzymes was attributed to the presumed internal accumulation of DHQ generated by the shikimate pathway, and provided the first *in vivo* evidence that the pools of DHQ and DHS produced by the quinate and shikimate pathways were not kept entirely separate, at least in these mutant strains [7,13]. Genetic analysis of the shikimate pathway mutants (designated *arom*) showed that the mutants lacking steps 2–6 in the shikimate pathway (see Fig. 1) were tightly linked, forming a 'cluster gene' [8,9,14].

Contemporary efforts to purify and characterize the AROM enzyme complex encoded by this cluster gene originally led to the proposal that the complex consisted of at least four separate polypeptides [15]. Later work carried out in the group led by Coggins showed that the AROM complex consisted of a dimer of identical subunits and that the former multipolypeptide model was an artefact caused by proteolysis during purification [16,17].

The observation that in wild-type strains the presence of shikimate-pathway-derived DHQ and DHS does not lead to internal induction of the *qut* pathway enzymes, taken in conjunction with the finding that the AROM enzyme consisted of two identical pentafunctional polypeptides, led to a channelling hypothesis. This hypothesis proposed that the AROM complex served as an efficient channelling mechanism to keep shikimate-pathway-derived DHQ and DHS separate from the quinate pathway [7]. The facts (a) that mutant AROM complex lacking the dehydroquinase activity leaks DHQ, and (b) that all five enzyme activities could be separately assayed *in vitro* using purified protein showed that, at least under these conditions, any channelling function could not be complete. It was, however, possible to propose the facile argument that any leakage of substrate/product off or on to the AROM protein was caused by either the nature of the dehydroquinase mutation or some non-characterized change caused by the purification protocol with wild-type protein.

It was later shown that one group was working with preparations of the *N. crassa* AROM protein that were subject to proteolytic degradation and were significantly deficient in zinc atoms, which are essential for the DHQ synthase activity of the AROM complex [18,19]. This same group promoted the channelling hypothesis of the AROM protein and in addition ascribed functions such as catalytic facilitation and co-ordinate activation [20–22]. These views were subsequently challenged by others who could find no *in vitro* evidence for a channelling function [23,24]. At this point, a more *in vivo* based approach to the whole question of metabolic flux and channelling was taken with work on *Aspergillus nidulans*.

Structural relationships between the proteins comprising the quinate and shikimate pathways in *A. nidulans* and prokaryotes

As will become apparent in succeeding sections, to fully appreciate the consequences of cross-pathway flux, it is necessary to have an overview of the structure and origins of the proteins involved in the two pathways. An extensive genetic analysis (Table 1) has identified a cluster of six genes involved in the catabolism of quinate and its regulation in wild-type strains. Three of the genes encode the necessary enzymes, one encodes a quinate permease, one a transcription activator protein and one a repressor protein. The complete *qut* gene cluster and the *aromA* gene (encoding the AROM protein) have been isolated by molecular cloning and the nucleotide sequences determined [3,25–30]. This exercise identified two new *qut* genes that had not been revealed by the mutational analysis [26,30].

Comparisons of all the deduced amino acid sequences with those of the monofunctional enzymes of the shikimate pathway in prokaryotes have revealed a long and complex evolutionary relationship between the two pathways (Fig. 2). In essence, the five genes encoding the monofunctional prokaryotic shikimate pathway enzymes have apparently become fused in the microbial eukaryote lineage to form a single large gene (for a review see [31]). Incidentally, it is also important to note that the order of the enzyme activities in the AROM protein deduced by sequence alignments matched the order deduced genetically by Case and Giles [9]. It is also evident that dehydroquinase activity has evolved independently in two separate lineages, forming type I and II dehydroquinases [32]. These enzymes bear no sequence similarity, have different reaction mechanisms and abstract water from DHQ with opposite stereochemistries [33–35]. *A. nidulans* utilizes a type I dehydroquinase as part of the AROM complex and a type II enzyme as part of the quinate pathway [31].

A further major surprise emerging from this comparison is that the proteins comprising the two pathways are made up from a small number of core modules that have become re-arranged and co-opted to new functions [31]. Indeed, almost certainly in keeping with its dispensable nature, the *qut* pathway proteins are almost all derived from modules present in the shikimate pathway, with the quinate permease almost certainly evolving from a

---

Fig. 2   **Modular structure of the enzymes and regulatory proteins comprising the quinate and pre-chorismate (shikimate) pathways in *A. nidulans***

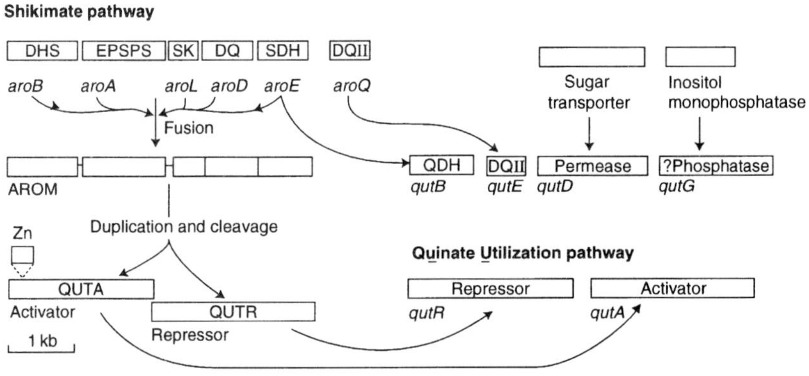

The boxes denoted *aro* designate genes from bacteria encoding monofunctional shikimate pathway enzymes: aroA, E. coli *5-enolpyruvylshikimate-3-phosphate synthase (EPSPS)*; aroB, E. coli *DHQ synthase (DHS)*; aroD, E. coli *type I 3-dehydroquinase (DQ)*; aroE, E. coli *shikimate dehydrogenase (SDH)*; aroL, E. coli *shikimate kinase (SK)*; aroQ, M. tuberculosis *type II 3-dehydroquinase (DQII)*. AROM designates the modular structure of the AROM protein of A. nidulans *which is specified by the* aromA *gene that arose by the fusion of the bacterial* aroA, aroB, aroD, aroE *and* aroL *genes. The boxes denoting the genes of the* qut *pathway are:* qutA, *activator;* qutB, *quinate/shikimate dehydrogenase (QDH);* qutD, *permease;* qutE, *type II 3-dehydroquinase (DQII);* qutG, *possibly a phosphatase;* qutR, *repressor. The genes encoding the quinate pathway activator and repressor proteins are proposed to have arisen by duplication of the* aromA *gene followed by cleavage in the DNA sequence specifying the C-terminus of the EPSPS domain (*aroA *equivalent). The* aromA *sequence encoding the DHQ synthase domain in the duplicated copy is proposed to have undergone an event in which the DNA sequence encoding a preformed zinc binuclear cluster motif (designated Zn) has become inserted into its N-terminus. The box denoted* aroQ *designates the type II 3-dehydroquinase from* Mycobacterium tuberculosis. *The arrows between boxes are there to indicate that genes denoted by the boxes are related to one another. We use* A. nidulans, E. coli *and* M. tuberculosis *to give specific examples, as the homologies between the various genes are evident across a wide range of species. Reprinted with permission from [31].*

---

sugar transporter [31,36]. The most extreme example of this sequential re-use and modification of a core modular design is represented by the quinate pathway transcription activator and repressor proteins, which are apparently homologous with the pentadomain AROM protein [28,37]. In this instance the repressor protein, which is homologous with the three C-terminal AROM domains, is proposed to have lost all enzyme activity towards its former substrates, which now apparently act as inducers of transcription [28,38].

Domain structure and function within the A. *nidulans* AROM protein

Domain structure and function within the A. *nidulans* AROM protein has been probed by expression studies in *Escherichia coli* shikimate pathway mutants (*aro⁻*) and by characterization of overproduced A. *nidulans* protein purified from *E. coli* [39]. Domain boundaries and the positions of possible linker regions between domains have been delineated by comparing the deduced amino acid sequence of the AROM protein with that of the five monofunctional non-aggregated prokaryotic shikimate pathway enzymes [40–44]. All possible linear combinations of mono-, bi-, tri- and penta-domain AROM protein have been overproduced in *E. coli* by placing the corresponding *aromA* sequences under the control of high-level promoters in commercially available *E. coli* expression plasmids. Of the overproduced AROM-derived proteins generated in this way only the N-terminal DHQ synthase domain and the 3-dehydroquinase domain are substantially soluble in *E. coli*. The DHQ synthase domain has been purified in bulk and shown to be an effective enzyme [45,46]. This domain has also been successfully crystallized and is currently the only DHQ synthase to produce crystals suitable for X-ray diffraction (K. Brown, J.D. Moore and A.R. Hawkins, unpublished work).

The AROM dehydroquinase has been purified as a monofunctional enzyme and as a bidomain fusion protein with the glutathione S transferase of *Schistosoma japonicum* attached to its N-terminus. The purified dehydroquinase domain has been shown to be monomeric but is in other respects a typical type I enzyme. The isolated dehydroquinase domain, in contrast to the N-terminal DHQ synthase domain, is a very poor enzyme with a greatly increased K_m/k_{cat} ratio compared with the native N. *crassa* AROM enzyme [47,48]. The remaining AROM domains are much less soluble; however, their characteristics and interactions have been probed by a very sensitive *in vivo* complementation assay. In this assay *aromA*-derived sequences are placed under the control of a prokaryotic promoter and expressed in *aro⁻* mutant *E. coli* strains (strains auxotrophic for the aromatic amino acids), with production of enzymically active protein being detected by the ability of the transformed *E. coli* strains to grow on minimal medium in the absence of aromatic amino acid supplementation [39,47].

Using this complementation assay, the penultimate N-terminal domain, 5-enolpyruvylshikimate-3-phosphate synthase, has been shown to be inactive as a monofunctional domain, but apparently is fully active when covalently attached to the N-terminal DHQ synthase domain. Covalent attachment of the two domains appears to be essential, as concomitant production of the two domains from two separate plasmids in the same cell does not stabilize the 5-enolpyruvylshikimate-3-phosphate synthase activity [49]. This stabilizing effect therefore appears to be specific and may possibly be due to interactions during the correct folding of the 5-enolpyruvylshikimate-3-phosphate synthase domain. Additionally, studies in which the three C-terminal domains of the AROM protein have been overproduced in *A. nidulans* have shown that the AROM protein can be divided into approximately two equal halves which can function independently of one another [49]. The picture that is emerging from these ongoing studies is that individual domains making up the AROM protein, with the exception of the N-terminal DHQ synthase domain, interact with one another at a gross structural level to stabilize and maximize enzyme activity.

Is the *A. nidulans* **AROM** protein leaky *in vivo*?

In order to address this question, the principles of Metabolic Control Analysis, in the form of *in vivo* modulation of enzyme activity in *A. nidulans*, have been applied in a set of reciprocal experiments. The early *in vivo* studies with the *N. crassa* AROM protein demonstrated that DHQ could leak from the AROM protein complex. The protein used was mutant (lacking dehydroquinase activity); therefore it was possible that the leak was a consequence of the mutation and that wild-type AROM protein may not leak DHQ at all.

In order to address this question a *qutE*⁻ mutant (lacking the *qut* pathway type II dehydroquinase and therefore unable to grow with quinate as sole carbon source) was transformed with the *aromA* gene under its native promoter. Transformants were selected by growth in minimal medium with quinate as sole carbon source, and biochemical analysis showed that they had elevated levels of the AROM protein in the range 2–5-fold over the wild-type value. These transformants grew poorly with quinate as carbon source and the simplest explanation for their growth characteristics is that *qut* pathway DHQ is taken up by the excess AROM protein, converted into DHS and released, thereby sidestepping the mutational block caused by the *qutE*⁻ mutation [50]. In a reciprocal experiment, an *aromA*⁻ mutant strain of *A. nidulans* (thereby unable to grow in minimal medium in the absence of aromatic amino acid supplementation) was transformed with the *aromA* gene under its own promoter and transformants selected by growth in minimal medium lacking aromatic amino acid supplementation. This experiment was repeated; however, in the second case the *aromA* gene had its native promoter replaced by a quinate-responsive *qut* promoter, placing its expression under the control of the QUTA activator protein. In these two cases, the range of overproduction of the AROM protein was much greater, with levels up to 30-fold over the wild-type level [50].

As expected, the overproduction of AROM protein in strains with the *aromA* gene under the control of the *qut* promoter was dependent on the presence of quinate. The copy number of the integrated transforming DNA was correlated with elevated specific activity of the AROM protein; however, transformants showed a striking response to the presence of quinate in the minimal medium. Transformants of both types (native or *qut* promoter for the transforming *aromA* DNA) containing AROM protein at levels 15–25-fold greater than in the wild type were unable to utilize quinate as sole carbon source. Further experiments with mixed carbon sources demonstrated that the inability to grow was not due to starvation for carbon due to reduced flux through the quinate pathway. The explanation for the inability of these transformants to grow in the presence of quinate was that the presence of quinate was toxic. The toxic effect is presumably because diversion of quinate-pathway-derived DHQ by the elevated levels of AROM protein caused an increase in shikimate pathway flux which led to toxic levels being produced of one or more shikimate pathway intermediates [50].

The toxicity hypothesis was tested in two ways. (1) If left for approx. 4 days, some AROM-overproducing strains were eventually able to produce sectors of vigorously growing mycelium. Upon purification, these sectors were found to have a reduced copy number of the transforming *aromA* DNA and a concomitant reduction in the level of the AROM protein. (2) AROM-overproducing transformants utilizing the *qut* promoter showed the quinate toxicity effect in mixed carbon sources with non-catabolite-repressing sources such as glycerol, but the effect was increasingly lessened with increasing concentrations of catabolite-repressing carbon sources such as glucose. The latter effect is most simply explained by the sensitivity to carbon catabolite repression displayed by the *qut* promoters [50].

Taken as a whole, these data demonstrate that wild-type AROM protein is leaky *in vivo* and that it is possible to shunt quinate-pathway-derived metabolites within and between the quinate and shikimate pathways by manipulating the *in vivo* concentration of the AROM protein. In order to further probe the *in vivo* accessibility of shikimate-pathway-derived DHQ and DHS to the quinate pathway enzymes, a series of reciprocal experiments was undertaken in which the *qut* pathway dehydroshikimate dehydratase enzyme concentration was modulated *in vivo* [51]. The basic question being addressed by this second series of experiments was: can the DHS dehydratase enzyme (which is at the bifurcation point between the quinate and shikimate pathways) divert flux of shikimate-pathway-derived DHS into the quinate pathway? (see Fig. 1). In order for this second series of experiments to be carried out, a triple mutant strain of *A. nidulans* was constructed. The strain had to carry the *qutR*^{c} mutation to allow the constitutive production of the three quinate pathway enzymes in the absence of exogenously added quinate. In addition the strain carried the *pyr-G* mutation, which allows for the selection of transformants able to grow in minimal medium without supplementation with uracil when transformed with plasmid DNA containing the *N. crassa pyr-4* gene as a selectable marker. Thirdly the recipient strain carried the *pcaE*$^-$ mutation, thereby lacking protocatechuic acid (PCA) oxygenase, and was consequently unable to grow with quinate as sole carbon source [51,52]. Mutant strains carrying the *pcaE*$^-$ mutation, if pre-grown with glucose as carbon source, are able to catabolize quinate to PCA which then subsequently leaks from the mycelium into the surrounding growth medium.

Preliminary experiments established that the PCA produced in this way could be accurately measured in liquid culture filtrates and that its rate of production was linear over a 24 h period. This allowed the rate of formation of extracellular PCA to be measured as a function of the *in vivo* flux in the quinate and shikimate pathways. Using this methodology, flux through the *qut* pathway was estimated to be 1.9 mM·h^{-1}·g of mycelium^{-1} and flux through the shikimate pathway to be 60 μM·h^{-1}·g of mycelium^{-1} [51]. The *qutC* gene (encoding DHS dehydratase) was subcloned into a plasmid containing the *pyr-4* selectable marker and used to transform the triple-mutant *A. nidulans* strain selecting for uracil-independence on minimal medium. A random sample of transformants was then purified and the specific activity of the DHS dehydratase enzyme determined in cell-free extracts. Transformants showing levels of DHS dehydratase 0.5–30-fold greater than the wild-type value were then selected to form the basis of the flux experiments. Mycelium was grown from conidiospores for 18 h using glucose as the carbon source, harvested, transferred to fresh medium lacking essential vitamins (thereby stopping mycelial growth), and the accumulation of PCA in the culture medium measured over a 12 h period. At this point the mycelium was re-harvested and the specific activity of the DHS dehydratase enzyme determined in cell-free extracts.

Fig. 3 shows the rate of production of PCA as a function of DHS dehydratase specific activity. For values up to 10-fold higher than wild type, an *n*-fold increase in DHS dehydratase concentration led to an *n*-fold increase in the rate of production of PCA [51]. In these experiments there was no exogenously supplied quinate, and the DHS dehydratase enzyme was produced constitutively due to the presence of the *qutR*^{c} mutation. Any PCA production under these conditions must therefore result from the quinate pathway DHS dehydratase diverting flux from the shikimate pathway, in the form of DHS from the AROM protein. These experiments show, therefore, that the wild-type AROM protein is extremely leaky *in vivo* and that under the conditions discussed here DHS dehydratase (up to 10-fold greater than wild type) has a shikimate pathway deviation control coefficient of -1 [51].

Fig. 3   **Rate of PCA production as a function of dehydroshikimate dehydratase concentration**

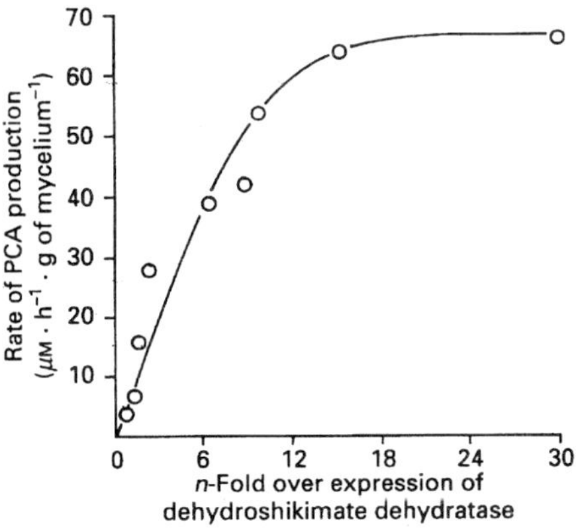

The rate of PCA production is shown as a function of the increase in dehydroshikimate dehydratase levels relative to wild type. Reprinted with permission from [51].

Control of flux within the quinate pathway

Empirical observations from as long ago as 1990 showed that, if the *in vivo* concentration of the *qutE*-encoded type II dehydroquinase was increased in an otherwise wild-type strain of *A. nidulans*, the minimal growth medium turned pink when the mycelium was grown with quinate as the carbon source [53]. The pink coloration was proposed to be due to the accumulation of PCA within the culture filtrate which subsequently formed a highly coloured complex with iron present in the essential salts component of the medium.

In retrospect, these observations were interpreted to indicate that the *qutE*-encoded dehydroquinase exerted a high degree of control over flux through the quinate pathway. As the *A. nidulans* strain used had a wild-type PCA oxygenase enzyme, it is reasonable to suggest that the secretion of PCA into the medium was due to increased flux through the pathway. If this suggestion is valid, it implies that in the wild-type strain DHS dehydratase has a lower flux control coefficient than the dehydroquinase. At the normal growth pH for *A. nidulans* (pH 6.5), quinate enters the mycelium with the aid of a specific permease; however, at lower pH ($\sim$ 3.5) significant amounts of quinate are protonated and enter the mycelium unaided. Previous reports had indicated that permeases exert a high degree of control over pathway flux [54]. A thorough investigation of the control of flux through the quinate pathway was undertaken utilizing the principles of Metabolic Control Analysis. The quinate pathway is a relatively simple three-step pathway that has a rate of relative flux approx. 30-fold higher than the shikimate pathway with which it shares the metabolites DHQ and DHS. This disparity in the relative rates of flux therefore allows the quinate pathway to be considered in isolation, even though under the special conditions discussed in the previous section the shikimate pathway DHQ and DHS is available to the quinate pathway enzymes [51].

The overall plan of the investigation was to empirically determine the flux control coefficients of the *qutB*-encoded quinate dehydrogenase (the first step) and the *qutE*-encoded type II dehydroquinase (the central step), and use the summation theorem to estimate the flux control coefficient of DHS dehydratase.

This calculation, however, would give a combined flux control coefficient for DHS dehydratase and quinate permease as, using the standard conditions under which we grow *A. nidulans*, a functional quinate permease is essential for growth. In order to gain some measure of the flux control coefficients for the permease and DHS dehydratase individually, a second strategy, that of determining the elasticity coefficients for the three quinate pathway enzymes with respect to their substrates and products, was pursued. The purpose behind this second strategy was to use the elasticity coefficients in conjunction with the connectivity theorem and the empirically determined value for the flux control coefficient of the dehydroquinase to estimate the flux control coefficient of DHS dehydratase.

Interpretation of the values estimated from these calculations is problematic, however, as in order for them to be valid, the *in vitro* values for the elasticity coefficients should be an accurate reflection of the *in vivo* values. The problems associated with relating the *in vitro* measurements of elasticity coefficients to their *in vivo* values and their use in calculating flux control coefficients has been comprehensively discussed [56]. It is of value to note that in at least one case elasticity coefficients have been measured *in vitro* and *in vivo* and been found to be in broad agreement, with the values determined making similar predictions about how enzymes in a pathway are likely to respond to changing metabolite concentrations [57].

In order to fully characterize the elasticity coefficients of all of the quinate pathway enzymes, the coding regions of all three enzyme-encoding genes were subcloned into commercially available *E. coli* plasmids, placing them under the control of high-level promoters. Overexpression and high-level overproduction of all three enzymes in *E. coli* was achieved and the three proteins were purified by combinations of ammonium sulphate fractionation, affinity chromatography and FPLC [48,55]. The substrate and product activation and inhibition profiles for the three enzymes were then determined empirically using purified proteins (see later: note added in proof).

The *qutE* gene was subcloned into an *A. nidulans* expression plasmid containing the *pyr-4* selectable marker and used to transform a quadruple mutant strain containing the *qutR*^{c}, *pyr-G*$^-$, *pcaE*$^-$ and *qutE*$^-$ mutations. Transformants were selected on the basis of uracil-independence using glucose as the carbon source, and transformants with type II dehydroquinase specific activities in the range 0.2–18-fold over the wild-type value were identified by assay of cell-free extracts. Transformants pre-grown with glucose as carbon source were transferred to fresh medium containing quinate as sole carbon source and the rate of PCA production was measured as a function of the dehydroquinase specific activity (see Note added in proof). The relationship between quinate pathway flux and dehydroquinase

---

Fig. 4   **Flux control coefficient of 3-dehydroquinase in growth medium at pH 6.5**

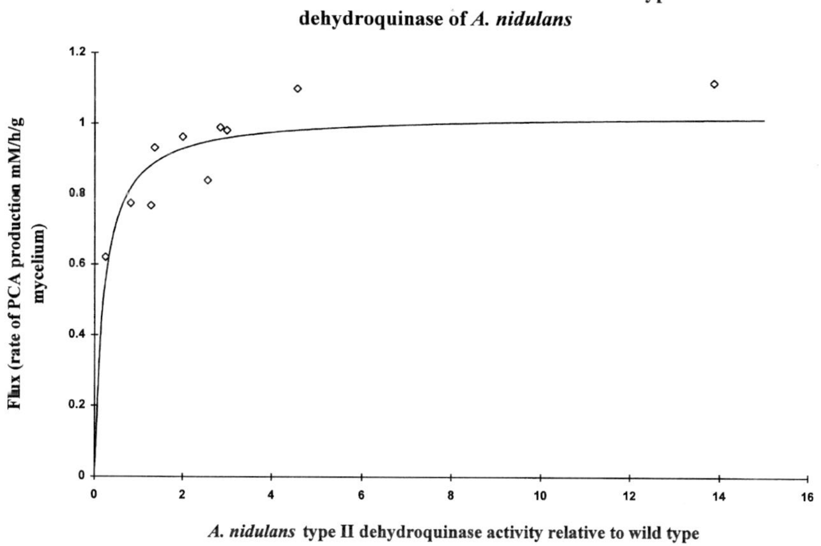

The rate of PCA accumulation is shown as a function of the increase in the qutE-encoded type II 3-dehydroquinase levels relative to wild type. The line was plotted using non-linear least-squares regression.

---

specific activity is shown in Fig. 4, where it can be seen that the *qutE*-encoded type II dehydroquinase has a flux control coefficient of 0.18 ± 0.03. Similar experiments in which the *qutB* gene encoding the quinate dehydrogenase was expressed *in vivo* estimated a value of 0.36 for the flux control coefficient of quinate dehydrogenase (see Note added in proof).

The use of the summation theorem shows that the combined flux control coefficient for DHS dehydratase and quinate permease is 0.46, implying that together they exert the greatest control over pathway flux. Calculations (using the elasticity coefficients measured *in vitro*) of how the relative values of the various flux control coefficients vary in response to changing metabolite concentrations predict that, in the range 0.05–0.30 mM dehydroshikimate, the relative value for the flux control coefficient of dehydroshikimate dehydratase will always be the lowest of the three quinate pathway enzymes (see Note added in proof). Starting at around a concentration of 0.40 mM dehydroshikimate, the elasticity coefficient measurements predict that the value of the flux control coefficient for dehydroshikimate dehydratase is larger than that for the dehydroquinase. Taking the situation where dehydroshikimate is at a concentration of 0.30 mM (the cross-over point where the value of the flux control coefficient for dehydroshikimate dehydratase starts to increase to a level comparable with that for dehydroquinase), the use of the elasticity coefficients in conjunction with the connectivity theorem predicts that the ratio of the flux control coefficient of dehydroquinase to that of dehydroshikimate dehydratase is 1.7:1. As the empirically determined value for the flux control coefficient of dehydroquinase is 0.18, this predicts a value of 0.11 for dehydroshikimate dehydratase under the standard growth conditions employed. In turn, application of the summation theorem implies that the flux control coefficient of quinate permease is approx. 0.35 (see Note added in proof).

Clearly these calculations are subject to the caveats discussed above and in greater detail by others [56] concerning the validity of extrapolating elasticity coefficients derived *in vitro* to make predictions about the situation *in vivo*. In this instance we believe that this approach has some validity, as the estimates about the hierarchy of control are in agreement with the independent *in vivo* biological evidence which implies that, under the standard growth conditions employed to grow *A. nidulans*, DHS dehydratase has the lowest flux control coefficient (see above).

There is, however, one other component of the *qut* pathway in wild-type *A. nidulans* that is proposed to interact with the pathway metabolites in a concentration-dependent manner, namely the *qutR*-encoded QUTR repressor protein. The QUTR repressor protein is proposed to mediate its repressor activity on transcription activation by a direct stoichiometric interaction with the QUTA transcription activator protein; however, this repressor activity is proposed to be negated by binding of one or more of the *qut* pathway metabolites [31]. As the repressor protein helps to determine the extent of transcription initiation, this will ultimately affect the rate of production of and/or steady-state levels of the *qut* pathway enzymes, and thereby the flux through the pathway. Any flux control coefficients associated with the repressor protein may therefore change rapidly from a high to a low value as the mycelium induces production of the *qut* pathway enzymes in response to the presence of quinate and the quinate pathway metabolites approach steady-state levels. In the experiments we report here, however, the repressor protein in the strains used was inactive due to the presence of the recessive *qutR*16 mutation. The value of the flux control coefficient calculated for the permease is therefore unlikely to have a component associated with the repressor protein, but it may have a minor term associated with the efflux of the PCA produced by the *qut* pathway.

These considerations lead us to the conclusion that, under the standard conditions employed to grow *A. nidulans* in our laboratory, quinate permease and quinate dehydrogenase exert approximately equal, and the greater, control over pathway flux, whereas DHS dehydratase exerts the least control.

If quinate permease really does exert the greatest control over pathway flux, then it should be possible to at least partly decouple or reduce this effect (thereby increasing the flux control coefficients of the quinate dehydrogenase and dehydroquinase enzymes) by carrying out the flux experiments at reduced pH. For example, at pH 3.5 significant quantities of quinate are protonated and are able to enter the mycelium via a concentration-driven diffusion gradient, independent of quinate permease. In order to test this prediction, the flux control coefficient of the *qutE*-encoded dehydroquinase was determined empirically at pH 3.5 and was found to have increased from a value of 0.18 to 0.28 (see Note added in proof).

Interpretation of these results is problematical, as growth at such a low pH may affect the internal pH of the mycelium, leading to differential effects on the activities of the various enzymes. *A. nidulans* is unusual in that it is able to grow in media as acidic as pH 3.5 or as basic as pH 9.0, and this ability to grow over such a wide pH range has been studied genetically and physiologically [57]. It has been shown that *A. nidulans* has an efficient pH homoeostatic mechanism so that non-secreted enzymes are required to act only over a narrow pH range [57]. Growth at pH 3.5 (instead of the usual growth pH of 6.5) has been shown to reduce the internal pH of the mycelium only to approx. pH 5.7 [57]. We have previously shown that growth of *A. nidulans* at a range of pH values varying from pH 6.5 to pH 3.5 does not increase the variation in the levels or relative ratios of the three quinate pathway enzymes over that observed when replicate samples of mycelium are grown at pH 6.5 [2,36]. These considerations suggest that flux through the quinate pathway at pH 3.5 is unlikely to be subject to major changes attributable to altered levels or relative activity ratios of the quinate pathway enzymes.

The 56% increase in the value of the flux control coefficient for the dehydroquinase in medium incubated at pH 3.5 is therefore consistent with a partial decoupling of the control over flux exerted by quinate permease.

Does the AROM protein have a channelling function?

The subject of metabolic channelling is an area rich in a rigorous debate that is firmly grounded in various chapters of this book. As should be clear from the content of this particular chapter, we are taking a biological, empirical approach to understanding the control of flux within and between the quinate and shikimate pathways, and do not feel qualified to comment on the mathematical development of the supporting theory. We do, however, wish to take this opportunity to raise a few biological observations which in the case of the AROM protein may help to illuminate the debate.

The data discussed in the preceding sections showed that the wild-type AROM protein is extremely leaky *in vivo* and that shikimate-pathway-derived DHQ and DHS are accessible to the quinate pathway enzymes. Indeed, the DHS dehydratase enzyme has a shikimate pathway flux deviation control coefficient of -1 and a quinate pathway flux control coefficient of less than 0.11. These data taken at face value can be simply explained by a mass action effect of enzymes on metabolites that approximate pool behaviour, without the necessity to impute a channelling function for the AROM protein [50,51].

There is, however, one other consequence of overproducing the DHS dehydratase enzyme in *A. nidulans* in the absence of exogenously supplied quinate. With an increasing *in vivo* concentration of DHS dehydratase under these conditions, there was a concomitant increase in a graded auxotrophic requirement for aromatic amino acids. This partial auxotrophic requirement under these circumstances is most simply interpreted in terms of flux through the shikimate pathway being decreased due to diversion into the quinate pathway [51]. Increasing the concentration of DHS dehydratase beyond 15-fold greater than the wild type causes the shikimate pathway flux control coefficient of this enzyme to drop to effectively zero (see Fig. 3), implying that, at this enzyme concentration and above, shikimate pathway DHS is being diverted into the quinate pathway at the maximum possible rate. If all the shikimate pathway DHS was being diverted into the quinate pathway then the auxotrophic requirement for aromatic amino acids in these strains should be absolute and the strains would fail to grow.

It is a fact, however, that strains overproducing DHS dehydratase up to 30-fold over the wild-type level have been isolated, and they are still able to grow in the absence of aromatic amino acid supplementation, albeit very poorly [51]. These observations therefore can be interpreted as reflecting a very low channelling effect due to the close juxtaposition and specific orientation of five sequential active sites maintaining an essential minimum level of flux through the shikimate pathway to prevent cell death. Under steady-state conditions in ideal laboratory conditions of optimal pH, aeration and nutrition supply, this possible channelling function is likely to be physiologically insignificant in wild-type strains.

Could this putative low-level channelling function have any physiological significance for the organism in its natural environment? *A. nidulans* will require solubilization of quinate before it can be utilized as a carbon source. The conditions for quinate solubilization may well be transient, causing quinate to enter the mycelium in pulses rather than at a constant steady state. The half-life of DHS dehydratase *in vivo* has been shown to be approx. 2 h in the absence of exogenously supplied quinate; therefore under conditions of quinate pulsing DHS dehydratase will deplete the shikimate pathway flux by diversion of DHS into the quinate pathway [51]. Under such conditions, any putative low-level channelling function associated with the AROM protein could become physiologically significant by maintaining a minimal flow of flux through the shikimate pathway to prevent cell death and/or facilitate conidiation. It is also worthy of note that strains displaying partial aromatic amino acid auxotrophy (due to increased concentrations of the DHS dehydratase enzyme) also show a strong correlation with an increase in the AROM protein concentration [51].

Thus the cell may have two mechanisms to protect the essential shikimate pathway from depletion by quinate pathway enzymes. The first, a protection against acute but transient depletion, could be accomplished by a putative low-level channelling function. The second, a mass action effect caused by increasing the AROM protein concentration, could be the cellular response to a more long-term chronic depletion of AROM pathway flux. Such a response has been well documented in yeast, where the molecular basis for this phenomenon is provided by a global control system positively mediated at the level of transcription regulation by the GCN4 protein [58].

In conclusion, however, we wish to highlight a possible contemporary physiological advantage in having a leaky AROM protein, although this will have no bearing on the forces driving the original fusion events. The model for the molecular control of transcription of the quinate gene cluster requires that there is always a low level of quinate permease present in the cell membrane, so that an autoregulatory circuit can be rapidly induced [38]. It is possible that this low-level background *qut* gene cluster transcription could be maintained by the DHQ and DHS leaking from the AROM protein interacting with the QUTR repressor protein, thereby negating the repressor activity of a significant population of the repressor modules.

Note added in proof

The flux control coefficient of the dehydroshikimate dehydratase enzyme has now been determined empirically and, under standard laboratory growth conditions applied to the whole of this study, the value has been shown to be less than 0.03. This value demonstrates that this enzyme exerts the least control over quinate pathway flux as predicted by the calculations discussed within the text of this chapter. The value is entirely consistent with the theoretical predictions made for the values of the flux control coefficients of the quinate permease and the dehydroshikimate dehydratase which were made by using the quinate pathway enzyme elasticity coefficients in conjunction with the connectivity theorem (see the text of this chapter). This observation gives some measure of confidence of the applicability of using *in vitro*-derived elasticity coefficients in conjunction with the connectivity theorem to make predictions about the hierarchy of control and how that control is proposed to shift in response to varying metabolite concentrations. The full information is now in press [59].

This research was supported by U.K. Research Council funding, and by The Wellcome Trust. We thank Sheila Gibbs-Barton for typing the manuscript.

References

1. Hawkins, A.R., Giles, N.H. and Kinghorn, J.R. (1982) Biochem. Genet. **20**, 271–286
2. Grant, S., Roberts, C.F., Lamb, H.K., Stout, M. and Hawkins, A.R. (1988) J. Gen. Microbiol. **134**, 347–358
3. Charles, I.G., Keyte, J.W., Brammar, W.J., Smith, M. and Hawkins, A.R. (1986) Nucleic Acids Res. **14**, 2201–2213
4. Bentley, R. (1990) Crit. Rev. Biochem. Mol. Biol. **25**, 307–384
5. Giles, N.H., Case, M.E., Baum, J., Geever, R., Huiet, L., Patel, V. and Tyler, B. (1985) Microbiol. Rev. **49**, 338–358
6. Case, M.E. and Giles, N.H. (1975) Proc. Natl. Acad. Sci. U.S.A. **72**, 553–557
7. Giles, N.H. (1978) Am. Nat. **112**, 641–657
8. Case, M.E. and Giles, N.H. (1968) Genetics **60**, 49–58
9. Case, M.E. and Giles, N.H. (1971) Proc. Natl. Acad. Sci. U.S.A. **68**, 58–62
10. Chaleff, R.S. (1974) J. Gen. Microbiol. **81**, 337–355
11. Giles, N.H., Partridge, C.W.H., Ahmed, S.I. and Case, M.E. (1967) Proc. Natl. Acad. Sci. U.S.A. **58**, 1930–1937
12. Giles, N.H. and Case, M.E. (1975) in Isozymes II: Physiological Function (Markert, C.L., ed.), pp. 865–876, Academic Press, New York
13. Case, M.E., Giles, N.H. and Doy, C.H. (1972) Genetics **71**, 337–348
14. Giles, N.H., Case, M.E., Partridge, C.W.H. and Ahmed, S.I. (1967) Proc. Natl. Acad. Sci. U.S.A. **58**, 1453–1460
15. Jacobson, J.W., Hart, B.A., Doy, C.H. and Giles, N.H. (1972) Biochim. Biophys. Acta **289**, 1–12
16. Lumsden, J. and Coggins, J.R. (1977) Biochem. J. **161**, 599–607
17. Lumsden, J. and Coggins, J.R. (1978) Biochem. J. **169**, 441–444
18. Gaertner, F.H. (1978) in Microenvironments and Metabolic Compartmentation (Srere, P.A. and Estabrook, R.W., eds.), pp. 345–353, Academic Press, New York
19. Lambert, J.M., Boocock, M.R. and Coggins, J.R. (1985) Biochem. J. **226**, 817–829
20. Welch, G.R. and Gaertner, F.H. (1975) Proc. Natl. Acad. Sci. U.S.A. **72**, 4218–4222
21. Gaertner, F.H., Ericson, M.C. and DeMoss, J.A. (1970) J. Biol. Chem. **245**, 595–600
22. Welch, G.R. and Gaertner, F.H. (1976) Arch. Biochem. Biophys. **172**, 476–489
23. Coggins, J.R. and Boocock, M.R. (1986) in Multidomain Proteins: Structure and Evolution (Hardie, D.G. and Coggins, J.R. eds.), pp. 259–281, Elsevier, Amsterdam
24. Coggins, J.R., Duncan, K., Anton, I.A., Boocock, M.R., Chaudhuri, S., Lambert, J.M., Lewendon, A., Millar, G., Mousdale, D.M. and Smith, D.D.S. (1987) Biochem. Soc. Trans. **15**, 754–759
25. Hawkins, A.R., Da Silva, A.J.F. and Roberts, C.F. (1985) Curr. Genet. **9**, 305–311
26. Hawkins, A.R., Lamb, H.K., Smith, M., Keyte, J.W. and Roberts, C.F. (1988) Mol. Gen. Genet. **214**, 224–231
27. Beri, R.K., Whittington, H., Roberts, C.F. and Hawkins, A.R. (1987) Nucleic Acids Res. **15**, 7991–8001
28. Hawkins, A.R., Lamb, H.K. and Roberts, C.F. (1992) Gene **110**, 109–114
29. Lamb, H.K., Hawkins, A.R., Smith, M., Harvey, I.J., Brown, J., Turner, G. and Roberts, C.F. (1990) Mol. Gen. Genet. **223**, 17–23
30. Lamb, H.K., Roberts, C.F. and Hawkins, A.R. (1992) Gene **112**, 219–224
31. Hawkins, A.R., Lamb, H.K., Moore, J.D., Charles, I.G. and Roberts, C.F. (1993) J. Gen. Microbiol. **139**, 2891–2899
32. Hawkins, A.R. (1987) Curr. Genet. **11**, 491–498
33. Kleanthous, C., Deka, R., Davis, K., Kelly, S.M., Cooper, A., Harding, S.E., Price, C., Hawkins, A.R. and Coggins, J.R. (1992) Biochem. J. **282**, 687–695
34. Harris, J., Kleanthous, C., Coggins, J.R., Hawkins, A.R. and Abell, C. (1993) J. Chem. Soc. Chem. Commun. **13**, 1080–1081

35. Shneier, A., Harris, J., Kleanthous, C., Coggins, J.R., Hawkins, A.R. and Abell, C. (1993) Bioorg. Med. Chem. Lett. **3**, 1399–1402
36. Whittington, H.A., Grant, S., Roberts, C.F., Lamb, H.K. and Hawkins, A.R. (1987) Curr. Genet. **12**, 135–139
37. Hawkins, A.R., Lamb, H.K., Moore, J.D. and Roberts, C.F. (1993) Gene **136**, 49–54
38. Hawkins, A.R., Lamb, H.K. and Roberts, C.F. (1994) in Genetics and Physiology of *Aspergillus nidulans* (Martinelli, S. and Kinghorn, J.R., eds.), pp. 195–220, Elsevier, Amsterdam
39. Kinghorn, J.R. and Hawkins, A.R. (1982) Mol. Gen. Genet. **186**, 145–152
40. Millar, G. and Coggins, J.R. (1986) FEBS Lett. **200**, 11–17
41. Millar, G., Lewendon, A., Hunter, M. and Coggins, J.R. (1986) Biochem. J. **237**, 427–437
42. Duncan, K., Lewendon, A. and Coggins, J.R. (1984) FEBS Lett. **170**, 59–63
43. Duncan, K., Chaudhuri, S., Campbell, M.S. and Coggins, J.R. (1986) Biochem. J. **238**, 475–483
44. Berlyn, M.B. and Giles, N.H. (1969) J. Bacteriol. **99**, 222–230
45. van den Hombergh, J.P.T.W., Moore, J.D., Charles, I.G. and Hawkins, A.R. (1992) Biochem. J. **284**, 861–867
46. Moore, J.D., Coggins, J.R., Virden, R. and Hawkins, A.R. (1994) Biochem. J. **301**, 297–304
47. Hawkins, A.R. and Smith, M. (1991) Eur. J. Biochem. **196**, 717–724
48. Hawkins, A.R., Moore, J.D. and Adeokun, A.M. (1993) Biochem. J. **296**, 451–457
49. Moore, J.D. and Hawkins, A.R. (1993) Mol. Gen. Genet. **240**, 92–102
50. Lamb, H.K., Bagshaw, C.R. and Hawkins, A.R. (1991) Mol. Gen. Genet. **227**, 187–196
51. Lamb, H.K., van den Hombergh, J.P.T.W., Newton, G.H., Moore, J.D., Roberts, C.F. and Hawkins, A.R. (1992) Biochem. J. **284**, 181–187
52. Kuswandi and Roberts, C.F. (1992) J. Gen. Microbiol. **138**, 817–823
53. Beri, R.K., Grant, S., Roberts, C.F., Smith, M. and Hawkins, A.R. (1990) Biochem. J. **265**, 337–342
54. Dykhuizen, D.F., Dean, A.M. and Hartl, D.L. (1987) Genetics **115**, 25–31
55. Moore, J.D., Lamb, H.K., Garbe, T., Servos, S., Dougan, G., Charles, I.G. and Hawkins, A.R. (1992) Biochem. J. **287**, 173–181
56. Fell, D.A. (1992) Biochem. J. **286**, 313–330
57. Caddick, M.X., Brownlee, A.G. and Arst, H.N. (1986) Mol. Gen. Genet. **203**, 346–353
58. Hinnebusch, A.G. (1988) Microbiol. Rev. **52**, 248–273
59. Wheeler, K.A., Lamb, H.K. and Hawkins, A.R. (1996) Biochem. J. **315**, 195–205

10

The urea cycle

Natalie S. Cohen*, Chia-Wei Cheung† and Luisa Raijman‡

Department of Biochemistry and Molecular Biology, University of Southern California School of Medicine, 2011 Zonal Avenue, Los Angeles, CA 90033, U.S.A.

Introduction

The liver and the intestinal mucosa are the two organs that contain all five pathway-specific enzymes required for the *de novo* synthesis of urea. The liver alone carries out the complete synthesis from HCO_3^- and NH_3 at rates sufficient to maintain normal ammonaemia, a fact which, at the physiological level, has been known for some 70 years [1]. The subjects we will discuss pertain to the pathway as it functions in the liver, and will focus on the channelling of some pathway-specific intermediates observed using isolated mitochondria and hepatocytes.

Throughout this chapter, channelling will be used to mean that a reactant is transferred between soluble enzymes with no or little diffusion into the bulk aqueous medium. Soluble enzymes are defined as those which are released into solution when cells or subcellular structures are disrupted in the absence of detergents.

Background

Two bodies of evidence led us to attempt to study the kinetic properties of the urea cycle enzymes *in situ*. The first has to do with specific characteristics of carbamoyl phosphate synthase (ammonia) (CPS) and ornithine trans-carbamylase (OTC) *in situ*, and the second with the nature of the mitochondrial matrix.

CPS

Several characteristics of the urea cycle *in vivo* appeared to be inconsistent with known properties of CPS in solution. Two of the major discrepancies

* *Present address: Department of Molecular Pharmacology and Toxicology, University of Southern California School of Pharmacy, 1985 Zonal Avenue, Los Angeles, CA 90033, U.S.A.*
† *Present address: Division of Biology, Beckman Research Institute of the City of Hope, 1450 East Duarte Road, Duarte, CA 91010, U.S.A.*
‡ *To whom correspondence should be sent, at present address: Department of Pathology, Anatomy and Cell Biology, Thomas Jefferson University, 1020 Locust Street, Room JAH271, Philadelphia, PA 19104, U.S.A.*

are in the effects of ornithine and of N-acetyl-L-glutamate on carbamoyl phosphate synthesis (see Fig. 1).

Ornithine stimulates urea synthesis in liver slices [5], perfused liver [6] and isolated hepatocytes [7]. The stimulation and its catalytic nature were logically attributed to ornithine being a substrate of OTC, and a product of arginase (Fig. 1). Experiments by Krebs, Hems and Lund [8], however, indicated that ornithine stimulates urea synthesis by an additional mechanism which involves a direct effect on CPS. This was surprising because, in solution, ornithine has no effect on the structural or kinetic properties of this enzyme.

We attempted to obtain direct evidence for the postulated effect of ornithine on CPS using a simpler system, i.e. isolated liver mitochondria synthesizing carbamoyl phosphate in the presence and absence of added ornithine. We observed that CPS undergoes a severe and sustained inhibition after 10–15 s of incubation without ornithine ([9]; see also [10]). Addition of ornithine relieves the inhibition nearly instantaneously. The inhibition in the absence of ornithine cannot be explained by the accumulation of reaction products such as carbamoyl phosphate and ADP, by a decrease in matrix acetylglutamate or by the deterioration of mitochondria [9,11]; rather, CPS *in situ* appears to have a low molecular activity in the absence of ornithine. These findings supported the proposal by Krebs et al. [8] that ornithine has a direct effect on matrix CPS.

The inhibition of CPS in the absence of ornithine occurs at low and at very high matrix content of acetylglutamate [11]. Stated differently, matrix CPS has a nearly absolute requirement for both ornithine and acetylgluta-mate. This is not observed in solution, and suggests that at least some important structural and kinetic characteristics of CPS are markedly different in the matrix. This working hypothesis invokes well established facts. Firstly, the structural and kinetic properties of CPS are affected by the nature of the environment in terms of content of low-molecular-mass compounds, ionic strength and protein concentration (both total and enzyme-specific). Secondly, regarding the variables just mentioned and in other respects, the mitochondrial matrix differs profoundly from the dilute aqueous solutions of simple composition in which enzymes are generally studied.

The liver mitochondrial matrix

The characteristics of the matrix, which make up the second body of evidence mentioned above, and the implications they may have on how enzymes function *in vivo* have been extensively discussed by Srere [12]. We will only refer briefly to those directly relevant to our topic.

Soluble proteins are at an extremely high concentration in the matrix, of the order of 500 μg/μl of matrix total water [12–14]. In State 3, about half of the total matrix water is free and the remainder is water of hydration [15,16]; the level of hydration of matrix proteins is likely to be not much greater than that of protein crystals [17].

Fig. 1   The pathway of urea synthesis

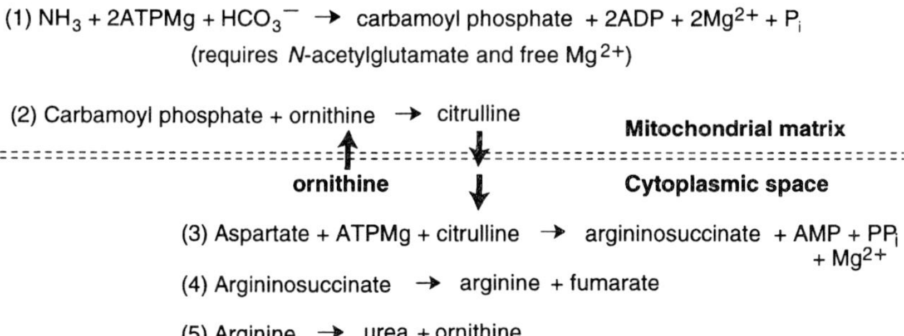

The pathway of urea synthesis in mammalian liver consists of five reactions catalysed by enzymes which operate in two cellular compartments; the first two reactions are catalysed by enzymes in the mitochondrial matrix [2,3], and the next three by enzymes in the cytoplasm [4]. Reactions (1)–(5) (not balanced for charge) are catalysed respectively by CPS (ammonia) (EC 6.3.4.16), OTC (EC 2.1.3.3), argininosuccinate synthase (EC 6.3.4.5), argininosuccinate lyase (EC 4.3.2.1) and arginase (EC 3.5.3.1). The broken lines represent the mitochondrial membranes.

Given the high concentration of protein in the mitochondrial matrix and the extensive surface area of the inner membrane, Srere calculated that matrix proteins must be in close proximity to one another, and that a substantial portion of them must be juxtaposed on to the membrane [18]. Experiments on the effects of various permeant cross-linkers on matrix proteins provided compelling evidence that soluble enzymes are indeed crowded in the matrix [19]. Enzymes which undergo little or no cross-linking in preparations of disrupted mitochondria cross-link readily and extensively in intact mitochondria [19]; identical observations were made in our laboratory (C.-W. Cheung and L. Raijman, unpublished work).

The conditions prevailing in the matrix are likely to influence the structure of individual enzymes, and may promote the formation of protein complexes. It is known that some pathway-related matrix enzymes have sufficient affinity for one another to form multiple-enzyme complexes in solution under favourable conditions [20,21]. One can conceive that weak associative forces that would not support complex-formation in solution may be sufficient to do so under the conditions prevailing in the matrix [22]. The crowding of macromolecules may give rise to the organization of soluble enzymes along metabolic pathways, by way of the formation of multiple-enzyme and enzyme–membrane complexes [23,24]. Kinetic and other properties inherent in such complexes would not be detectable in dilute solutions.

Given the sensitivity of the structural and kinetic properties of CPS to the nature of its environment, we could not ignore the possibility that the observations we had made on the effects of ornithine reflect properties inherent in CPS *in situ*.

Other characteristics of the CPS and OTC systems in the matrix

The CPS system is unusual in several respects. CPS is by far the most abundant soluble enzyme of liver mitochondria, constituting about 15% of the total matrix protein of mitochondria from rats fed a normal diet [3,25,26] (this trait is also found in human and other mammalian livers). Its concentration is about 80 μg (0.5 nmol of CPS monomer) per μl of matrix total water. With respect to some of its substrates, CPS is present in stoichiometric rather than catalytic amounts; for example, the amount of CPS monomer (mol per μl of matrix water) is about the same as that of NH_4^+, or about 100-fold greater than that of its true substrate, NH_3 [27]. At its highest, the amount (mol) of acetylglutamate *in vivo* is the same as that of CPS [28]; most of the matrix acetylglutamate may be enzyme-bound.

OTC is also present at a high concentration, about 0.12 nmol of monomer per μl of matrix total water [11]. In mitochondria synthesizing citrulline *de novo*, the amount of carbamoyl phosphate (mol) generally exceeds that of OTC by one order of magnitude (the steady-state concentration of carbamoyl phosphate varies as a function of the activity of CPS, but it is usually not greater than 3–4 nmol/μl of matrix total water [9,11]). In the absence of ornithine the concentration of newly synthesized matrix carbamoyl phosphate increases at first, as would be expected since it cannot be utilized by OTC, and then decreases (by leakage from mitochondria) to levels similar to those observed in the presence of ornithine [9]. The relationship between OTC and the matrix content of ornithine is discussed in detail below.

The cytoplasmic compartment

The protein content of the cytoplasmic compartment does not reach the level in the mitochondrial matrix but it is also high, of the order of 200 mg per ml of water [29]. This compartment contains membranous structures and a vast filamentous network with which specific proteins are known to associate [29,30]. The cytoplasmic enzymes of the urea cycle appear to be among the soluble proteins which are associated with membranes *in vivo* (see below).

Attempts at determining simple kinetic parameters *in situ*

Among the kinetic parameters of enzymes which may differ *in situ* and in dilute solution is their affinity for substrates; for example, CPS in the matrix appears to have greater affinity for NH_3 than the enzyme in solution [27].

We now give a summary of work aimed at measuring some of the K_m values of CPS and OTC in isolated mitochondria.

OTC

We attempted to measure the K_m of matrix OTC for ornithine in mitochondria synthesizing carbamoyl phosphate at different rates [31]. Low and medium rates (10–30 nmol/min per mg) were obtained in mitochondria incubated with 0.2 and 10 mM NH_4Cl [31] respectively; higher rates (about 50 nmol/min per mg) in mitochondria preincubated with glutamate, acetyl-carnitine and ATP in order to increase their content of acetylglutamate [32]; and the highest rates (80–100 nmol/min per mg) in uncoupled mitochondria preincubated with acetylglutamate [11]. The external concentration of ornithine ranged from 0.03 to 2.0 mM, which encompasses both the *in vivo* concentration in liver (0.18–0.44 μmol/g wet weight, depending on the nutritional state [28]) and the K_m of OTC in solution for ornithine at pH 7.4 (about 0.4 mM; see [33–35] and below). In this concentration range, ornithine entry into the matrix is mediated by a transporter [2]. The rates of total carbamoyl phosphate and citrulline synthesis, and the matrix content of ornithine and citrulline, were measured under all conditions. The experimental conditions and analytical methods used are described in detail in [31].

At rates of carbamoyl phosphate synthesis between 10 and 50 nmol/min per mg, OTC was not fully saturated with carbamoyl phosphate, and the rate of citrulline synthesis was determined by CPS. External ornithine at 0.2 mM was nearly saturating for citrulline synthesis, yet ornithine was undetectable in the matrix even when the external concentration was as high as 0.5–1.0 mM. We established that the absence of ornithine from the matrix was not the result of limitation by the transporter, or of a transport mechanism involving a compulsory ornithine–citrulline exchange [36]. Together, these facts imply that only as much ornithine entered the matrix as was used for citrulline synthesis [31].

At very high rates of carbamoyl phosphate synthesis (80–100 nmol/min per mg), the rate of citrulline synthesis was limited either by OTC or by ornithine transport. The $S_{0.5}$ for external ornithine was about 0.4 mM, similar to the K_m of OTC for ornithine in solution at pH values between 7.37 and 7.90 [33–35]. OTC functioned as if it were exposed to the external concentration of ornithine, as though a continuum existed from the external medium through the ornithine transporter to OTC in the matrix [31].

The possibility that matrix OTC preferentially uses external ornithine was studied using mitochondria preloaded with ornithine. This was feasible because, when present at high external concentration, ornithine bypasses the transporter [2] and reaches matrix concentrations virtually identical to those in the suspension medium [31]. Mitochondria were preincubated with 20 mM ornithine for 5 min, and then incubated for 10 and 15 s under optimum conditions for carbamoyl phosphate and citrulline synthesis in a medium containing 40 μCi (2 nmol) of L-[2,3-^{3}H]ornithine per ml. The final concentration of ornithine in the incubation medium was about 2 mM, owing to carry-over from the mitochondrial suspension used to start the reactions. Incubations were ended, and mitochondria were deproteinized, by rapid centrifugation through a layer of silicone oil into an underlying layer of $HClO_4$. The amount and specific radioactivity of ornithine and citrulline in the mitochondrial extracts and in the medium were measured by ion-exchange HPLC and liquid scintillation counting of eluted fractions [31].

Table 1   Channelling of extramitochondrial ornithine into citrulline by mitochondria preloaded with ornithine

	Specific radioactivity (c.p.m./nmol)			Orn_{in} (nmol/μl)	Total Orn_{in} (nmol)	Total citrulline (nmol)
	Citrulline	Orn_{out}	Orn_{in}			
Expt. 1						
Experimental	8493	8508	956	4.19	25.1	76.1
Control	–	–	–	5.95	35.6	0
Expt. 2						
Experimental	8640	8433	1295	3.52	24.2	69.0
Control	–	–	–	6.05	41.6	0

Specific radioactivities are shown for total citrulline and for ornithine in the medium (Orn_{out}) and in the matrix (Orn_{in}). Counting efficiency for ^3H was 55%. Expts. 1 and 2 were done at 23 and 30 °C respectively. Data from [31].

The results of these experiments are summarized in Table 1. The specific radioactivity of citrulline was virtually identical to that of the ornithine in the incubation medium. Conversely, the specific radioactivity of matrix ornithine at the end of the incubations was very low, indicating that the external and the matrix pools of ornithine mixed very slowly. It was crucial to these experiments that the amount of unlabelled ornithine present in the matrix was sufficient to decrease the specific radioactivity of citrulline if matrix and external ornithine were both used by OTC. Indeed, the amount of matrix ornithine at the start of the incubations was more than half of the total amount of citrulline synthesized, and most of it was still in the matrix at the end of the incubations. Virtually no matrix ornithine was used for citrulline synthesis.

These findings are direct evidence that external ornithine is tightly channelled to matrix OTC. The methodology used in this work allows the detection of stable channelling only, such as would be mediated by stably associated entities. In this case, the association would involve OTC and components of the mitochondrial inner membrane required for the transport of ornithine.

Organization of CPS and OTC *in situ*

We have already discussed some of the special properties that CPS exhibits in the matrix. Some characteristics of OTC also differ *in situ* and in solution. For example, matrix OTC does not readily use added carbamoyl phosphate and is poorly inhibited by δ-N-phosphonacetyl-L-ornithine (PALO, a bifunctional transition state analogue [37]) despite the fact that these compounds permeate into the matrix and reach concentrations which would be saturating for OTC in solution [11]. The binding of the added compounds to OTC in the matrix is hindered, perhaps as a result of interactions between it and CPS.

The characteristics of CPS and OTC were studied in greater detail in experiments using mitochondria made permeable to low-molecular-mass compounds. Mitochondria treated with toluene as described in [38] were freely permeable to sucrose and citrulline, while retaining 89% of their CPS and OTC activity [39]. They carried out *de novo* carbamoyl phosphate and citrulline synthesis from ammonia, bicarbonate, ornithine and ATP in the presence of added acetylglutamate, as well as citrulline synthesis from added carbamoyl phosphate and ornithine.

The apparent K_m values of OTC for added substrates were higher than those of the soluble enzyme in the same medium; for carbamoyl phosphate the difference was 8-fold, and for ornithine it was 2-fold. PALO was less inhibitory for OTC *in situ* than for the enzyme dissolved in the same medium. Of more interest, PALO was much less inhibitory when carbamoyl phosphate was generated endogenously than when it was added to the medium. Wanders et al. [40] reported a comparable observation on the effects of added norvaline; this compound inhibits citrulline synthesis from endogenous carbamoyl phosphate less than from added carbamoyl phosphate.

Ornithine had no effect on CPS in permeabilized mitochondria, but it affected the distribution of carbamoyl phosphate between mitochondria and medium during *de novo* synthesis [39]. In the absence of ornithine, carbamoyl phosphate levels in the matrix and the medium were the same during *de novo* synthesis. In the presence of ornithine, however, about 80% of carbamoyl phosphate synthesized *de novo* was converted into citrulline in the matrix; the concentration of carbamoyl phosphate in the mitochondria was more than 10 times higher than that in the medium, despite the full permeability of the organelles to added molecules of this size. We cannot explain this observation. The concentration of citrulline was the same in the matrix and the external medium under all conditions.

The possibility that OTC *in situ* uses endogenously formed carbamoyl phosphate preferentially was tested by using $[^{14}C]HCO_3^-$ as a substrate for carbamoyl phosphate synthesis and examining the effect of added unlabelled carbamoyl phosphate on the incorporation of radioactivity into citrulline. Nearly 60% of carbamoyl phosphate synthesized *de novo* was converted into citrulline within the matrix. Addition of a 40- or 200-fold excess of unlabelled carbamoyl phosphate (1 or 5 mM) decreased the percentage of labelled carbamoyl phosphate that was converted into citrulline in the matrix by only 13 or 18% respectively. These findings were not duplicated when lysed mitochondria were used in otherwise identical experiments.

In all, this work indicates that endogenously generated carbamoyl phosphate is channelled to OTC. Partial channelling of carbamoyl phosphate in intact mitochondria had been suggested by Wanders et al. [40]. These authors considered that newly formed and existing carbamoyl phosphate equilibrate sufficiently rapidly so as to constitute a single pool; our findings, on the contrary, indicate slow mixing of endogenous and added carbamoyl phosphate.

Partial channelling of endogenous carbamoyl phosphate, poor utilization of added carbamoyl phosphate and a diminished effectiveness of PALO are observed in both intact and permeabilized mitochondria [11] and cannot, therefore, be attributed to permeability barriers. The lack of an ornithine effect on CPS in permeabilized mitochondria, on the other hand, may reflect the disruption of an association between OTC and membrane regions involved in ornithine transport [31], which we had postulated on the basis of work using intact mitochondria.

Arginase

We attempted to carry out simple kinetic studies on the synthesis and utilization of arginine using isolated hepatocytes permeabilized with α-toxin. This agent creates a pore in the plasma membrane by a well defined mechanism [41]; previous work by others [42] indicated that fully permeable yet sufficiently stable cells could be obtained. Under the conditions described in [43], α-toxin treatment yielded cells which were stable beyond the time required to carry out our experiments. The cells were freely permeable to low-molecular-mass compounds such as neutral, anionic and cationic amino acids, but not to inulin (5000–5500 Da), and retained 80–90% of their soluble enzymes (with respect to the activities in intact cells) after incubation. The cells were metabolically competent to the extent that they synthesized urea *de novo* at good rates, a process which requires the proper functioning of several synthetic and transport processes.

We tested the possibility that endogenously generated arginine did not mix with arginine in the bulk aqueous phase of the cell; the experimental approach consisted of examining the pattern of incorporation of $[^{14}C]HCO_3^-$ into urea, arginine and citrulline, and the effect on that pattern of non-labelled arginine added in large excess. Cells were incubated in media containing $[^{14}C]HCO_3^-$, NH_4Cl, ornithine and aspartate, with succinate as the respiratory substrate. In most experiments urea accounted for 40–50% of the total $(NH_3 + $ ornithine)-dependent radioactivity incorporated, citrulline for about 30% and arginine for less than 10%; the remainder was assumed to be in argininosuccinate. The addition of a 200-fold excess of unlabelled arginine (1 mM) had no effect on the total or the percentage of radioactivity fixed in urea, or on the percentage of radioactivity recovered as arginine (Table 2), even though a substantial portion of the added unlabelled arginine

Table 2   Effects of added arginine on urea synthesis from endogenously synthesized substrates by permeabilized hepatocytes

Substrates used	Additions	$(NH_3 + Orn)$-dependent (c.p.m.)	Urea		Arginine		Citrulline		Total in urea + Arg + citrulline (%)
			(c.p.m.)	(% of total)	(c.p.m.)	(% of total)	(c.p.m.)	(% of total)	
Expt. 1									
None	0	740	310	–	100	–	330	–	–
NH$_4$Cl + Orn	0	13950	3750	27	1020	7	6470	46	80
NH$_4$Cl + Orn	1 mM Arg	16180	3950	24	1070	7	8930	55	86
NH$_4$Cl + Orn	5 mM Arg	15530	2130	14	940	6	11470	74	94
Expt. 2									
None	0	> 620	620	–	0	–	N.D.	–	–
NH$_4$Cl + Orn	0	9330	4690	50	650	7	2490	27	84
NH$_4$Cl + Orn	1 mM Arg	9030	4740	52	750	8	3100	34	94
NH$_4$Cl + Orn	5 mM Arg	9270	3090	33	520	6	4890	53	92

The results of two separate experiments are shown. In each, the total counts fixed from $[^{14}C]HCO_3^-$/min per ml of incubation mixture, as well as the number of counts recovered in urea, arginine and citrulline, were measured. There were always some counts fixed in the absence of added NH$_4$Cl and ornithine (Orn); about 20% of these were usually accounted for by urea, arginine and citrulline. The total counts fixed were corrected for counts fixed in the absence of added NH$_4$Cl and ornithine in compounds other than those of the urea cycle; these corrected values are shown as $(NH_3 + Orn)$-dependent c.p.m. The specific radioactivity of the $[^{14}C]HCO_3^-$ was 530 and 1070 c.p.m./nmol in Expts. 1 and 2 respectively; counting efficiency for ^{14}C was 96%. Added NH$_4$Cl was 0.5 mM, and added ornithine was 0.2 mM. N.D., not determined. From [43].

was hydrolysed within the permeabilized cells. If the added arginine and the labelled arginine synthesized endogenously had mixed freely, the specific radioactivity of the arginine pool would have decreased 200-fold, and labelled urea would have been undetectable. There was no isotopic dilution of endogenous arginine.

These observations were not the result of a kinetic effect brought about by the addition of 1 mM arginine to the medium. Finally, the results could not be reproduced in solution using liver homogenates incubated under otherwise identical conditions.

The addition of a 1000-fold excess of unlabelled arginine (5 mM) caused a decrease in the total and the percentage of radioactivity in urea, but the label was not recovered in arginine, as would have been the case if the added and the endogenous arginine had simply mixed. Instead, the label was recovered quantitatively in citrulline, owing to the partial inhibition of argininosuccinate synthase by the added 5 mM arginine. Once again, there was no isotopic dilution of endogenous arginine by added arginine. Taken together, these observations show that, in permeabilized cells, arginine is tightly channelled between argininosuccinate lyase and arginase.

Argininosuccinate lyase

The experimental approach used in studies of this enzyme and of argininosuccinate synthase (see the next section) was the same as that described above for arginase.

The addition of a 200-fold excess of unlabelled argininosuccinate (2 mM) to the incubation mixtures resulted in a decrease of about 25% in the percentage of radioactivity recovered in urea compared with control conditions (Table 3). Had added and endogenously synthesized argininosuccinate mixed freely, the radioactivity in urea would have been undetectable [43]. These findings are indicative of channelling of argininosuccinate between argininosuccinate synthase and argininosuccinate lyase.

Argininosuccinate synthase

For this enzyme the same variables were measured as in the preceding work. In addition, since citrulline is synthesized in mitochondria but utilized in the cytoplasmic compartment, the distribution of citrulline between the two compartments was determined. Cells and media were separated following incubation under the standard conditions for *de novo* urea synthesis, and citrulline was measured in each fraction. About half of the citrulline present at the end of incubation was in mitochondria, and the remainder was presumably distributed throughout the aqueous medium.

The addition to incubation mixtures of 0.3 mM unlabelled citrulline, which was about 20 times the amount of citrulline released from mitochondria in the course of the incubations, had no effect on the labelling pattern (Table 3). The addition of 2 mM unlabelled citrulline resulted in an increase in the percentage of total radioactivity recovered as citrulline and a 60%

Table 3 **Effects of urea cycle intermediates on urea synthesis from endogenously synthesized substrates by permeabilized hepatocytes**

Substrates added	Additions	$(NH_3 + Orn)$-dependent (c.p.m.)	Urea		Arginine		Citrulline		Total in urea + Arg + citrulline (%)
			(c.p.m.)	(% of total)	(c.p.m.)	(% of total)	(c.p.m.)	(% of total)	
Expt. 3									
None	0	1110	510	–	180	–	420	–	–
$NH_4Cl + Orn$	0	8220	3300	40	360	4	2720	33	77
$NH_4Cl + Orn$	2 mM Cit	11790	2010	17	650	6	6620	56	79
$NH_4Cl + Orn$	2 mM Argsucc	12690	3910	31	510	4	5320	42	77
$NH_4Cl + Orn$	2 mM Arg	14490	5700	39	1190	8	5860	43	90
Expt. 4									
None	0	1510	1060	–	170	–	280	–	–
$NH_4Cl + Orn$	0	26460	10270	39	3770	14	7630	29	82
$NH_4Cl + Orn$	0.3 mM Cit	37440	15830	42	2590	7	11530	31	80
$NH_4Cl + Orn$	1 mM Cit	40760	12110	30	2700	7	15190	37	74
$NH_4Cl + Orn$	2 mM Cit	41130	7340	18	1630	4	21660	53	75

The results of two separate experiments are shown. The collection and treatment of the data are described in the legend of Table 2. The specific radioactivity of the $[^{14}C]HCO_3^-$ was 1300 c.p.m /nmo . Orn, ornithine; Cit, citrulline; Argsucc, argininosuccinate. From [43].

decrease in that in urea. This is indicative of partial mixing of endogenous and added citrulline (radioactivity in urea would have been undetectable if these two pools had fully mixed). Citrulline is channelled, but not as tightly as arginine or argininosuccinate [43]. In this case, channelling involves OTC in the mitochondrial matrix, the mitochondrial membranes and argininosuccinate synthase in the cytoplasmic compartment.

In all, these experiments demonstrate that, in permeabilized cells, the cytoplasmic enzymes of the urea cycle, which are soluble proteins (with the exception of a small fraction of arginase [32]), are not randomly distributed but are organized in such a way that pathway-specific intermediates are transferred from the synthesizing to the utilizing enzyme without mixing with the bulk aqueous medium. Since citrulline is channelled to argininosuccinate synthase across the mitochondrial membranes, the three cytoplasmic enzymes must be organized around mitochondria [43].

Heterogeneity of liver arginase

Liver mitochondria isolated in low-salt media contain a substantial amount of arginase; about 90% of it is dissociated by washing with 0.15 M KCl but the remainder is tightly associated with the mitochondrial outer membrane [32]. Such profoundly different solubility properties suggested that the soluble and the mitochondrial arginases are isoenzymes. This notion is supported by recent work from our laboratory.

Immunoblots of intact, permeabilized and 'nude' [44] hepatocytes, and of isolated mitochondria, contain two sharp arginase bands of slightly different molecular mass. Judging by the intensity of the bands, the ratio of the larger to the smaller species was approximately 2:1 in intact and permeabilized hepatocytes, and 1:1 in nude hepatocytes and isolated mitochondria, owing to the partial loss of the larger species.

Contact sites are regions where the mitochondrial inner and outer membranes appear to be tightly juxtaposed, and are characterized by high activities of marker enzymes of both the inner and outer membranes. Preparations obtained as described in [45] were enriched in cytochrome *c* oxidase and monoamine oxidase (inner and outer membrane markers respectively), and they also contained arginase and OTC at higher specific activities than in other membrane fractions. Immunoblots revealed that only the arginase of lower molecular mass was present (N.S. Cohen, C.-W. Cheung and L. Raijman, unpublished work); this is presumably the arginase associated with the outer membrane [32].

Immunocytochemical localization of CPS and OTC

Yokota and Mori [46] described studies at the electron microscopic level which showed that OTC is predominantly located in the immediate vicinity of the mitochondrial inner membrane. Powers-Lee et al. [47] confirmed these findings, and obtained evidence that CPS is also located in the vicinity of the inner membrane, though its distribution does not exactly parallel that of OTC.

Immunocytochemical localization of argininosuccinate synthase and argininosuccinate lyase at the electron microscopic level

The following work was carried out using liver from a rat that had been fed a diet containing 60% protein for 8 days to induce higher levels of argininosuccinate synthase and argininosuccinate lyase proteins [48]. Thin slices of tissue were fixed in paraformaldehyde, and then in paraformaldehyde/glutaraldehyde; 1 mm^3 cubes were embedded in LR white resin [49]. Thin sections were treated with antibodies to argininosuccinate synthase or argininosuccinate lyase, exposed to goat anti-rabbit–biotin, treated with streptavidin/gold (10 nm) and counterstained in uranyl acetate. The electron micrographs were quantified by morphometric analysis. The relative amounts ('densities') of the mitochondrial matrix, mitochondrial outer membrane, endoplasmic reticulum and nuclei were determined by the point counting method [50], and the total numbers of gold particles and their location were scored to obtain the 'relative frequency' of gold over each structure. Random background gold particles generate a ratio of relative frequency to density of 1.0 or lower, whereas ratios greater than 1.0 indicate that there is a preferential association of the signal with the structure in question [50]. Gold particles which were directly over, immediately adjacent to or within 30 nm of the mitochondrial membrane were scored as mitochondrial-membrane-associated.

Analysis of 10 micrographs for each of the two enzymes showed that mitochondrial-membrane-associated gold particles were present at much higher frequency than would be expected from the density of the membranes. The mean enrichment ratio for outer membrane was 1.59 ± 0.07 for argininosuccinate synthase and 1.77 ± 0.18 for argininosuccinate lyase (means $\pm$ S.E.M.). In contrast, for all other structures the mean ratios were ≤ 1.0, indicating that the presence of gold particles over those structures was the result of random background distribution. For control sections treated with rabbit IgG instead of specific antibody, the number of gold particles was too low to conduct any quantitative analysis.

These findings [51a] are direct evidence that most of the argininosuccinate synthase and argininosuccinate lyase in intact liver is located just outside the mitochondrial outer membrane, confirming the findings of our previous biochemical work.

Localization of argininosuccinate lyase mRNA

The immunocytochemical findings just described raised compelling questions regarding the cellular mechanisms whereby this localization is accomplished. To address this, *in situ* reverse transcription-PCR studies at the electron microscope level were performed (N.S. Cohen, unpublished work), using a method based on those currently in use for paraffin sections [51]. This work used thin sections from the liver of a rat fed a 60% protein diet for 8 days; levels of argininosuccinate lyase mRNA in liver have been shown to increase about 6-fold under these conditions [52]. The liver was fixed in 4% paraformaldehyde/0.1% glutaraldehyde and embedded in Lowicryl [53]. The oligonucleotide primers targeted a region of 150 nucleotides of the coding sequence of rat argininosuccinate lyase [54]. The label employed was digoxigenin-dUTP, and it was detected with anti-digoxigenin coupled to 1 nm gold, followed by silver enhancement.

Morphometric evaluation of the electron micrographs showed that most silver grains were near the mitochondria. In controls in which reverse transcription was omitted, or the 5′ (sense) primer was used for reverse transcription, or the digoxigenin-dUTP was omitted, only small, non-localized background silver grains were observed. These results suggest that argininosuccinate lyase mRNA is located in the vicinity of mitochondria [54a]. Targeting of mRNAs for a number of cellular components of the cytoskeleton [55,56] and myofibrils [57,58] has been described in a variety of vertebrate cell models, and it has been pointed out that this is a mechanism whereby locally high concentrations of newly synthesized proteins could be achieved [59,60]. It is possible that the first step of the mechanism whereby the cytoplasmic urea cycle enzymes are organized is the targeting of the specific mRNA species to ribosomes in the vicinity of mitochondria.

Some comments

The findings that we have summarized describe a metabolic pathway within which pathway-specific intermediates are channelled from enzyme to succeeding enzyme, and from the mitochondrial matrix to the cytoplasmic compartment and back. The structural basis of the channelling appears to be the association of the urea-cycle enzymes with membranes in mitochondria and in the cytoplasmic compartment.

The evidence that the catalytic intermediates of the urea cycle are channelled in isolated rat liver mitochondria and in permeabilized hepatocytes is strong and direct; the experiments were exacting and the results unambig-uous. The immunocytochemical evidence on the location of CPS, OTC, argininosuccinate synthase and argininosuccinate lyase in liver is consistent with the requirements for channelling, in that it shows that these enzymes are adjacent to membranes in the intact liver. This suggests that channelling may occur *in vivo*, but as yet there is no direct evidence that this is the case.

As of now, channelling within the pathway of urea synthesis has been demonstrated only for carbamoyl phosphate, ornithine, citrulline, argininosuccinate and arginine. It is not known whether aspartate, HCO_3^- and NH_3 are also channelled. Meijer et al. [61] established that mitochondria are the net source of aspartate for the synthesis of argininosuccinate; this by no means implies, nor did those authors claim [61], that mitochondrial aspartate is channelled to cytoplasmic argininosuccinate.

The occurrence of channelling is not an insurmountable barrier to the net removal of intermediates. The evidence that we have described indicates that the channelling of urea-cycle intermediates is tight overall, but not leak-proof. Since these intermediates are not suicide inhibitors of the pathway enzymes, it is expected that when the rate of synthesis of an intermediate exceeds that of the utilizing enzyme, the excess compound will leak from the channel and accumulate [9,11,43]. The mere accumulation of intermediates when unphysiologically high concentrations of precursors are used (such as 10 mM ammonia, as in [62]) conveys no information about whether or not they are channelled (cf. [62]).

If channelling occurs *in vivo*, mechanisms must exist to replenish the catalytic reactants of the urea cycle, given that some loss of intermediates is bound to occur. The most likely mechanism is the net input of liver cytoplasmic ornithine arising either from dietary arginine (we have shown that arginine is readily hydrolysed outside the urea cycle in hepatocytes [43]) or from arginine synthesized in the kidney from citrulline of intestinal origin [63,64], depending on the nutritional state.

Unlike citrulline and argininosuccinate, which are reactants only in the pathways of arginine and urea synthesis, ornithine and arginine are reactants in other pathways which function in the same cellular compartment in which their channelling occurs. Questions arise, therefore, about how they are distributed among pathways. How, for example, does ornithine become available to ornithine aminotransferase in the mitochondrial matrix? Arginine is not an essential amino acid for most adult mammals; it is synthesized in the kidney from citrulline synthesized *de novo* in the intestinal mucosa [63,64] and transported to the liver, where it is available for protein and other syntheses. In view of this, it is possible that little or no arginine generated within the urea cycle escapes channelling under normal conditions.

The organization of soluble enzymes and the occurrence of channelling are factors that must be considered in quantitative analyses of kinetically regulated pathways. The possibility that the kinetic constants of enzymes differ *in situ* and in solution cannot be ignored, nor can the need to use pertinent reactant concentrations. The fact that the cytoplasmic concentration of ornithine, not its bulk concentration in the matrix, is the relevant one for OTC, is a case in point.

It is a pleasing thought that, 60 years after its discovery, the urea cycle still offers information not only about its regulation *in vivo* but about a mode of metabolic organization which may be representative of a basic feature of cells.

The rabbit antisera used for the immunocytochemical studies were generously donated by Dr. William O'Brien. Antiserum to rat liver arginase was a gift from Dr. Stephen Cederbaum. Tissue preparation and electron microscopy were done by Ms. Aileen Kuda, Department of Cell and Neurobiology, USC.

References

1. Bollman, J.L., Mann, F.C. and Magath, T.B. (1924) Am. J. Physiol. **69**, 371–392
2. Gamble, J.D. and Lehninger, A.L. (1973) J. Biol. Chem. **248**, 610–618
3. Clarke, S. (1976) J. Biol. Chem. **251**, 950–961
4. Ratner, S. (1976) Adv. Enzymol. **39**, 1–90
5. Krebs, H.A. and Henseleit, K. (1932) Hoppe-Seyler's Z. Physiol. Chem. **210**, 33–66
6. Hems, R., Ross, B.D., Berry, M.N. and Krebs, H.A. (1966) Biochem. J. **101**, 284–292
7. Krebs, H.A., Cornell, N.W., Lund, P. and Hems, R. (1974) Alfred Benzon Symp. **4**, 549–564
8. Krebs, H.A., Hems, R. and Lund, P. (1973) Adv. Enzyme Regul. **11**, 361–377
9. Cohen, N.S., Cheung, C.-W. and Raijman, L. (1980) J. Biol. Chem. **255**, 10248–10255
10. Glasgow, A.M. and Chase, H.P. (1976) Biochem. J. **156**, 301–307
11. Cohen, N.S., Cheung, C.-W., Kyan, F.S., Jones, E.E. and Raijman, L. (1982) J. Biol. Chem. **257**, 6898–6907
12. Srere, P.A. (1987) Annu. Rev. Biochem. **56**, 89–124
13. Hackenbrock, C.R. (1968) Proc. Natl. Acad. Sci. U.S.A **61**, 598–605
14. Hoppel, C.L. (1972) J. Biol. Chem. **247**, 832–841
15. Garlid, K.D. (1979) in Cell-Associated Water (Drost-Hansen, W. and Clegg, J., eds.), pp 293–361, Academic Press, New York
16. Raijman, L.R., Cohen, N.S. and Cheung, C.-W. (1991) FASEB J. **5**, 4764
17. Srere, P.A. (1981) Trends Biochem. Sci. **6**, 4–6
18. Srere, P.A. (1982) Trends Biochem. Sci. **7**, 375–378
19. Henslee, J.G. and Srere, P.A. (1979) J. Biol. Chem. **254**, 5488–5497
20. Fahien, L.A., Kmiotek, E.H., Woldegiorgis, G., Evenson, M., Shrago, E. and Marshall, M. (1985) J. Biol. Chem. **260**, 6069–6079
21. Datta, A., Merz, J.M. and Spivey, H.O. (1985) J. Biol. Chem. **260**, 15008–15012
22. McConkey, E.H. (1982) Proc. Natl. Acad. Sci. U.S.A. **79**, 3236–3240
23. Minton, A.P. and Wilf, J. (1981) Biochemistry **20**, 4821–4826
24. Minton, A.P. (1983) Mol. Cell. Biochem. **55**, 119–140
25. Raijman, L. and Jones, M.E. (1976) Arch. Biochem. Biophys. **175**, 270–278
26. Raijman, L. (1976) in The Urea Cycle (Grisolia, S., Baguena, R. and Mayor, F., eds.), pp. 243–254, John Wiley and Sons, New York
27. Cohen, N.S., Kyan, F.S., Kyan, S.S., Cheung, C.-W. and Raijman, L. (1985) Biochem. J. **229**, 205–211
28. Beliveau Carey, G., Cheung, C.-W., Cohen, N.S., Brusilow, S. and Raijman, L. (1993) Biochem. J. **292**, 241–247
29. Clegg, J.S. (1984) Am. J. Physiol. **246**, R133–R151
30. Knull, H.R. and Walsh, J.L. (1992) Curr. Top. Cell. Regul. **33**, 15–30
31. Cohen, N.S., Cheung, C.-W. and Raijman, L. (1987) J. Biol. Chem. **262**, 203–208
32. Cheung, C.-W. and Raijman, L. (1981) Arch. Biochem. Biophys. **209**, 643–649
33. Snodgrass, P.J. (1968) Biochemistry **7**, 3047–3051
34. Marshall, M. and Cohen, P.P. (1972) J. Biol. Chem. **247**, 1654–1668
35. Lusty, C.J., Jilka, R.L. and Nietsch, E.H. (1979) J. Biol. Chem. **254**, 10030–10036

36. Bradford, N.M. and McGivan, J.D. (1980) FEBS Lett. **113**, 294–298
37. Hoogenraad, N.J. (1978) Arch. Biochem. Biophys. **188**, 137–144
38. Lof, C., Cohen, M., Vermeulen, L.P., Van Roermund, C.W.T., Wanders, R.J. and Meijer, A.J. (1983) Eur. J. Biochem. **135**, 251–258
39. Cohen, N.S., Cheung, C.-W., Sijuwade, E. and Raijman, L. (1992) Biochem. J. **282**, 173–180
40. Wanders, R.J.A., Van Roermund, C.W.T. and Meijer, A.J. (1984) Eur. J. Biochem. **142**, 247–254
41. Fussle, R., Bhakdi, S., Sziegoleit, A., Tranum-Jensen, J., Kranz, T. and Wellensiek, H.J. (1981) J. Cell Biol. **91**, 83–94
42. McEwen, B.F. and Arion, W.J. (1985) J. Cell Biol. **100**, 1922–1929
43. Cheung, C.-W., Cohen, N.S. and Raijman, L. (1989) J. Biol. Chem. **264**, 4038–4044
44. Katz, J. and Wals, P.A. (1985) J. Cell. Biochem. **28**, 207–228
45. Ardail, D., Privat, J-P., Egret-Charlier, M., Levrat, C., Lerme, F. and Louisot, P. (1990) J. Biol. Chem. **265**, 18797–18802
46. Yokota, S. and Mori, M. (1986) Histochem. J. **18**, 451–457
47. Powers-Lee, S.G., Mastico, R.A. and Bendayan, M. (1987) J. Biol. Chem. **262**, 15683–15688
48. Schimke, R.T. (1962) J. Biol. Chem. **237**, 459–468
49. Geiger, B., Dutton, A.H., Tokuyasu, K.T. and Singer, S.J. (1981) J. Cell Biol. **91**, 614–628
50. Weibel, E.R. and Bolender, R.P. (1973) in Principles and Techniques of Electron Microscopy: Biological Applications (Hayat, M.A., ed.), vol. 3, pp. 239–312, Van Nostrand Reinhold, New York
51. Nuovo, G.J., Lidonnici, K., MacConnell, P. and Lane, B. (1993) Am. J. Surg. Pathol. **17**, 683–690
51a. Cohen, N.S. and Kuda, A. (1996) J. Cell. Biochem. **60**, 334–340
52. Morris, S.M., Jr., Moncman, C.L., Rand, K.D., Dizikes, G.J., Cederbaum, S.D. and O'Brien, W.E. (1987) Arch. Biochem. Biophys. **256**, 343–353
53. Fischer, D., Weisenberger, D. and Scheer, U. (1992) in Boehringer Mannheim Nonradioactive In Situ Hybridization Application Manual, pp. 56–58
54. Amaya, Y., Matsubasa, T., Takiguchi, M., Kobayashi, K., Saheki, T., Kawamoto, S. and Mori, M. (1988) J. Biochem. (Tokyo) **103**, 177–181
54a. Cohen, N.S. (1996) J. Cell. Biochem. **61**, 81–96
55. Sundell, C.L. and Singer, R.H. (1990) J. Cell Biol. **111**, 2397–2403
56. Kislauskis, E.H., Li, Z., Singer, R.H. and Taneja, K.L. (1993) J. Cell Biol. **123**, 165–172
57. Isaacs, W.B. and Fulton, A.B. (1987) Proc. Natl. Acad. Sci. U.S.A. **84**, 6174–6178
58. Morris, E.J. and Fulton, A.B. (1994) J. Cell Sci. **107**, 377–386
59. Bassell, G.J., Powers, C.M., Taneja, K.L. and Singer, R.H. (1994) J. Cell Biol. **126**, 863–876
60. Kislauskis, E.H., Zhu, X. and Singer, R.H. (1994) J. Cell Biol. **127**, 441–451
61. Meijer, A.J., Gimpel, J.A., Deleeuw, G., Tischler, M.E., Tager, J.M. and Williamson, J.R. (1978) J. Biol. Chem. **253**, 2308–2320
62. Geissler, A., Kanamori, K. and Ross, B.D. (1992) Biochem. J. **287**, 813–820
63. Windmueller, H.G. and Spaeth, A.E. (1981) Am. J. Physiol. **241**, E473–E480
64. Wakabayashi, Y. and Jones, M.E. (1983) J. Biol. Chem. **258**, 3865–3872

11

Channelling in the Krebs tricarboxylic acid cycle

Paul A. Srere*†¶, A. Dean Sherry‡§, Craig R. Malloy*‡ and Balazs Sumegi‖

*Department of Veterans Affairs Medical Center, 4500 South Lancaster Rd., Dallas, TX 75216, †Biochemistry Department and ‡Rogers NMR Center, University of Texas Southwestern Medical Center, Dallas, TX, §Chemistry Department, University of Texas at Dallas, Dallas, TX, U.S.A., and ‖Biochemistry Department, University Medical School, Pècs, Hungary

Introduction

The proposal of cycles of sequential metabolic enzymes first made by Krebs for urea biosynthesis and later for the oxidation of acetyl groups was an important conceptual innovation not only for the detailed knowledge of those particular metabolic pathways but for the conceptual simplification of many metabolic elements into that of a single entity. This affords a decrease in complexity and an increase in our ability to consider metabolic interactions. There was no associated structural idea connected with this functional insight. Krebs, however, did state "...all essential metabolic phenomena are bound to cell structure..." [1]. It was Green and his co-workers who first promulgated the idea of a structural complex of Krebs tricarboxylic acid (TCA) cycle enzymes with their studies of the cyclophorase system [2]. This putative complex of Krebs TCA cycle enzyme activities proved to be the mitochondria of the cell [3]. Subsequently the suborganellar structure of mitochondria and mitochondrial enzyme distribution were investigated, and it was demonstrated that almost all (with the exception of succinate dehydrogenase) of the Krebs TCA cycle (Fig 1) enzymes appeared as soluble entities in the matrix fraction of mitochondrial extracts. Thus the cycle activity was tacitly assumed to be the result of the activities of randomly distributed soluble enzymes within the mitochondrial matrix.

The concept of channelling of metabolic substrates is rather an old one, and evidence presented for it is found in a variety of systems, including microbial glycolysis, polyamine synthesis, amino acid metabolism, protein synthesis and nucleic acid synthesis to name a few (see [4] for a review, and also other chapters of this book).

¶*To whom correspondence should be addressed.*

The hypothesis that oxaloacetate (OAA), one substrate for citrate synthase (CS), is directly transferred to CS from mitochondrial malate dehydrogenase (mMDH) was introduced to explain some kinetic calculations on this system concerning the apparently very low concentration of OAA within the mitochondrial matrix [5]. Somewhat earlier it was realized that enzymes of the Krebs TCA cycle and of glycolysis, as well as other enzymes of major metabolic pathways, exist in their cellular spaces at quite high concentrations [6,7]. Thus, depending upon the tissue, CS could reach mitochondrial concentrations of 10^{-4}–10^{-5} M. This observation, coupled with the fact that total OAA in the matrix was measured at about 10^{-6}–10^{-5} M after one considers all the binding sites available for OAA, means the *free* OAA concentration was about 10^{-9} M. Since the K_m for OAA in the CS reaction was about 5×10^{-6} M, the rate of the CS reaction could be calculated to be at least one order of magnitude lower than the rate of the Krebs TCA cycle. One possible explanation for this apparent discrepancy was

---

Fig. 1   The Krebs TCA cycle

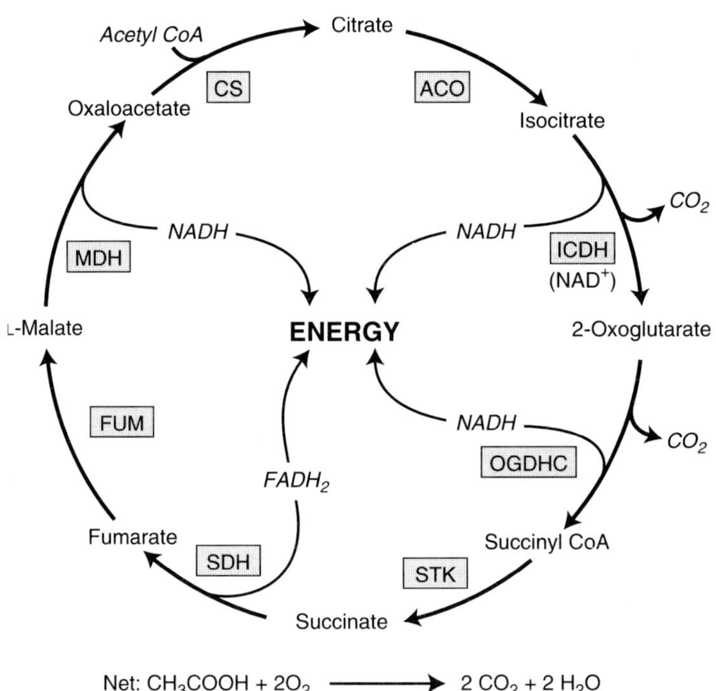

Abbreviations: ACO, aconitase; OGDHC, 2-oxoglutarate (α-ketoglutarate) dehydrogenase complex; STK, succinyl thiokinase; SDH, succinate dehydrogenase; FUM, fumarase; ICDH, isocitrate dehydrogenase; MDH, malate dehydrogenase.

that the OAA was passed directly from MDH to CS, i.e. it was out of diffusion equilibrium or, in common biochemical parlance, it was channelled. Other possible explanations for this phenomenon, such as differences in V_{max} and K_m values *in situ*, were tested and no differences between *in vitro* and *in vivo* kinetic constants for CS were found [8].

At this point the hypothesis of enzyme–enzyme interactions was tested in a number of different ways which will be discussed below. It should be remembered that interactions *per se* do not constitute either necessary or sufficient support for the channelling of Krebs TCA cycle intermediates. For the testing of channelling, different methods have been devised, and these are also described below.

Interactions of Krebs TCA cycle enzymes

Justification for approach

Fractionation of disrupted mitochondria identified the matrix compartment to be the subcellular location of the Krebs TCA cycle enzymes CS, aconitase (ACO), (NAD^+)isocitrate dehydrogenase $[(NAD^+)ICDH]$, the 2-oxoglutarate (α-ketoglutarate) dehydrogenase complex, succinyl thiokinase, succinate dehydrogenase (which is bound firmly to the inner membrane), fumarase and MDH. The consensus of experiments was that the seven enzymes (excluding succinate dehydrogenase) existed free in the mitochondrial matrix. It should be noted that several studies did appear in the literature that reported some binding of one or other of the 'soluble' enzymes to the mitochondrial membranes, but little attention was given to these results.

The low OAA concentration in mitochondrial matrices (see above) encouraged us to investigate possible complexes and interactions between enzymes of the Krebs TCA cycle. We were also persuaded to use this approach when calculations revealed that the quantity of Krebs TCA cycle enzymes correlated extremely well with the area of the inner surface of the mitochondrial inner membrane and not with the matrix volume [5]. A second important observation was that the protein concentration of the mitochondrial matrix was 50% [9]. The surface area/enzyme concentration observation would support the concept of enzyme–enzyme interactions since the Krebs TCA cycle enzymes must produce electrons for the electron transport system which is located in the mitochondrial inner membrane. One cannot get continuous oxidation in the Krebs TCA cycle without the regeneration of oxidized nucleotides by the electron transport system. Thus one can envision the existence of interactions and bindings between the dehydrogenases in the Krebs TCA cycle and the electron transport proteins of the inner membrane.

The high protein concentration of the matrix would lead to the enhancement of weak protein–protein interactions (see Chapters 2 and 3 of the current volume). Minton and his colleagues have demonstrated that, under conditions of volume exclusion that can be achieved with proteins and other polymers, activity coefficients of interacting ligands change in a way that enhances complex formation [10]. Thus, when mitochondria are disrupted in a buffer, a significant lowering of both the concentrations of the ligands and the total volume-excluding effect occurs so that interactions with a K_d of 10^{-6} M or greater would be difficult to observe in the diluted mitochondrial extract.

Interaction of consecutive enzymes

For the reasons listed above, we chose to examine the interaction of CS and MDH in the presence of the volume excluder poly(ethylene glycol). We showed that CS and mMDH would interact to form a precipitate in 14% poly(ethylene glycol). When cytosolic MDH (cMDH), serum albumin and many other proteins were substituted for mMDH, no precipitate was observed [11]. Other techniques have subsequently been employed to establish this interaction between CS and mMDH. These include a change in anisotropy of fluorescently labelled CS when titrated with mMDH [12], binding of CS to immobilized mMDH [13], and agarose gel electrophoresis [14].

Some of these techniques were used to show specific interactions between metabolically sequential enzymes of the Krebs TCA cycle. CS has been shown to interact with two auxiliary Krebs TCA cycle enzymes, the pyruvate dehydrogenase complex (PDHC) [15] and 3-oxoacyl-CoA thiolase [16]. CS also interacts with mitochondrial aconitase (mACO) [17] and with the citrate transporter [18] of mitochondrial inner membranes. Aconitase interacts with (NAD^+)ICDH but not with $(NADP^+)$ICDH [17]. (NAD^+)ICDH interacts with the 2-oxoglutarate dehydrogenase complex, which in turn interacts with succinyl thiokinase [19]. Finally, interaction of mMDH and fumarase has been shown using several techniques [13].

Fahien and his co-workers have shown that auxiliary enzymes of amino acid metabolism, which are metabolically sequential to Krebs TCA cycle enzymes, interact with the appropriate Krebs TCA cycle enzyme [20,21]. Recently Fahien has shown that the auxiliary Krebs TCA cycle enzyme pyruvate carboxylase interacts with mMDH and that this complex interacts with CS [22] (see also Chapter 16 in the current volume).

Interaction of Krebs TCA enzymes with inner membrane protein

The next level of interaction studied was that of the Krebs TCA cycle enzymes with the inner surface of the mitochondrial inner membrane. All seven of the Krebs TCA cycle enzymes bound specifically to the inner membrane [23]. Thus mMDH and mACO bound to mitochondrial inner membranes, whereas cMDH, cACO and the mitochondrial non-TCA cycle enzyme $(NADP^+)$ICDH [17] did not. The enzymes did not bind to the outer surface of the mitochondrial inner membrane, nor did they bind to liposomes made from lipids of the mitochondrial inner membrane. Similar results have been reported for the mitochondrial amino acid-metabolizing enzymes [21]. The conclusion drawn from these observations is that the Krebs TCA cycle enzymes are bound to mitochondrial inner membrane proteins exposed on the matrix side of the inner membrane.

The dehydrogenases of the Krebs TCA cycle have been shown to bind to liposomes containing Complex I [24]. In addition, cross-linking experiments have indicated that the Krebs TCA cycle enzymes are located close to the matrix surface of the mitochondrial inner membrane [25].

When mitochondria are gently sonicated, a disrupted mitochondrial preparation is obtained which is open to high-molecular-mass proteins (antibodies) and which contains most of the Krebs TCA cycle enzymes in a bound form [26]. We have termed this preparation a metabolon [27], and its kinetic characteristics are described below.

Kinetic evidence for channelling in the Krebs TCA cycle

Studies on the kinetics of the MDH/CS coupled reaction

As indicated above, the first indication that channelling may occur in the Krebs TCA cycle came from calculations of the rate *in situ* of rat liver CS ($\sim$ 0.1 μmol/min per g) compared with the QO_2 of rat liver (1 μmol/min per g). The calculated low rate of CS activity was due to the apparently low concentration of OAA in mitochondria ($< 10^{-8}$ M). This paradox could be explained if one assumed a compartmentalization of the total OAA in the microenvironment of CS. This would in effect be a channelling of OAA from MDH to CS.

The effect on the kinetics of the coupled reaction of MDH and CS was examined by immobilizing MDH and CS to Sepharose and by entrapping these enzymes in acrylamide [28]. The MDH/CS systems were studied with and without the addition of lactate dehydrogenase. The latter enzyme when included in the immobilization mixture would act by re-oxidizing the NADH formed. This addition of lactate dehydrogenase, producing a three-enzyme immobilized system, yielded the most striking kinetic results in which the transient time for the coupled immobilized system was shorter than the transient time (lag phases) of an identical system of free enzymes. Similar but not as dramatic results were seen with the immobilized two-enzyme system of CS and MDH. The decrease of transient times in such a system has been shown to be a hallmark of channelled behaviour [29].

For the immobilized enzyme systems [28], calculations of the number of enzyme molecules immobilized and the areas (or volumes in the case of bead entrapment) involved indicated that the enzymes were immobilized at a distance from each other (if random immobilization occurred) so that direct passage of OAA from site to site was improbable. If this is indeed the case, one postulated mechanism to explain the observations was that an unstirred layer effect allowed the OAA to diffuse two-dimensionally and accounted for the channelling effect.

Using a different experimental approach, Spivey and his co-workers co-precipitated MDH and CS with poly(ethylene glycol) and examined the coupled reaction of the conversion of malate into citrate [30]. The precipitated enzymes had an overall rate about one-quarter that of the enzymes in solution. To test for channelling of the intermediate OAA, an external trap of aspartate aminotransferase and glutamate was used. When added in a 100-fold excess the aspartate aminotransferase system should trap a freely diffusible OAA intermediate. When the enzymes were in solution, almost complete trapping of OAA occurred so that little or no citrate was formed. This indicated that the OAA diffused freely into the bulk medium. When the same trapping system was used with the solid-state precipitate of CS and MDH, then no decrease in citrate formation was observed. Calculations by these authors did not enable them to distinguish between a direct transfer mechanism between the two enzymes or an unstirred layer effect, but the channelling was clearly demonstrated by these experiments.

A third approach to examine the possibility of channelling of OAA from MDH to CS has recently been published [31,32]. The cDNA for yeast mitochondrial CS (CS1) was fused via a short linker (Gly-Ser-Gly) to the cDNA for yeast mMDH (MDH1). A plasmid containing this cDNA was used to transform CS⁻ *Escherichia coli* cells. The fusion protein of the C-terminus of CS1 linked to the N-terminus of MDH1 (CS1–MDH1) was overproduced by recombinant techniques in *E. coli* and isolated as a pure active soluble fusion protein. The kinetics for CS1 activity in the CS1–MDH1 fusion protein were essentially unchanged from those of CS1. The V_{max} values for the forward and reverse directions for MDH1 of pure MDH1 and of CS1–MDH1 were the same; however, the K_m values for all four substrates of MDH1 were reduced by a factor of two in the fusion protein [32].

When the fusion protein (CS1–MDH1) was compared with a free enzyme control system using the aspartate aminotransferase trap for the OAA intermediate as described by Spivey, we found that production of citrate from malate by the fusion protein system was inhibited ∼30%, whereas the system using the free enzymes was inhibited ∼75%. This therefore indicated that the intermediate OAA was not equilibrating as well with the bulk solution when fusion protein catalysed the reaction as when free enzymes were used. In addition, it was determined that the transient time for the fusion-protein-catalysed reaction is shorter than the transient time for the free-enzyme-catalysed reaction. By these two criteria the fusion protein CS1–MDH1 is channelling the intermediate OAA between the two active sites of the fusion protein. This approach eliminates the possibility of surface effects, as was possible in the immobilization and solid-state experiments, although it seems probable that the latter two approaches may be a better model for the matrix of a mitochondrion than is a pure solution model.

Tompa et al. [12] have shown that although the addition of free MDH had no effect on the free CS reaction, in the reverse case an effect was observed. They reported that, on addition of CS to a reaction in which OAA was being reduced by MDH and NADH, an increase in rate was observed that was dependent on the CS concentration.

Channelling in other reactions of the Krebs TCA cycle

Kinetic effects on other coupled TCA cycle reactions have been reported. One of the first of these studies by Sumegi et al. [15] showed that in the specific complex of PDHC and CS, the K_m for CoA in the PDHC reactions decreased from 10 μM for the free enzymes to 1.5 μM for the complex of the two enzymes. For the CS enzyme alone they reported a K_m for acetyl-CoA of 12 μM, whereas in the PDHC–CS complex the K_m for acetyl-CoA was 3 μM. One possible explanation for these results is that channelling of CoA and acetyl-CoA is occurring in the PDHC–CS complex. Förster and Staib [33] have presented evidence that PDHC in mitochondria probably interacts with some Krebs TCA cycle enzymes. This evidence was based on the non-linearity of Hill plots in the presence of C_2 and C_4 substrate analogues for PDHC substrates.

D'Souza and Srere [23] have shown that Krebs TCA cycle enzymes bind to proteins on the inner surface of the mitochondrial inner membrane (see above). These authors showed that the dehydrogenases of the Krebs TCA cycle bound to Complex I [24]. These studies were confirmed by several additional studies (see above). Fukushima et al. [34] and Ovàdi et al. [35] showed that channelling of NADH to Complex I occurred when a complex of MDH and Complex I was formed. Using the enzyme buffering technique Ushiroyama et al. [36] were able to show that direct transfer of NADH to Complex I occurred.

Three different enzyme couples of the TCA cycle have been tested for channelling using a gently sonicated mitochondrial preparation which contained bound TCA cycle enzymes [26]. The rates of coupled reactions tested were higher in the preparation containing the bound enzymes, the so-called metabolon, than in the preparations that contained unbound enzymes. The reactions of the Krebs TCA cycle that were tested in this mitochondrial preparation included (1) fumarate oxidation, which involves fumarase, MDH, Complex I and the remainder of the electron transport system [26], (2) isocitrate oxidation, which involves (NAD$^+$)ICDH, the 2-oxoglutarate dehydrogenase complex, Complex I and the electron transport system [37], and (3) malate conversion into citrate, which involves MDH and CS [26].

Still another indication that channelling may occur in the mitochondrial matrix was derived from early experiments which suggested that non-mixing pools of acetyl-CoA existed in the mitochondrion, one presumably from glucose metabolism and one being derived from fatty acid oxidation [38].

In summary, several different kinetic studies of the Krebs TCA cycle indicate that channelling of intermediates occurs. This channelling results in increased rates of reactions and reduced transient times. Westerhoff and Welch [29] have shown how important the reduced transient times can be in a long metabolic sequence which achieves new steady states rapidly.

NMR data and orientation conserved transfer (OCT) in the Krebs TCA cycle

Metabolic channelling of an intermediate can be defined as the passage of a common intermediate between two enzymes. The intermediate is localized and out of equilibrium with the bulk solution. One of the classic methods used to detect channelling is to start with a labelled substrate and determine the label in the product of the metabolic pathway being examined

---

Scheme 1   Use of radiolabelling to detect channelling

(1) $A^* \rightarrow B^* \rightarrow C^* \rightarrow D^* \rightarrow E^*$ Determine specific radioactivity of E^*

     Add unlabelled 10-fold excess of C, and if there is no channelling of C

(2) $A^* \rightarrow B^* \rightarrow C^\circ \rightarrow D^\circ \rightarrow E^\circ$ Specific radioactivity of E° is $\frac{1}{10}$ that of E^* in (1)
             $\updownarrow$
             C

     If there is complete channelling of C

(3) $A^* \rightarrow B^* \rightarrow C^* \rightarrow D^* \rightarrow E^*$ Specific radioactivity of E^* same as that of E^* in (1)
             $\nparallel$
             C

(Scheme 1). One then adds an excess of a proposed channelled intermediate and re-examines the label in the product. If complete mixing of the intermediate with the bulk solution occurs, then the label in the product will be decreased according to the relative amount of labelled intermediate compared with the added unlabelled intermediate. If complete channelling of the intermediate occurs, then the label in the product will be unaffected by the added unlabelled intermediate (Scheme 1).

Of course, it is possible to obtain results intermediate between these two examples. The experiment can also be performed using an exogenous labelled intermediate and unlabelled substrates and observing the label in the product. No channelling in this case would yield a highly labelled product, and complete channelling would yield a product with decreased label.

There are several other experimental methods that can be used to identify a channelled reactant (see also Chapters 4–6 in the current volume). One of these depends on measuring the transient time in the sequence of reactions in which channelling may be occurring. A decrease in transient time is indicative of a channelled pathway. In some instances there is an increase in the rate of a coupled immobilized system over that of a system where the enzymes are free in solution (see above). In terms of kinetics, channelling would be indicated in a sequence of reactions where the total concentration of an intermediate(s) is lower than that which would be necessary to attain the rates that are observed. However, by computer modelling one can find specific conditions where this latter statement is not true.

Orientation conserved transfer (OCT)

It has been known for many years that metabolism of asymmetrical Krebs TCA cycle intermediates results in a phenomenon loosely termed 'scrambling', or randomization of the carbon atoms in these intermediates. This means, for example, that *methyl*-^{13}C-labelled acetyl-CoA yields 2-[4-^{13}C]oxoglutarate followed by [3-^{13}C]succinyl-CoA and succinate labelled in its methylene carbon. Succinate is an achiral symmetrical molecule, so if it is allowed to be free in a bulk solution then rotational diffusion, which is rapid, would lead to binding by succinate dehydrogenase of both

---

Scheme 2   **Rotational diffusion of succinate**

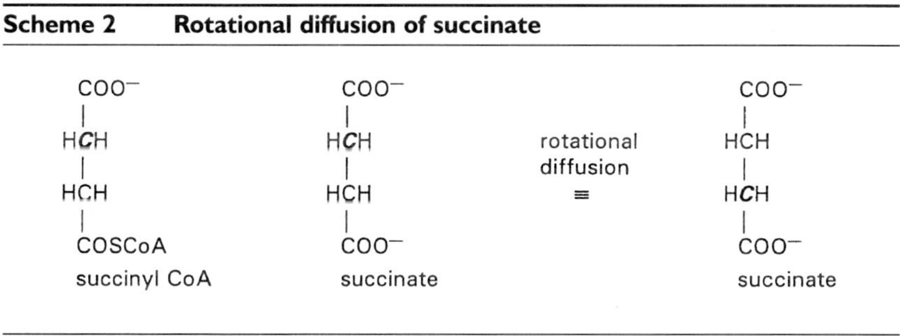

See the text for details.

---

orientations (Scheme 2). Fumarase would then add water stereospecifically to fumarate to produce two differently labelled malates (Scheme 3). Thus both of the methylene carbons appear to be labelled but, as a matter of fact, in a single turn of the Krebs TCA cycle, individual molecules have only a single

Scheme 3   Production of malate from fumarate

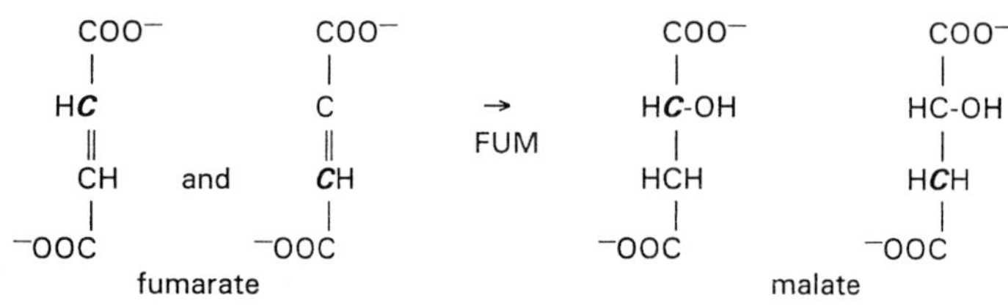

FUM, fumarase. See the text for details.

labelled methylene carbon. After one turn of the cycle, a difference in the enrichment of C-2 relative to C-3 of malate would suggest OCT. Equal labelling after numerous turns of the cycle (i.e. as it approaches steady state) might be interpreted as evidence favouring full randomization. Indeed, over the years a host of experiments of many different types using labelled Krebs TCA cycle intermediates and following their incorporation into other metabolites, such as glucose, indicated that C-2 and C-3 in malate were equally enriched [39–41]. The problem is, as explained above, that the OCT pathway (Fig. 2) also provides a mechanism for equal labelling in C-2 and C-3. Thus, in experiments where the label enters as acetyl-CoA on each turn and whose duration is longer than several turns of the cycle, the observation of 'scrambled' carbons does not distinguish between the OCT pathway and randomization.

Bernhard and Tompa [42] were the first to attempt to detect OCT in the Krebs TCA cycle. They incubated [5-^{13}C]glutamate with rat liver mitochondria and after 10 min showed that equal ^{13}C labelling appeared in C-1 and C-4 of aspartate. They concluded that this ruled out OCT. It would appear from their metabolic data that their mitochondria were severely damaged, since O_2 consumption decreased rapidly from the beginning of the experiment.

Sumegi et al. [43] used labelled [3-^{13}C]propionate in yeast cells to test for OCT. Since in most cells propionate is metabolized through the Krebs TCA cycle, a singly labelled propionate could be introduced into the Krebs TCA cycle as singly labelled succinyl-CoA using the pathway shown (Fig. 3A). In these experiments little aspartate was observed, but alanine was found as a product obtained from succinate, as shown in Fig. 3(B). If one started with either [3-^{13}C]propionate or [2-^{13}C]propionate and molecular rotation occurred at the succinate and fumarate level, then both the C-2 and C-3 of alanine should be equally labelled. If the pathway were as shown in Fig. 3 and little or no molecular rotation of either succinate or fumarate occurred (i.e. OCT), then the ^{13}C-3/^{13}C-2 ratio of alanine would differ from 1 depending upon which labelled propionate was used. The direction of deviation of this ratio from unity would depend on the stereochemistry of the addition of water in the fumarase step. It was found that when [3-^{13}C]propionate is used the [3-^{13}C]alanine/[2-^{13}C]alanine ratio is greater than 1, and when [2-^{13}C]propionate is used this ratio is less than 1. Thus OCT appears to be occurring in the mitochondria of yeast cells under these conditions.

In the initial experiments using [3-^{13}C]propionate the C-3/C-2 ratio of ^{13}C alanine was 2.4. When 50 mM malonate (an inhibitor of succinate dehydrogenase) was added, the ratio decreased to 1.3. When Sumegi et al. [43] used [3-^{13}C]propionate in a quinone-deficient yeast strain the C-3/C-2 ratio in ^{13}C alanine was 1.0; on addition of quinone to the deficient yeast cells this ratio increased to 1.8. Thus in two separate ways the proper operation of the Krebs TCA cycle was shown to be necessary for experimental results which indicated OCT of symmetrical intermediates in yeast cells.

Fig. 2   **Transfer of Krebs cycle intermediates**

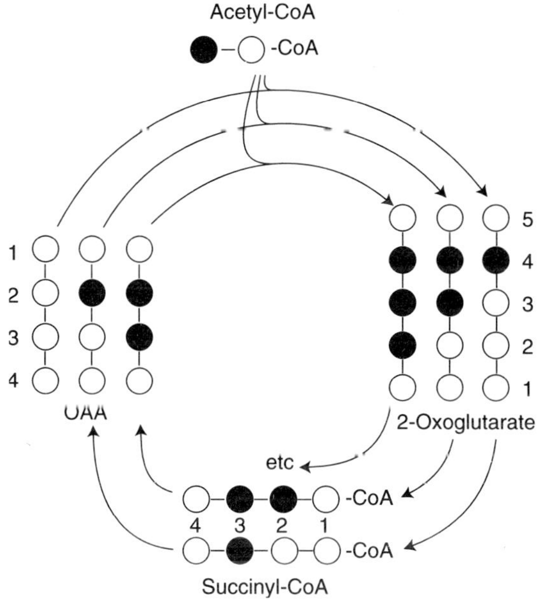

Schematic diagram which illustrates that the fractional ^{13}C enrichment of glutamate C-2 and C-3 becomes equal after three turns through the cycle pools if the symmetrical intermediates are passed from one enzyme to another via orientation 1. Note that the number of turns required to achieve equal enrichment would increase if the ^{13}C enrichment of the acetyl-CoA methyl carbon was not 100 and the pool sizes were not infinitesimally small. The figure illustrates that the glutamate C-3/C-2 ratio would be < 1 only very early during isotopic turnover. Reprinted with permission from [47].

Subsequent to the appearance of the paper by Sumegi et al. [43], two letters appeared in *Trends in Biochemical Science* which objected to the interpretation of channelling [44,45]. The two main objections were: (1) earlier data showed randomization, and (2) a possible direct conversion of

---

Fig. 3   **Conversion of propionate into alanine**

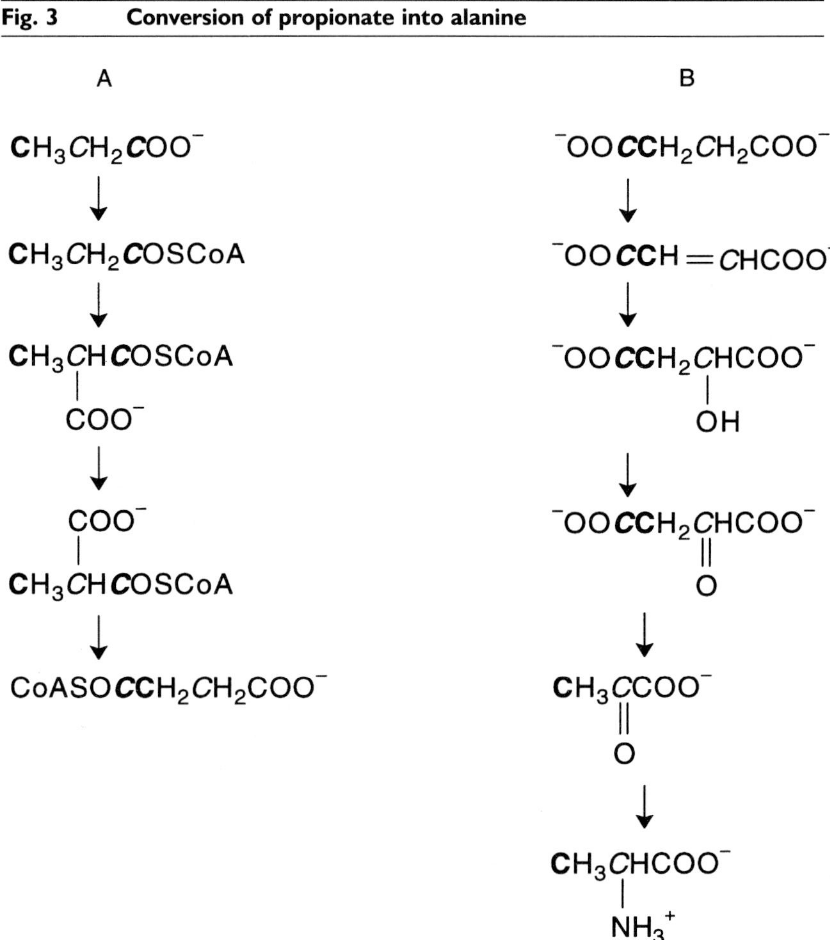

The propionate carbons are labelled as follows: C-1 = **C** (bold and italics); C-2 = C (italics); C-3 = **C** (bold). (A) The conversion of propionate into succinyl-CoA through methylmalonate. It can be seen that the relative position of C-1 is changed in the B_{12}-catalysed mutase reaction. (B) The conversion of the labelled succinate from (A) into alanine. The original C-1 of propionate is lost in the conversion of oxalacetate into pyruvate. The C-3 of propionate and the C-2 of propionate maintain their relative positions as the C-3 and C-2 of alanine in this pathway. It should be noted that if C-1-, C-2- and C-3-labelled propionate is used, alanine labelled at only C-2 and C-3 is obtained. This means that if ^{13}C labelling is used the resonance of C-2 of propionate yields a quartet and its product, the C-2 of alanine, yields a doublet (see the text).

propionate into pyruvate was not considered. We have already answered point 1 (see above), and the published paper and other papers negate the second possibility of a direct pathway. This point will be discussed later in this chapter.

In a second paper by Sumegi et al. [46], the study of channelling and OCT in yeast was expanded by using substrates other than propionate. In the first set of experiments, [4-^{13}C]glutamate was incubated with yeast cells and the ^{13}C resonances in C-2 and C-3 of aspartate were observed. If the OCT and the stereochemistry observed in the propionate occurred with glutamate, one would expect a C-2/C-3 ratio of ^{13}C in aspartate ratio greater than 1. In two experiments ratios of 1.4 and 1.1 were observed. When fluoroacetate was added to the yeast strain in order to slow the Krebs TCA cycle, then the ratios were increased to 1.5 and 1.8. In another experiment [2-^{13}C]acetate was used as the carbon source in yeast, and again the C-2/C-3 ratio of ^{13}C in aspartate was examined; a ratio of 1.5 was found at 2 min, which decreased to 1.0 after 10 min.

Thus in yeast the metabolism of singly labelled substrates showed asymmetrical labelling in products derived from labelled acetate, glutamate and propionate. The asymmetrical labelling was shown to be dependent on efficient running of the Krebs TCA cycle and was time-dependent.

In another series of experiments, Sherry et al. [47] used [2-^{13}C]-, [3-^{13}C]- and [1,2,3-^{13}C]propionate in mammalian tissues. Once again asymmetrical labelling in lactate, alanine and aspartate was seen using 2-^{13}C- and 3-^{13}C-labelled propionate, thus supporting the yeast data which indicated a lack of randomization in the Krebs TCA cycle. This was confirmed when [1,2,3-^{13}C]propionate was used in perfused rat liver. The NMR spectrum of metabolites derived from this compound provides more information than with singly labelled propionate. If the conversion occurred through a direct propionate conversion, then the lactate obtained would be mainly [1,2,3-^{13}C]lactate, with some [2,3-^{13}C]lactate possible after multiple turns of the cycle. In this case the NMR spectrum would show a larger quartet (from the [1,2,3-^{13}C]lactate) and a smaller doublet (from [2,3-^{13}C]lactate) in the C-2 resonance of lactate. If propionate is oxidized through the Krebs TCA cycle with randomization, one would see 50% [1,2,3-^{13}C]lactate and 50% [2,3-^{13}C]lactate. If, however, OCT occurs with the same orientation as shown by singly labelled propionates, then one would see more [2,3-^{13}C]lactate than [1,2,3-^{13}C]lactate. Thus it is possible to distinguish between direct conversion, Krebs TCA cycle with randomization and Krebs TCA cycle with OCT. In a series of experiments the doublet seen in lactate C-2 was always greater than the quartet in perfused liver extracts, in perfusates from perfused livers and in hepatocytes.

The temporal dependence of ^{13}C appearing in glutamate C-3 versus C-2 and in glutamate C-4 versus C-3 was also monitored at 3 min in hearts perfused with [2-^{13}C]acetate. These area ratios were 2.0 and 2.1 respectively. Both ratios progressively decreased towards 1.0 with time, and in the steady state glutamate C-2, C-3 and C-4 were equally labelled. When the temperature of perfusion was lowered in an attempt to slow Krebs TCA cycle activity, then the C-2/C-3 ratio of ^{13}C of glutamate was increased.

These data for mammalian tissues are consistent with the data obtained in yeast cells. [1,2,3-^{13}C]Propionate provides a novel way of distinguishing between OCT and randomization in the Krebs TCA cycle.

In studies of glioma cell metabolism of [1-^{13}C]glucose, Portais et al. [48] concluded that channelling occurred in the Krebs TCA cycle in the succinyl-CoA/succinate/fumarate part of the cycle, confirming the results of Sumegi et al. [46] and Sherry et al. [47]. However, the stereochemistry of the addition of water to fumarate to form malate catalysed by fumarase was opposite to that reported for yeast, rat liver and rat heart.

In a series of papers studying the Krebs TCA cycle in humans, Magnusson et al. [49] and Schumann et al. [50] used [3-^{14}C]lactate and [2-^{14}C]acetate. They measured the ^{14}C content of each carbon of glutamate and glucose. No asymmetry in the labelling of the carbons of these two compounds was observed, and these workers concluded that no channelling of Krebs TCA intermediates occurred in the human liver. However, all of their experiments were long term and, as indicated above, no differentiation can be made between OCT and randomization in the Krebs TCA cycle in long-term experiments.

In a recent paper, Landau et al. [51] used [^{14}C]propionate in humans to examine hepatic metabolism. They analysed the ^{14}C distribution in glucose and glutamate in order to study gluconeogenesis and Krebs TCA cycle flux. One of their conclusions was that there was no channelling of succinyl-CoA in liver mitochondria. These results are in disagreement with the studies of propionate metabolism in liver reported by Sherry et al. [47]. However, the two studies differed in one important aspect: one used tracer quantities of propionate whereas the other used quantities which contributed significantly to the net production of glucose and glutamate. No conclusions can be drawn from these differences at the present time.

Let us now consider the possibility that the results of propionate metabolism indicating OCT reflect direct conversion of propionate into pyruvate. In yeast there are two points that are relevant to this possible explanation. A pathway known as the methylcitrate cycle (Fig. 4) has been described in *Saccharomyces cerevesiae* under conditions of growth on glucose and propionate [52]. Also it was reported that yeasts do not contain co-B$_{12}$ or the methylmalonyl-CoA mutase enzyme [53]. However, we have found considerable quantities of B$_{12}$ in our yeast cells (P.A. Srere and B. Sumegi, unpublished work) and in the absence of B$_{12}$ and HCO$_3$, two requirements of Krebs TCA cycle utilization of propionate, no propionate metabolism occurs (P.A. Srere, A.D. Sherry, C.R. Malloy and B. Sumegi, unpublished work).

The ^{13}C NMR data in yeast show that the asymmetry observed from propionate to alanine is dependent upon Krebs TCA cycle activity. Even if there was a secondary dependence on Krebs TCA cycle activity for the direct conversion pathway, it would be impossible to explain why the asymmetry disappears. In any direct pathway the amount of asymmetry should remain constant; only the amount of conversion should change.

Similar arguments apply to the propionate data in mammalian tissues. However, no direct pathway for the conversion of propionate into pyruvate has ever been described in mammals. We also know that these tissues contain the enzymes necessary for propionate conversion into succinyl-CoA. In addition, the experiment in mammalian tissue with [1,2,3-^{13}C]propionate provides an independent and sensitive test for distinguishing between OCT and randomization in the Krebs TCA cycle.

Fig. 4   The methylcitric acid cycle of propionate metabolism

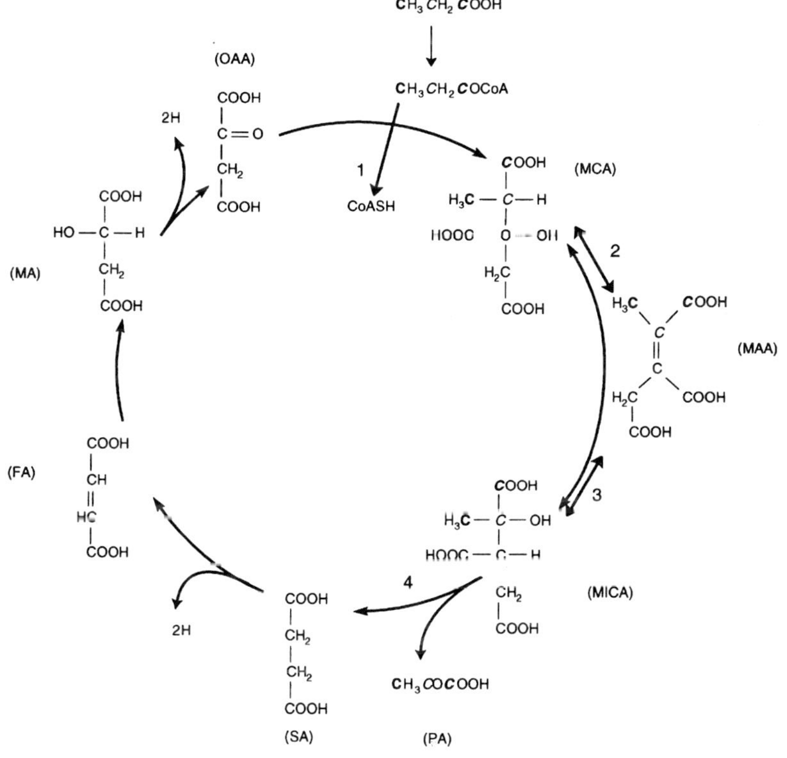

Carbons are labelled as follows: C-1 = **C** (bold and italics); C-2 = C (italics); C-3 = **C** (bold). Enzymes: 1, methylcitrate synthase; 2, methylcitrate dehydratase; 3, methylisocitrate dehydratase; 4, methylisocitrate lyase. Abbreviations: FA, fumarate; MA, malate; MAA, methylaconitate; MCA, methylcitrate; MICA, methylisocitrate; PA, pyruvate; SA, succinate.

Conclusions

It has recently been noted that [54], in spite of all the evidence to the contrary, biochemists consider the reactions of metabolism in a linear fashion. In addition, in spite of all the evidence there is continued thinking about the cell and its reactions as a 'bag of enzymes'. It does not seem likely, if in fact the metabolic pathways of cells are organized in fluctuating channelled pathways, that any important insights will come from overly simplistic metabolic models.

The evidence reviewed in this chapter indicates by several different experimental approaches that channelling does exist in the Krebs TCA cycle. The metabolic importance of these observations in intact animals remains to be examined.

We thank Penny Kerby for manuscript preparation and colleagues who are cited in references herein. This work was supported by grants from the Department of Veterans Affairs (P.A.S. and C.R.M.), the National Science Foundation (MCB-9117385) (P.A.S.), the NIH National Center for Research Resources (P41–02584) (C.R.M.), and NIH grant RO1-HL34557 (A.D.S.).

References

1. Krebs, H.A. and Henseleit, K. (1932) Z. Physiol. Chem. **210**, 33–66
2. Green, D. (1949) Sci. Am. **181**, 48–50
3. Kennedy, E.P. and Lehninger, A.L. (1949) J. Biol. Chem. **179**, 957–972
4. Srere, P.A. (1987) Annu. Rev. Biochem. **56**, 89–124
5. Srere, P.A. (1972) in Energy Metabolism and the Regulation of Metabolic Processes in Mitochondria (Mehlman, M.A. and Hanson, R.W., eds.), pp. 79–91, Academic Press, New York
6. Srere, P.A. (1967) Science **158**, 936–937
7. Srere, P.A. (1970) Biochem. Med. **4**, 43–46
8. Matlib, A.M., Finkelstein, M.B., and Srere, P.A. (1978) Arch. Biochem. Biophys. **191**, 426–430
9. Hackenbrock, C.R. (1968) Proc. Natl. Acad. Sci. U.S.A. **61**, 598–605
10. Zimmerman, S.B. and Minton, A.P. (1993) Annu. Rev. Biophys. Biomol. Struct. **22**, 27–65
11. Halper, L.A. and Srere, P.A. (1977) Arch. Biochem. Biophys. **184**, 529–534
12. Tompa, P., Batke, J., Ovádi, J., Welch, G.R. and Srere, P.A. (1987) J. Biol. Chem. **262**, 6089–6092
13. Beeckman, S. and Kanarek, L. (1981) Eur. J. Biochem. **117**, 527–535
14. Ashmarina, L.I., Pshezhetsky, A.V., Spivey, H.O. and Potier, M. (1994) Anal. Biochem. **219**, 349–355
15. Sumegi, B., Gyocsi, L. and Alkonyi, I. (1980) Biochim. Biophys. Acta **616**, 158–166
16. Sumegi, B., Gilbert, H.F. and Srere, P.A. (1985) J. Biol. Chem. **260**, 188–190
17. Tyiska, R.L., Williams, J.S., Brent, L.G., Hudson, A.P., Clark, B.J., Robinson, J.B., Jr. and Srere, P.A. (1986) NATO Ser. **127**, 177–189
18. Persson, L.-O. and Srere, P.A. (1992) Biochem. Biophys. Res. Commun. **183**, 70–76
19. Porpaczy, Z., Sumegi, B., and Alkonyi, I. (1983) Biochim. Biophys. Acta **749**, 172–179

20. Fahien, L.A., Kmiotek, E.H., MacDonald, M.J., Fibich, B. and Mandic, M. (1988) J. Biol. Chem. **263**, 10687–10697
21. Fahien, L.A., MacDonald, M.J., Teller, J.K., Fibich, B. and Fahien, C.M. (1989) J. Biol. Chem. **264**, 12303–12312
22. Fahien, L.A., Davis, J.W. and Laboy, J. (1993) J. Biol. Chem. **268**, 17935–17942
23. D'Souza, S.F. and Srere, P.A. (1983) J. Biol. Chem. **258**, 4706–4709
24. Sumegi, B. and Srere, P.A. (1984) J. Biol. Chem. **259**, 15040–15045
25. D'Souza, S.F. and Srere, P.A. (1983) Biochim. Biophys. Acta **724**, 40–51
26. Robinson, J.B., Jr. and Srere, P.A. (1985) J. Biol. Chem. **262**, 10800–10805
27. Srere, P.A. (1985) Trends Biochem. Sci. **10**, 109–110
28. Srere, P.A., Mattiasson, B. and Mosbach, K. (1973) Proc. Natl. Acad. Sci. U.S.A. **70**, 2534–2538
29. Westerhoff, H.V. and Welch, G.R. (1992) Curr. Top. Cell. Regul. **33**, 361–390
30. Datta, A., Merz, J.M. and Spivey, H.O. (1985) J. Biol. Chem. **260**, 15008–15012
31. Lindbladh, C., Brodeur, R.D., Small, W.C., Lilius, G., Bülow, L., Mosbach, K. and Srere, P.A. (1994) Biochemistry **33**, 11684–11691
32. Lindbladh, C., Rault, M., Hagglund, C., Small, W.C., Mosbach, K., Bülow, L., Evans, C. and Srere, P.A. (1994) Biochemistry **33**, 11692–11698
33. Förster, M. and Staib, W. (1990) Int. J. Biochem. **22**, 773–778
34. Fukushima, T., Decker, R.V., Anderson, W.M. and Spivey, H.O. (1989) J. Biol. Chem. **264**, 16483–16488
35. Ovàdi, J., Huang, Y. and Spivey, H.O. (1994) J. Mol. Recognit. **7**, 265–272
36. Ushiroyama, T., Fukushima, T., Styre, J.D. and Spivey, H.O. (1992) Curr. Top. Cell. Regul. **33**, 291–307
37. Sumegi, B., Porpaczy, Z., McCammon, M.T., Sherry, A.D., Malloy, C.R. and Srere, P.A. (1992) Curr. Top. Cell. Regul. **33**, 249–260
38. Von Glutz, G. and Walter, P. (1975) Eur. J. Biochem. **60**, 147–152
39. Lorber, V., Lifson, V., Sakami, W. and Wood, H.G. (1950) J. Biol. Chem. **183**, 531–538
40. Grunnet, N. and Katz, J. (1978) Biochem. J. **172**, 595–603
41. Badar-Goffer, R.S., Bachelard, H.S. and Morris, P.G. (1990) Biochem. J. **266**, 133–139
42. Bernhard, S.A. and Tompa, P. (1990) Arch. Biochem. Biophys. **276**, 191–198
43. Sumegi, B., Sherry, A.D. and Malloy, C.R. (1990) Biochemistry **29**, 9106–9110
44. Shulman, R.J. (1991) Trends Biochem. Sci. **16**, 171
45. Rognstad, R. (1991) Trends Biochem. Sci. **16**, 172
46. Sumegi, B., Sherry, A.D., Malloy, C.R. and Srere, P.A. (1993) Biochemistry **32**, 12725–12729
47. Sherry, A.D., Sumegi, B., Miller, B., Cottam, G.L., Gavva, S., Jones, J.G. and Malloy, C.R. (1994) Biochemistry **33**, 6268–6275
48. Portais, J.-C, Schuster, R., Merle, M. and Canioni, P. (1993) Eur. J. Biochem. **217**, 457–468
49. Magnusson, I., Schumann, W.C., Bartsch, G.E., Chandramouli, V., Kumaran, K., Wahren, J. and Landau, B.R. (1991) J. Biol. Chem. **266**, 6975–6984
50. Schumann, W.C., Magnusson, I., Chandramouli, V., Kumaran, K., Wahren, J. and Landau, B.R. (1991) J. Biol. Chem. **266**, 6985–6990
51. Landau, B.R., Schumann, W.C., Chandramouli, V., Magnusson, I., Kumaran, K. and Wahren, J. (1993) Am. J. Physiol **265**, E636–E647
52. Pronk, J.T., van der Linden-Beuman, A., Verduyn, C., Scheffers, W.A. and van Dijken, J.P. (1994) Microbiology **140**, 717–722
53. Ledley, F.D., Crane, A.M., Klish, K.T. and May, G.S. (1991) Biochem. Biophys. Res. Commun. **177**, 1076–1081
54. Buxbaum, R.E. (1995) Nature (London) **373**, 567–568

12

Kinetic advantages of multienzyme complexes involving aminotransferases

Leonard A. Fahien*‡ and Michal C. Chobanian†

Departments of *Pharmacology and †Pediatrics, University of Wisconsin Medical School, Madison, WI 53706, U.S.A.

Introduction

Mitochondrial aspartate aminotransferase (AspAT) catalyses the reactions:

Glutamate + AspAT-PLP $\rightleftharpoons$ AspAT-PMP + 2-oxoglutarate

OAA + AspAT-PMP $\rightleftharpoons$ AspAT-PLP + aspartate

where AspAT-PLP and AspAT-PMP are the pyridoxal-phosphate and pyridoxamine-phosphate forms respectively of the aminotransferase, and OAA is oxaloacetate. The enzyme is important because of the pivotal position in metabolism of its substrates and products and the ability of these compounds to enter many pathways of metabolism. A rather unique feature of the AspAT reaction in intact liver mitochondria is that the free concentration of the substrate OAA has been estimated to be only 0.04 μM [1], and in the mitochondria of most organs the concentrations of AspAT and a major supplier of OAA, malate dehydrogenase (MDH), are both high, respectively, and considerably higher than the concentration of OAA [1–3]. In addition, the reaction in liver mitochondria is not readily reversible; Duszynski et al. [4] found that the aspartate generated readily enters the cytosol, where it functions as a metabolic precursor of glucose and/or urea. In the mitochondria of most organs, glutamate generated by glutaminase and glutamate itself primarily reacts with AspAT instead of glutamate dehydrogenase (GDH) [5]. This is because of the higher concentrations of AspAT than GDH activity, the unfavourable K_{eq} of the GDH compared with the AspAT reaction and the marked inhibition of GDH by its products H^+, NADH and the 2-oxoglutarate generated by AspAT [6–8a]. In this chapter we will present evidence that AspAT forms multienzyme complexes with other enzymes that have shared substrates or products, and describe kinetic advantages of these interactions. We will also discuss the consequences of these interactions in

‡*To whom correspondence should be addressed.*

regulating the production of ammonia, glucose and urea, and in regulating acid–base homoeostasis.

Association of mitochondrial AspAT with other enzymes and with the mitochondrial inner membrane (IMM)

In 1969 we found that pure AspAT readily associates with pure GDH [9]. Since that time, interactions between several other mitochondrial enzymes which are functionally related or share a common substrate have been demonstrated [1,2,9–29]. Organization of mitochondrial enzymes might be especially favoured by the dehydrated state (0.7 g of protein per ml of water [30]) of the matrix, which results in the mitochondrial concentrations of some enzymes being orders of magnitude higher than their K_D values in heteroenzyme complexes [2]. Another factor favouring organization in mitochondria is that some enzymes can associate with both specific sites on the IMM and other enzymes in the matrix [22,26,31–34]. Sumegi and Srere [31] and Fukushima et al. [33] found that Complex I provides the binding site for several mitochondrial dehydrogenases, and we have purified an IMM protein which apparently functions as the IMM binding site for AspAT [34].

In addition to associating with GDH, which has a molecular mass of at least 340 kDa [35], AspAT associated with pyruvate carboxylase (PC) and the 2-oxoglutarate (α-ketoglutarate) dehydrogenase complex (OGDHC), which are also high-molecular-mass mitochondrial enzymes that have a substrate or product in common with AspAT [2,10,11,25,26,36–39]. Carbamoyl phosphate synthase I (CPS) and the pyruvate dehydrogenase complex (PDHC) were exceptions in that they are high-molecular-mass mitochondrial enzymes which associated with AspAT but do not have a substrate or product in common with it. However, the interaction between AspAT and PDHC would not be expected to hinder the interaction between AspAT and GDH, OGDHC, PC or CPS in liver mitochondria, where the concentration of PDHC is only 0.3 μM compared with considerably higher concentrations of GDH, OGDHC, PC and CPS [2]. AspAT did not associate with other high-molecular-mass mitochondrial enzymes (fumarase, ornithine transcarbamylase) without a common substrate. AspAT associated only weakly with low-molecular-mass enzymes with a common substrate [citrate synthase (CS), MDH], and did not associate at all with any of the other mitochondrial or cytosolic enzymes tested [2,10,11,21,25,26,36–39].

Binding of GDH, OGDHC, CPS and PC to AspAT was also specific in that PC and CPS did not associate with each other and also did not associate with GDH or OGDHC [2,10,11,21,25,26,36–39]. However, we found that GDH had a high affinity for OGDHC [2,10], and others [31,33] found that OGDHC had a high affinity for Complex I. GDH, OGDHC, PC and CPS either did not associate at all with any of the other proteins tested, or in the few cases where there was an interaction, it was considerably weaker than the interaction with AspAT [2,21,25,26]. An exception was that PC also associated with MDH [36].

The methods used by us and others to study these heteroenzyme complexes included: (1) finding that the enzyme pairs had a considerably higher molecular mass, as measured by light scattering, than the sum of the molecular masses of each enzyme alone; (2) cross-linking the enzyme pairs with a 12 Å bridge-length cross-linker; (3) co-sedimenting the enzyme pairs; (4) finding that one enzyme altered the fluorescence of a fluorescent probe attached to a second enzyme; (5) use of a gel filtration equilibrium method; and (6) co-precipitation of the enzymes in the presence of poly(ethylene glycol) (PEG) [2,10,21,25,26,38–43].

We measured the numbers of binding sites (n) and the dissociation constants (K_D) of binary complexes between AspAT and PC, OGDHC, CPS or GDH by titrating one enzyme against another in PEG [2]. This is a valid method because, under the conditions employed, an equilibrium concentration of heteroenzyme complex was formed rapidly (the concentration was the same at 2 min as at 20 min). Furthermore, it has been shown by Sumegi and Alkonyi [44] and us [34] that the exact same K_D and n values can be obtained in similar systems in the presence and absence of PEG. We also calculated the concentrations of these enzymes in liver mitochondria [2] using the ratio of the specific activity of the enzyme in the mitochondrial extract (prepared using several different methods) with the specific activity of the pure enzyme and a previously obtained value of 1 μl of mitochondrial water per mg of mitochondrial protein [30,45]. These calculations were consistent with AspAT, GDH, OGDHC, PC and CPS concentrations of 140, 70, 2, 18 and 400 μM respectively in liver mitochondria [2]. By multiplying the enzyme concentration by the value of n, it was found that the concentration of AspAT-binding sites in liver mitochondria on these four high-molecular-mass enzymes would be over two times higher than the concentration of AspAT (140 μM). In addition, we found that the concentrations of AspAT and AspAT-binding enzymes were considerably higher than the K_Ds of the heteroenzyme complexes with AspAT, which were 0.5, 0.1, 0.01 and 0.4 μM with CPS, GDH, PC and OGDHC respectively. Therefore, in liver mitochondria, these binary complexes would be expected to be stable, and there would be a more than adequate concentration of AspAT-binding sites to accommodate all of the AspAT.

LaNoue's group [4] found that aspartate generated by AspAT is transported out of liver mitochondria without mixing with the aspartate in the matrix, indicating that the AspAT is localized in the vicinity of the IMM. This is consistent with our experiments [26,34], which demonstrated that the inverted IMM has a high affinity (K_D 1 μM) and capacity (8 nmol of AspAT bound per mg of IMM protein) for AspAT. Furthermore, other enzymes which have a high affinity for the IMM, such as CS and fumarase, did not inhibit binding of AspAT to the IMM [34]. AspAT decreased binding of MDH to the IMM, but the reverse was not the case.

Although membrane lipids facilitated binding of AspAT to the IMM, a specific protein also played a role. We solubilized an IMM protein which had a high affinity for AspAT. This protein, which had a molecular mass of 45 kDa, was purified on a Sephacryl S-300 column, followed by further purification on an AspAT affinity column. MDH did not associate with this protein but, unlike AspAT, MDH associated with high-molecular-mass fractions from the Sephacryl column, which also contained Complex I activity. Others [31] found that, on the intact IMM, Complex I provided the binding site for MDH, whereas we [34] found that AspAT readily dissociated MDH from the IMM, indicating that the AspAT-binding protein is in close proximity to Complex I on the IMM.

Others [31,33] found that OGDHC associates with isolated Complex I and the IMM. The number of OGDHC- and AspAT-binding sites on the IMM was found to be sufficiently high and the K_Ds of both of these enzymes for the IMM sufficiently low so that a large fraction of AspAT and AspAT/OGDHC could be associated with their respective binding sites on the IMM. In addition, AspAT could be localized in the vicinity of the IMM as a result of OGDHC associating with Complex I and AspAT associating with the IMM-bound OGDHC. Either structure could facilitate the delivery of NADH from OGDHC to Complex I (as has been demonstrated *in vitro* [33]) and the delivery of aspartate from AspAT through the mitochondrial membrane and into the cytosol (as has been demonstrated in intact mitochondria [4]).

Addition of MDH to heteroenzyme complexes

The heteroenzyme complexes which contain AspAT would be rather inactive without a supply of OAA for AspAT. MDH is a mitochondrial enzyme which can supply OAA to AspAT [5,46]. However, in mitochondria the transfer of OAA from MDH to AspAT probably requires that these two enzymes are in close proximity to each other. This is because, at physiological pH, the equilibrium of the MDH reaction is quite unfavourable [47] and MDH has a high affinity for OAA [29]. Thus, since we found the concentration of OAA-binding sites on MDH to be 280 μM in liver mitochondria [2], a significant fraction of the OAA generated by MDH would remain bound to MDH. In addition, the concentration of free OAA is only 0.04 μM [1] in liver mitochondria, considerably lower than the concentration of matrix proteins which bind OAA [48–50]. Consequently there would be a high concentration of OAA-binding sites in competition with AspAT for OAA. The requirement of enzymes which generate or react with OAA to be in close proximity to each other could be why MDH has been found by others to associate with [1] and channel [17] OAA into CS, and why we [36] found that PC can associate with either MDH or AspAT.

We [2,10] found that MDH neither readily associates with nor channels OAA to AspAT. Therefore there are probably some mitochondrial structures which can associate simultaneously with both MDH and AspAT and thus place these two enzymes in close proximity to each other. The IMM could not fulfil this role, since others [33] found that 0.1–1.0 mM NAD^+ or malate facilitates the dissociation of MDH from Complex I, and we found that AspAT, citrate and high ionic strength dissociate MDH from the IMM [26,34]. However, we found that, although MDH does not have a high affinity for OGDHC, GDH or CPS, MDH readily associates with complexes between these high-molecular-mass enzymes and AspAT without displacing AspAT [2,10,11]. Consequently AspAT and MDH could be in close proximity to each other in these ternary complexes. In the presence of AspAT, the K_{DS} of MDH for GDH and OGDHC were 0.3 μM and 1.2 μM respectively, and GDH and OGDHC had 1 and 10 MDH binding sites respectively. Therefore, since the concentrations of MDH, GDH and OGDHC were found to be 140, 70 and 2 μM respectively in liver mitochondria, a significant fraction of the total mitochondrial MDH could be incorporated into these complexes [?]

Binding of MDH to complexes between AspAT and these high-molecular-mass enzymes was specific. With the exception of PC, and to a much lesser extent CS, other proteins tested did not associate with MDH. Other proteins tested also did not associate with binary complexes between AspAT and GDH, OGDHC or CPS [2,10,11,36].

GDH probably plays the major role in liver mitochondria in placing MDH in close proximity to AspAT. This is because GDH has a higher affinity than CPS for AspAT, and in liver mitochondria the concentration of GDH is considerably higher than that of OGDHC [2]. Furthermore, formation of the MDH–GDH–AspAT complex does not exclude PC, OGDHC or CPS from MDH and AspAT, since MDH–GDH–AspAT was found to associate with PC, OGDHC or CPS [2,10,21,36]. Association of PC with MDH–GDH–AspAT might be the only way that PC could be in close proximity to both MDH and AspAT, since AspAT decreased binding of MDH to PC, rather than enhancing it. However, although PC did not associate with GDH, it associated with AspAT–GDH, and MDH associated with PC–AspAT–GDH [36]. Quaternary complexes of these types could be formed, as the supporting enzymes are large. Thus one subunit of the AspAT dimer could associate with one and the other subunit could associate with the other high-molecular-mass supporting enzyme. This might enhance the affinity of one or the other supporting enzyme for MDH. We [26,34] found that GDH and NAD^+–MDH do not readily associate with the IMM. However, as shown in Fig 1, these two enzymes could be localized in the vicinity of the IMM as a result of GDH associating with AspAT–OGDHC–IMM and NAD^+–MDH then associating with the bound GDH.

All of the heteroenzyme interactions described above were stable in the presence of even higher than physiological concentrations of the substrates of the component enzymes [2,11,25,26,51,52] (physiological concentrations were obtained from the data of [53]) and thus, as discussed below, the complexes are catalytically active. One exception was high concentrations of 2-oxoglutarate, which inhibited binding of MDH to AspAT–OGDHC. However, this could be a feedback type of inhibition so that, when the concentration of 2-oxoglutarate is sufficiently high to supply OGDHC, generation of 2-oxoglutarate from the combined MDH–AspAT reaction would not be required.

Physiological concentrations of Mg^{2+} promoted dissociation of AspAT from its IMM site, but did not alter the interaction between OGDHC and AspAT [11,26,34]. Thus Mg^{2+} would favour AspAT assoc-

---

Fig. 1   **Organization of AspAT in liver mitochondria**

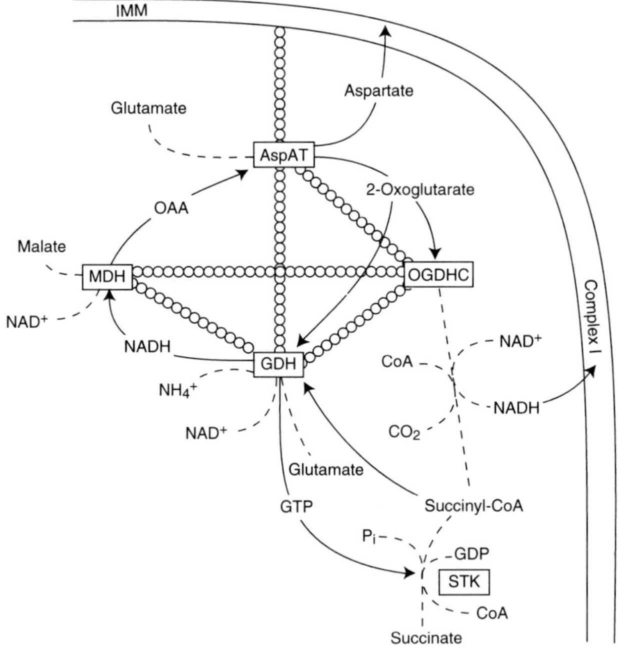

Aspects depicted are the association of AspAT with the IMM or OGDHC, which in turn is associated with Complex I. This permits facilitated transfers of aspartate and 2-oxoglutarate from AspAT to the cytosol and OGDHC respectively, and the facilitated transfer of NADH from OGDHC to Complex I. Also depicted are the binding of MDH and GDH to AspAT–OGDHC. This permits the facilitated transfer of oxaloacetate from MDH to AspAT and of NADH between GDH and MDH. The facilitated transfer of GTP from GDH to succinate thiokinase is also shown. The latter, which is not discussed in the text, results in GTP (a potent inhibitor of GDH) being replaced on GDH by succinyl-CoA (an activator of GDH [10]).

iating with OGDHC–IMM over binding of AspAT to the IMM in the vicinity of OGDHC. Mg^{2+} could also promote formation of MDH–GDH–AspAT–OGDHC–IMM, since we [26,34] found that Mg^{2+} favoured formation of GDH–AspAT, which provides a binding site for NAD^+–MDH.

Although 2-oxoglutarate and Mg^{2+} were found to weaken some of the bonds of the heteroenzyme system, it is unlikely that they would completely dissociate the organized system of enzymes, for the following reasons: (a) not all of the bonds were dissociated by 2-oxoglutarate or Mg^{2+} [2,11,34]; (b) the experiments were performed with concentrations of the pure enzymes in the range of the K_D of the enzyme complexes, while *in vivo* the concentration of enzyme can be two orders of magnitude higher [2]; and (c) ligands would not be expected to markedly physically displace one enzyme from the vicinity of another enzyme because of the slow diffusion rate of an enzyme in the mitochondrial matrix [50]. Ligands could, however, enable the system to be flexible and dynamic enough to undergo the necessary ultrastructural transformations [54].

The heteroenzyme interactions described above were found to be specific. With the exception of the interactions noted below, other proteins tested did not interact with CPS, PC, GDH, OGDHC, MDH, AspAT, AspAT–GDH, AspAT–CPS, AspAT–MDH–OGDHC or AspAT–GDH–MDH [2,10,11,26,34,37,51]. Halper and Srere [1] and we [51] found that CS associates with MDH and AspAT. Also, OGDHC was found by Porpaczy et al. [12,14] to associate with succinate thiokinase and with (NAD^+)isocitrate dehydrogenase, while we [11] found OGDHC to associate with CS. However, in liver mitochondria these complexes would be expected to be less abundant than those described above, since we found that they were weaker *in vitro* [2,11], and the concentrations of these enzymes in liver [CS (25 μM), succinate thiokinase (60 μM) and (NAD^+)isocitrate dehydrogenase (4 μM)] would be too low to displace the enzymes in complexes with AspAT described above. Other known heteroenzyme interactions with high-molecular-mass enzymes, such as ornithine transcarbamylase–CPS [19], GDH–alanine aminotransferase [55] and GDH–thiolase [24], would not be expected to inhibit binding of AspAT to GDH or binding of MDH to AspAT–GDH or AspAT–CPS, as in liver the mitochondrial concentrations of ornithine transcarbamylase (34 μM), alanine aminotransferase (8 μM) and thiolase (40 μM) are considerably lower than the concentrations of CPS (400 μM) and GDH (70 μM).

Facilitated transfer of OAA from MDH to AspAT by 2-OGDHC

We found that when malate oxidation by MDH (0.1 μg/ml) was coupled with glutamate plus an excess of AspAT (2 μg/ml), the addition of low (16 μg/ml) concentrations of OGDHC activated the MDH reaction as a result of markedly decreasing the K_m of malate. The V_{max} and K_m values of NAD$^+$ were not altered [11]. OGDHC was not active catalytically in these assays, which were performed in the absence of CoA. Therefore, in agreement with direct binding experiments which demonstrated that AspAT can associate with OGDHC and that MDH can associate with AspAT–OGDHC, these kinetic results indicate that OGDHC can play a structural role by placing MDH and AspAT in close proximity to each other so that a transfer of OAA from MDH to AspAT is facilitated (Fig. 2).

The MDH reaction is known to be an ordered Bi-Bi reaction [56,57], as shown in Fig. 2. The additional steps shown in Fig. 2 are binding of the complex between AspAT-PMP (E_2') and OGDHC (E_3) to the NADH–MDH–OAA complex (QE_1P), followed by the OAA bound to MDH reacting with AspAT-PMP within the trienzyme complex ($QE_1RE_2E_3$) to yield aspartate (R) plus PLP-AspAT. In this reaction, AspAT-PMP could either react directly with OAA bound to MDH or enhance dissociation of OAA from MDH so that OAA can react with AspAT-PMP before it leaves the heteroenzyme system. After this reaction, the NADH–MDH complex (E_1Q) dissociates from the trienzyme complex and PMP–AspAT–OGDHC ($E_2'E_3$) is regenerated, as depicted in and discussed in the legend to Fig. 2. The steady-state rate equation for this mechanism in the absence of $E_2'E_3$ and the presence of saturating concentrations of $E_2'E_3$ are shown in eqns (1) and (2) respectively of Fig. 3. In these equations, v is the initial velocity of the MDH reaction, E_{1t} is the total concentration of MDH catalytic sites and the other terms are those shown in Fig. 2. In deriving these equations it was assumed that the concentrations of NADH and OAA together would be too low to reverse the reaction and that the concentration of aspartate would be low compared with its product inhibition constants. The latter would be expected to be the case in the vicinity of the heteroenzyme complex in intact mitochondria, since aspartate generated by AspAT readily enters the cytosol [4]. For this reason, the term $k_{12}[RE_2E_3]$ was also considered to be equal to zero. The steps involving the dissociation of 2-oxoglutarate from or binding of glutamate to AspAT free of MDH were also omitted because AspAT was in excess over MDH; consequently these steps would not influence MDH activity. Terms containing $k_5 + k_7$ were converted to k_5 because it is known [56,57] that k_7 is the rate constant for the rate-limiting step in the MDH reaction (dissociation of NADH from MDH). Similarly, terms containing $k_7 + k_{11}$ were converted to k_{11} because the V_{max} of the MDH reaction was not altered by OGDHC, indicating that k_7 is also rate-limiting in the heteroenzyme system and low compared with k_{11} (the rate constant for dissociation of the NADH–MDH complex from the trienzyme complex).

According to eqns. (1) and (2), and consistent with experimental results, the heteroenzyme interactions shown in Fig. 2 would not alter the K_m of NAD$^+$, since this equals k_7/k_1 in both the presence and the absence of OGDHC. However, in the absence of heteroenzyme interactions the K_m of malate equals $k_7(k_4 + k_5)/k_3k_5$, compared with k_7/k_3 in the presence of

Fig. 2   Activation of MDH activity by the AspAT–OGDHC complex

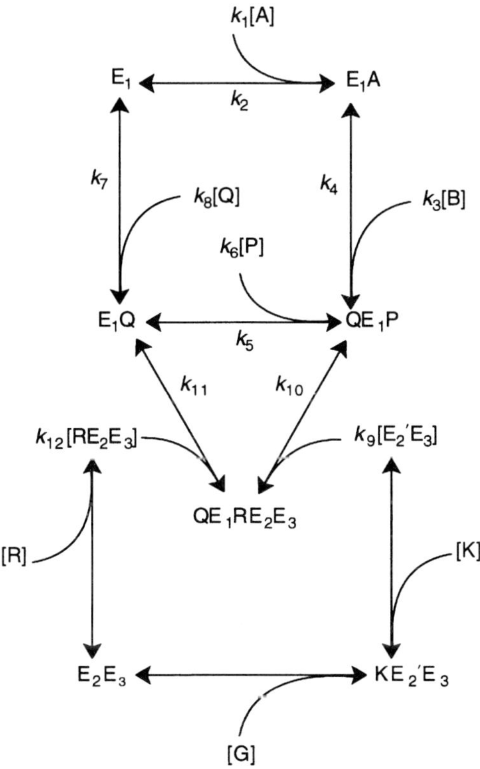

Depicted is the classical MDH (E_1) Bi-Bi reaction, where NAD$^+$ (A) adds to MDH before malate (B), and OAA (P) dissociates from MDH before NADH (Q). The additional steps are binding of AspAT-PMP–OGDHC ($E_2'E_3$) to NADH–MDH–OAA (QE$_1$P) followed by the OAA bound to MDH reacting with AspAT-PMP within the trienzyme complex to yield aspartate (R) plus AspAT-PLP. NADH–MDH (E_1Q) then dissociates from the trienzyme system and aspartate dissociates from AspAT-PLP–OGDHC (E_2E_3). AspAT-PMP–OGDHC is then rejuvenated by glutamate (G) reacting with AspAT-PLP–OGDHC followed (in the absence of CoA) by 2 oxoglutarate (K) dissociating from AspAT-PMP–OGDHC. Although AspAT–OGDHC can associate with free MDH, NAD$^+$–MDH and NADH–MDH, only binding of AspAT–OGDHC to NADH MDH OAA is shown. This is because in these assays, which are discussed in the text, the concentration of AspAT-PMP–OGDHC is sufficiently high so that it only associates with NADH–MDH–OAA, a complex which has an extremely high affinity for AspAT-PMP–OGDHC.

heteroenzyme interactions. The rate constant for the dissociation of malate from the NAD$^+$–MDH complex (k_4) is much higher than the rate constant of dissociation of OAA from the NADH–MDH–OAA complex (k_5) [36]. Thus the K_m of malate in the absence of heteroenzyme interaction is higher by a factor of k_4/k_5 than in its presence. Therefore OGDHC, by playing an

Fig. 3   **Steady-state rate equations for the mechanism shown in Fig. 2**

Absence of E_2E_3

$$\frac{\vartheta}{[E_{1t}]} = \frac{k_7}{1 + \dfrac{k_7}{k_1[A]} + \dfrac{k_7(k_4+k_5)}{k_3k_5[B]} + \dfrac{k_2k_7(k_4+k_5)}{k_1k_3k_5[A][B]} + \dfrac{k_2k_4k_6[P]}{k_1k_3k_5[A][B]} + \dfrac{k_6[P]}{k_5} + \dfrac{k_4k_6[P]}{k_3k_5[B]} + \dfrac{k_2k_8(k_4+k_5)[Q]}{k_1k_3k_5[A][B]} + \dfrac{k_8[Q]}{k_1[A]}} \tag{1}$$

Saturation of E_2E_3

$$\frac{\vartheta}{[E_{1t}]} = \frac{k_7}{1 + \dfrac{k_7}{k_1[A]} + \dfrac{k_7}{k_3[B]} + \dfrac{k_2k_7}{k_1k_3[A][B]} + \dfrac{k_6[P]}{k_{11}} + \dfrac{k_2k_4[P]}{k_1k_3[A][B]} + \dfrac{k_8[Q]}{k_1[A]}} \tag{2}$$

Eqn. (1) is the equation for the MDH reaction in the absence of AspAT–OGDHC. Eqn. (2) is the equation for the case when the concentration of AspAT-PMP–OGDHC is sufficiently high to saturate NADH–MDH–OAA. The rate constants are those for the steps in the mechanism shown in Fig. 2. The terms [A], [B], [P] and [Q] are the concentrations of NAD^+, malate, OAA and NADH respectively. The terms v and E_{1t} refer to the initial velocity of the MDH reaction and the total concentration of MDH active sites respectively. The simplifications used in deriving these equations are given in the text.

organizational role, markedly decreases the K_m of malate and provides a channelling mechanism for the transfer of OAA from MDH to AspAT.

Also according to eqns. (1) and (2) in Fig. 3, heteroenzyme interaction as a result of bypassing the dissociation of OAA from free MDH markedly decreases product inhibition of the MDH reaction by OAA. In the presence of heteroenzyme interaction (eqn. 2), product-inhibition terms involving the concentration of OAA plus malate or OAA plus NAD^+ and malate are eliminated. Also, the term $k_6[P]/k_5$ in eqn. (1) is replaced by the term $k_6[P]/k_{11}$ in eqn. 2. As mentioned above, at physiological pH k_5 is quite low, and the specific activity of pure MDH with malate as a substrate is much lower than that of pure AspAT with glutamate as a substrate. Therefore k_{11} must be considerably higher than k_5, which would further diminish product inhibition of the heteroenzyme system by OAA.

The concentrations of the MDH dimer, AspAT dimer and OGDHC oligomer used in these experiments were 1.4, 20 and 6 nM respectively, indicating that PMP–AspAT–OGDHC has a high affinity for NADH–MDH–OAA.

Facilitated transfer of 2-oxoglutarate from AspAT to 2-OGDHC or GDH

AspAT-PMP was found to inhibit both OGDHC and GDH when added to assays of these dehydrogenases with low (20 μM) concentrations of

2-oxoglutarate. However, inhibition was much less than expected on the basis of the V_{max} and K_m values of free 2-oxoglutarate in the OGDHC and GDH reactions and the ability of 2-oxoglutarate to associate and react with AspAT-PMP [10]. Thus when OGDHC or GDH is bound to AspAT-PMP they can apparently react directly with 2-oxoglutarate bound to AspAT-PMP. Another possible explanation is that binding of OGDHC or GDH to AspAT-PMP facilitates dissociation of 2-oxoglutarate from AspAT-PMP, so that 2-oxoglutarate can react with GDH or OGDHC without having to diffuse from the heteroenzyme complex. In the case of GDH (OGDHC was not tested), both of these possibilities would also be consistent with stopped-flow experiments performed by Salerno et al. [58]. However, when similar kinetic experiments were performed by adding AspAT-PMP to assays of MDH with a low (20 μM) concentration of OAA, inhibition by AspAT-PMP was exactly as predicted on the basis of the V_{max} and K_m values of free OAA in the MDH reaction and the ability of OAA to associate and react with AspAT-PMP [10]. Thus, as discussed in the preceding section, facilitated transfer of OAA between MDH and AspAT would require binding of both MDH and AspAT to OGDHC or GDH so that MDH and AspAT could be in close proximity to each other.

The facilitated transfer of 2-oxoglutarate from AspAT to GDH or OGDHC discussed above indicates that the coupled reaction between AspAT and GDH or OGDHC could take place as shown in Fig. 4. That is, in addition to the classical aminotransferase Ping-Pong mechanism [59], the complex between GDH or OGDHC and their substrates (E_2X) would associate with AspAT-PMP–2-oxoglutarate. This would be followed by conversion of 2-oxoglutarate into compound G, which is glutamate when E_2 is GDH and succinyl-CoA when E_2 is OGDHC.

The steady-state rate equation for the mechanism shown in Fig. 4 (again derived for the case when the concentration of aspartate is low and the term $k_{12}[GE_2Y]$ equals zero) reveals that a significant advantage of catalysis by the heteroenzyme system is that bypassing dissociation of 2-oxoglutarate from the aminotransferase results in a complete elimination from the denominator of the rate equation of product-inhibition terms which contain [2-oxoglutarate]/[glutamate][OAA]. This is a quite significant factor because the K_m and K_D values of glutamate and OAA are both considerably higher than their physiological concentrations in mitochondria [1,6,36,60]. Consequently, in mitochondria, 2-oxoglutarate is a potent inhibitor of free AspAT [5,8,8a]. However, when AspAT is in a complex with OGDHC or GDH, inhibition of AspAT by 2-oxoglutarate would be markedly diminished at the same time that OGDHC and GDH are being supplied directly with 2-oxoglutarate.

In liver mitochondria the concentrations of glutamate and AspAT are so high that the functional concentration of AspAT-PMP–2-oxoglutarate could be 200 μM, whereas the K_D of AspAT–OGDHC is no higher than 0.4 μM [2,10]. Since the K_m of free 2-oxoglutarate is 20–80 μM (depending on conditions), a quite high concentration of free 2-oxoglutarate would be required for it to compete successfully with AspAT-PMP–2-oxoglutarate for OGDHC. Consequently the heteroenzyme system could be the preferred pathway for the delivery of 2-oxoglutarate from AspAT to OGDHC in liver mitochondria. When GDH is also associated with MDH–AspAT–OGDHC, the facilitated transfer of 2-oxoglutarate from AspAT to GDH would inhibit ammonia production by GDH. However, we [10] also found a facilitated transfer of NADH from GDH to MDH. Consequently, when PC is the source of OAA, and MDH is reacting with and competing with AspAT for the limiting concentrations of free OAA, ammonia production would be enhanced as a result of less 2-oxoglutarate production by AspAT (which would relieve GDH of product inhibition by 2-oxoglutarate) and a facilitated transfer of NADH from GDH to MDH (which would relieve GDH of product inhibition by NADH). Thus, since CPS can also associate with MDH–GDH–AspAT, it would be localized in liver mitochondria, where ammonia production is regulated by heteroenzyme interaction.

Fig. 4   Catalysis of the coupled reactions between AspAT and GDH or OGDHC

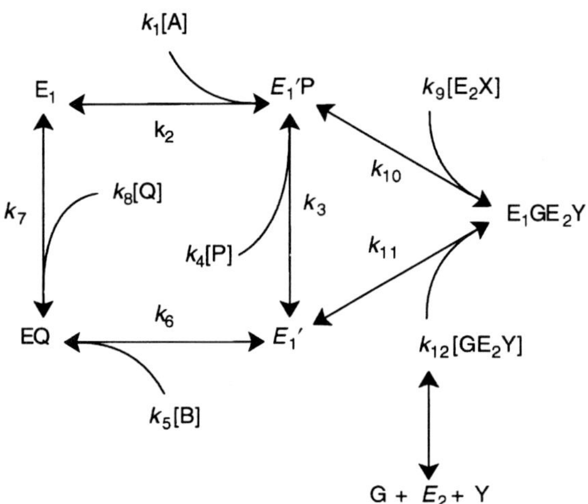

Depicted is the classical AspAT Ping-Pong reaction where glutamate (A) adds to AspAT-PLP (E_1), followed by dissociation of 2-oxoglutarate (P) from AspAT-PMP [E_1'], binding of OAA (B) to AspAT-PMP and dissociation of aspartate (Q) from AspAT-PLP. The additional steps are binding of either NADPH–GDH–NH_4^+ or NAD^+–OGDHC–CoA (E_2X) to AspAT-PMP–2-oxoglutarate ($E_1'P$). In the resultant bienzyme complex, 2-oxoglutarate is then either reductively aminated when GDH is E_2 or undergoes oxidative decarboxylation when OGDHC is E_2. This is followed by dissociation of AspAT-PMP from the bienzyme complex and regeneration of E_2. When E_2 is GDH, G is glutamate and Y is $NADP^+$. When E_2 is OGDHC, G is succinyl-CoA and Y is $NADH + CO_2$.

The facilitated transfers mentioned above have a high probability of occurring and being significant in liver mitochondria for the following reasons: (a) the concentrations of interacting enzymes are considerably higher than required for interactions *in vitro* [2]; (b) the mitochondrial concentrations of active sites of the donating enzyme would be sufficiently high compared with the concentration of the transferred product and the receiving enzyme, so that a significant amount of product could be transferred within the heteroenzyme complex [2,48]; (c) the heteroenzyme complexes are stable in the presence of substrates and products [2,10,11,26] and thus the complex between the donating enzyme and its product would not have to diffuse to the receiving enzyme; and (d) all of these transfers would decrease the potent product inhibition of the donating enzyme. Furthermore, with the possible exception of the transfer of 2-oxoglutarate from AspAT to OGDHC, the turnover rate of the pure donating enzyme is considerably lower than that of the pure receiving enzyme [2], and the final product of the receiving enzyme has a much lower affinity for the heteroenzyme system than the transferred product of the donating enzyme [48,56,57,60,61]. Thus the receiving enzyme could rapidly convert a potent product inhibitor of the donating enzyme into a product which readily dissociates from the heteroenzyme system.

Facilitated transfers in intact mitochondria

As mentioned above, the concentration of AspAT in liver mitochondria is about 140 μM, which is 70-fold higher than the concentration of OGDHC and orders of magnitude higher than the K_D of the complex between pure AspAT and pure OGDHC. Thus it would be expected that in liver mitochondria essentially all of the OGDHC would be associated with AspAT, and OGDHC might react preferentially with 2-oxoglutarate bound to AspAT instead of free 2-oxoglutarate. This has been found to be the case by LaNoue's group [7,8,8a]. In experiments performed by adding both [^{3}H]glutamate and 2-[^{14}C]oxoglutarate to intact liver mitochondria, it was found that although transport of 2-oxoglutarate into the mitochondria was not rate limiting, OGDHC used 2-oxoglutarate generated within the mitochondria by transamination in preference to transported 2-oxoglutarate. This was the case even when the fractional ^{3}H specific radioactivity of the ultimate products of the OGDHC reaction (malate and succinate) was quite high compared with the fractional specific radioactivity of intramitochondria 2-oxoglutarate generated from [^{3}H]glutamate, indicating a clear preference of OGDHC for 2-oxoglutarate generated by transamination. Furthermore, although H$^+$ ions activated isolated liver OGDHC, they inhibited 2-oxoglutarate flux through OGDHC in liver mitochondria, indicating that H$^+$ inhibits AspAT–OGDHC.

When LaNoue's group performed the same type of experiments with kidney mitochondria, it was found that 2-[^{3}H]oxoglutarate flux through OGDHC represented a much smaller proportion of total OGDHC flux, the fractional ^{3}H specific radioactivity of malate and succinate compared with that of intramitochondria 2-oxoglutarate generated from [^{3}H]glutamate was considerably lower, and H$^+$ enhanced 2-oxoglutarate flux through OGDHC. This is apparently because in kidney mitochondria the amount of OGDHC is 7-fold higher and the amount of AspAT almost 2-fold lower than in liver mitochondria [2,7]. Therefore in kidney mitochondria a significant amount of OGDHC could be free of AspAT. Consequently, when kidney mitochondria were incubated with AspAT, thus increasing the concentration of the enzyme, it was found that H$^+$ changed from an activator into an inhibitor of OGDHC flux [7].

Physiological advantages of multienzyme complexes

Ammonia metabolism in both mammalian kidney and liver is involved in systemic, organ and cellular acid–base metabolism. The link between the two organs and the ammonia pathway is the metabolic fate of L-glutamine. When an animal is provided with an acid load either naturally in the diet or unnaturally by administering HCl, L-glutamine availability to the kidney increases, and that to the liver decreases. This complementary response is essential for acid to be neutralized and excreted in that bicarbonate, the main systemic buffer, must be reabsorbed, reclaimed and regenerated. This is accomplished by processes involving both organs, with L-glutamine metabolism as the common link. The primacy of the kidney's role in this process over that of the liver is moot, considering the importance of both organs in the disposal of acid equivalents and the maintenance of systemic pH [62].

At normal physiological pH, the liver both produces and extracts L-glutamine [63]. If the substrate is delivered to phosphate-dependent glutaminase (PDG), either urea or another amino acid is generated. Conversely, the liver can convert ammonia into either urea or amino acids, including L-glutamine [64]. It is well established that liver PDG can be activated consistently by ammonium ions, alkaline pH or directly by bicarbonate [65–68]. Extraction of L-glutamine under normal physiological conditions has been found by some, but not all, investigators [69–74]. When an acid load is introduced to an animal, the extraction of L-glutamine or its production by the liver can be altered. These findings are consistent in either an acute or a chronic acidic state [69–76]. Furthermore, these effects can be attributed directly to low pH inhibiting both L-glutamine uptake [63,77] and PDG inactivation [65,78] in liver mitochondria. As the studies of LaNoue's group [7,8] suggest, in liver mitochondria acidosis decreases OGDHC flux, leading to increased concentrations of 2-oxoglutarate and inhibition of AspAT, GDH and PDG by 2-oxoglutarate. This results in decreased gluconeogenesis and ureagenesis (secondary to decreased aspartate and ammonia production), and reduced CPS activity. Reduced CPS activity would in turn result in HCO_3^- being spared in order to buffer H^+.

The response of the kidney to a change in systemic pH involves both acute and chronic adaptations. A fall in systemic pH leads to a fall in cellular pH and, in turn, acts as the primary signal to enhance ammonia production in the renal proximal tubule. The enzymic response to this fall in pH involves increasing PDG activity and L-glutamine uptake into the mitochondria [84–86]. However, acute changes, in contrast to chronic ones, cannot be accounted for solely by those involving PDG or L-glutamine transport. A consistent finding with an acute fall in systemic or cellular pH is a decline in both glutamate and 2-oxoglutarate concentrations in the kidney cortex [87,88]. As stated previously, these findings are a result of the activation of free OGDHC (decreased K_m) by a fall in the kidney mitochondrial pH, which increases the flux of 2-oxoglutarate to succinate [89]. This is turn would cause a fall in the mitochondrial 2-oxoglutarate concentration and relieve GDH, AspAT and PDG of inhibition by 2-oxoglutarate. The increase in the rate of glutamate deamination and transamination results in a fall in the mitochondrial glutamate concentration [90]. Hypothetically, then, a fall in pH is the primary signal to stimulate deamination and transamination of glutamate from the PDG reaction, ultimately resulting in enhanced ammonia and glucose production. Chronic adaptation to a fall in pH has firmly established mitochondrial glutamine transport/deamidation as a key regulatory site [91]. Whether glutamate is preferentially channelled to GDH in chronic acidosis [92] remains to be determined. Beyond the GDH reaction, mitochondrial concentrations of 2-oxoglutarate fall chronically, as they do acutely, in response to a decrease in pH. However, this change is insufficient to fully explain the adaptation to chronic acidosis, as flux through OGDHC remains high in mitochondria isolated from acidotic rats and incubated at normal pH with high 2-oxoglutarate concentrations [93]. Increased conversion of 2-oxoglutarate into succinate as a result of an acute fall in pH appears to be the potential mechanism for this adaptation [89,92,94].

Because of the importance of determining the fate of the L-glutamine carbon skeleton in acidosis and its association with increased glucose production, many investigations have focused upon the tricarboxylic acid (TCA) cycle as a regulatory site [79]. A common inhibition of ammonium production from L-glutamine occurs when most TCA cycle intermediates or precursors are added to the incubation medium. The likely point of inhibition involves a change in metabolites within the mitochondria at the level of 2-oxoglutarate or glutamate. When inhibitors of TCA cycle enzymes or mitochondrial substrate transporters are used, metabolites accumulate and negatively or positively influence ammonia production [80,81,95]. These reactions also apply in principle to actions of polypeptide hormones upon renal ammonia metabolism [80,81] and, in turn, can be influenced by changes in intracellular calcium, as well as pH. We and others have shown that nearly all polypeptide hormones enhance ammonia production independent of glucose metabolism, but remain tightly coupled to changes in intracellular pH or Ca^{2+} [80,81,83,96–100]. Because OGDHC is known to be activated by H^+ and Ca^{2+} and the control of ammonia metabolism by hormones can be mediated in part by changes in pH or Ca^{2+}, it is appealing to propose that hormonal regulation of ammoniagenesis occurs at the level of OGDHC [7,8,100] and involves the channelling of 2-oxoglutarate from AspAT. Therefore it would appear that understanding the roles that multienzyme complexes involving aminotransferases play in regulating acid–base metabolism and its de-regulation in diabetes mellitus, starvation, the cachexia of cancers, burns or sepsis is most critical.

References

1. Halper, L.A. and Srere, P.A. (1977) Arch. Biochem. Biophys. **184**, 529–534
2. Fahien, L.A. and Teller, J.K. (1992) J. Biol. Chem. **267**, 10411–10422
3. Pette, D., Klingenberg, M. and Bücher, T.H. (1962) Biochem. Biophys. Res. Commun. **7**, 425–431
4. Duszynski, J., Mueller, G. and LaNoue, K. (1978) J. Biol. Chem. **253**, 6149–6157
5. Wanders, R.J.A., Meijer, A.J., Green, A.K. and Tager, J.M. (1983) Eur. J. Biochem. **133**, 245–254
6. Fahien, L.A. and Strmecki, M. (1969) Arch. Biochem. Biophys. **130**, 456–467
7. Smith, B.C., Hyatt, D.L., Cheung, J.Y. and LaNoue, K.F. (1994) Contrib. Nephrol. **110**, 158–169
8. Smith, B.C., Clotfelter, L.A., Cheung, J.Y. and LaNoue, K.F. (1992) Biochem. J. **204**, 819–826
8a. Strzelecki, T., Strzelecka, D., Koch, C.D. and LaNoue, K.F. (1988) Arch. Biochem. Biophys. **264**, 310–320
9. Fahien, L.A. and Smith, S.E. (1969) Arch. Biochem. Biophys. **135**, 136–151
10. Fahien, L.A., MacDonald, M.J., Teller, J.K., Fibich, B. and Fahien, C.M. (1989) J. Biol. Chem. **264**, 12303–12312
11. Fahien, L.A., Kmiotek, E.H., MacDonald, M.J., Fibich, B. and Mandic, M. (1988) J. Biol. Chem. **263**, 10687–10697
12. Porpaczy, Z., Sumegi, B. and Alkonyi, I. (1987) J. Biol. Chem. **262**, 9509–9514
13. Beeckmans, S. and Kanarek, L. (1981) in The Organization of Cell Metabolism (Welch, G.R. and Srere, P.A., eds.), pp. 199–208, Plenum Press, New York and London
14. Porpaczy, Z., Sumegi, B. and Alkonyi, I. (1983) Biochim. Biophys. Acta **749**, 172–179
15. Sumegi, B., Gyocsi, L. and Alkonyi, I. (1980) Biochim. Biophys. Acta **616**, 158–166
16. Sumegi, B., Gilbert, H.F. and Srere, P.A. (1985) J. Biol. Chem. **260**, 188–190
17. Merz, J.M., Webster, T.A., Appleman, J.R., Manley, E.R., You, H.A., Datta, A., Ackerson, B.J. and Spivey, H.O. (1987) Arch. Biochem. Biophys. **258**, 132–142
18. D'Souza, S.F. and Srere, P.A. (1983) Biochim. Biophys. Acta **724**, 40–51
19. Powers-Lee, S.G., Mastico, R.A. and Bendayan, M. (1987) J. Biol. Chem. **262**, 15683–15688
20. Cheung, G.W., Cohen, N.S. and Raijman, L. (1989) J. Biol. Chem. **264**, 4038–4044
21. Fahien, L.A., Kmiotek, E.H. and Marshall, M. (1984) Arch. Biochem. Biophys. **230**, 213–221
22. Kispal, G., Sumegi, B. and Alkonyi, I. (1986) J. Biol. Chem. **261**, 14209–14213
23. Sumegi, B. and Srere, P.A. (1984) J. Biol. Chem. **259**, 8748–8752
24. Schwerdt, G., Moller, U. and Huth, W. (1991) Biochem. J. **280**, 353–357

25. Fahien, L.A. and Kmiotek, E. (1979) J. Biol. Chem. **254**, 5983–5990
26. Fahien, L.A., Kmiotek, E., Woldegiorgis, G., Evenson, M., Shrago, E. and Marshall, M. (1985) J. Biol. Chem. **260**, 6069–6079
27. Hearl, W.G. and Churchich, J.E. (1984) J. Biol. Chem. **259**, 11459–11463
28. Salerno, C., Ovádi, J., Keleti, T. and Fasella, P. (1982) Eur. J. Biochem. **121**, 511–517
29. Teller, J.K., Fahien, L.A. and Davis, J.W. (1992) J. Biol. Chem. **267**, 10423–10432
30. Halestrap, A.P. (1989) Biochim. Biophys. Acta **973**, 355–382
31. Sumegi, B. and Srere, P.A. (1984) J. Biol. Chem. **259**, 15040–15045
32. D'Souza, S.F. and Srere, P.A. (1983) J. Biol. Chem. **258**, 4706–4709
33. Fukushima, T., Decker, R.V., Anderson, W.M. and Spivey, H.O. (1989) J. Biol. Chem. **253**, 16483–16488
34. Teller, J.K., Fahien, L.A. and Valdivia, E. (1990) J. Biol. Chem. **265**, 19486–19494
35. Smith, E.L., Lanon, M., Piskiewicz, D., Brattin, W.J., Langley, T.J. and Melamed, M.D. (1970) Proc. Natl. Acad. Sci. U.S.A. **67**, 724–730
36. Fahien, L.A., Davis, J.W. and Laboy, J. (1993) J. Biol. Chem. **268**, 17935–17942
37. Fahien, L.A., Kmiotek, E. and Smith, L. (1979) Arch. Biochem. Biophys. **192**, 33–46
38. Fahien, L.A., Ruoho, A.E. and Kmiotek, E. (1978) J. Biol. Chem. **253**, 5745–5751
39. Fahien, L.A. and Smith, S.E. (1974) J. Biol. Chem. **249**, 2696–2703
40. Fahien, L.A. and Van Engelen, D.L. (1976) Arch. Biochem. Biophys. **176**, 298–305
41. Salerno, C., Churchich, J.E. and Fasella, P. (1975) Ital. J. Biochem. **25**, 351–359
42. Churchich, J.E. and Lee, Y.H. (1976) Biochem. Biophys. Res. Commun. **68**, 409–416
43. Churchich, J.E. (1978) Biochem. Biophys. Res. Commun. **83**, 1105–1110
44. Sumegi, B. and Alkonyi, I. (1983) Biochim. Biophys. Acta **749**, 163–171
45. Quinlin, P.T., Thomas, A.P., Armston, A.E. and Halestrap, A.P. (1983) Biochem. J. **214**, 395–404
46. Moreadith, R.W. and Lehninger, A.L. (1984) J. Biol. Chem. **259**, 6215–6221
47. Burton, K. and Wilson, T.H. (1953) Biochem. J. **54**, 86–92
48. Spivey, H.O. and Merz, T.M. (1989) BioEssays **10**, 127–130
49. Srere, P.A. (1987) Annu. Rev. Biochem. **56**, 89–124
50. Srere, P.A. (1976) in Gluconeogenesis (Hanson, R.W. and Melman, M.A., eds.), pp. 153–161, John Wiley and Sons, New York
51. Fahien, L.A. and Kmiotek, E.H. (1983) Arch. Biochem. Biophys. **220**, 386–397
52. Fahien, L.A., Kmiotek, E. and Kajawara, K. (1981) Arch. Biochem. Biophys. **209**, 143–151
53. Tischler, M.E., Freidrichs, D., Coll, K. and Williamson, J.R. (1977) Arch. Biochem. Biophys. **184**, 222–236
54. Chazotte, B. and Hackenbrock, C.R. (1991) J. Biol. Chem. **266**, 5973–5979
55. Fahien, L.A., Hsu, S.L. and Kmiotek, E. (1977) J. Biol. Chem. **252**, 1250–1256
56. Silverstein, E. and Suleke, G. (1969) Biochemistry **8**, 2543–2549
57. Silverstein, E. and Suleke, G. (1969) Biochim. Biophys. Acta **18**, 297–303
58. Salerno, C., Ovádi, J., Keleti, T. and Fasella, P. (1982) Eur. J. Biochem. **121**, 511–517
59. Henson, C.P. and Cleland, W.W. (1964) Biochemistry **3**, 338–344
60. Michuda, C.M. and Martinez-Carrion, M. (1969) J. Biol. Chem. **244**, 5920–5927
61. Rife, T.F. and Cleland, W.W. (1980) Biochemistry **19**, 2321–2326
62. Halperin, M.L., Jungas, R.L., Cheema-Dhadli, S. and Brosnan, J.T. (1987) Trends Biochem. Sci. **12**, 197–199
63. Haussinger, D. (1989) Metabolism (Suppl. 1) **38**, 14–17
64. Tannen, R.L. and Sastrasinh, S. (1984) Kidney Int. **25**, 1–10
65. Haussinger, D., Akerboom, T.P.M. and Sies, H. (1980) Hoppe Seylers Z. Physiol. Chem. **361**, 995–1001
66. Joseph, S.K. and McGivan, J.D. (1978) Biochem. J. **176**, 837–844
67. McGivan, J.D., Lacey, J.H. and Joseph, S.K. (1980) Biochem. J. **192**, 537–542
68. Verhoeven, A.J., Van Iwaarden, J.F., Joseph, S.K. and Meijer, A.J. (1983) Eur. J. Biochem. **133**, 241–244
69. Addae, S.K. and Lotspeich, W.D. (1968) Am. J. Physiol. **215**, 269–277
70. Aikawa, T., Matsutako, H., Yamomoto, H., Okuda, T., Ishikawa, E., Kawano, T. and Matsumura, E. (1973) J. Biochem. (Tokyo) **74**, 1003–1017
71. Fine, A. (1982) Kidney Int. **21**, 439–444
72. Fine, A. (1982) Biochem. J. **202**, 271–273
73. Schrock, H. and Goldstein, L. (1981) Am. J. Physiol. **240**, E519–E525

74. Welbourne, T.C., Phromphetcharat, V., Gwens, G. and Joshi, S. (1986) Am. J. Physiol. **250**, E457–E463
75. Heitmann, R.M. and Bergmann, E.N. (1978) Am. J. Physiol. **234**, E197–E203
76. Heitmann, R.M. and Bergmann, E.N. (1980) Am. J. Physiol. **239**, E248–E254
77. Lenzen, C., Soboll, S., Sies, H. and Haussinger, D. (1987) Eur. J. Biochem. **166**, 483–488
78. Lueck, J.D. and Miller, L.L. (1970) J. Biol. Chem. **254**, 5491–5497
79. Pitts, R.F. (1966) Physiologist **9**, 97–109
80. Tannen, R.L. (1993) in Handbook of Physiology, Section 8: Renal Physiology, 2nd edn. (Windhager, E., ed.), pp. 1017–1059, Open University Press, Oxford and New York
81. Schoolwerth, A.C. (1991) Kidney Int. **40**, 961–973
82. Chobanian, M.C., Julin, C.M., Molteni, K.H. and Brazy, P.C. (1992) Am. J. Physiol. **262**, F878–F884
83. Sastrasinh, S. and Sastrasinh, M. (1986) Am. J. Physiol. **250**, F667–F673
84. Curthoys, N. and Lowry, O.H. (1973) J. Biol. Chem. **248**, 162–168
85. Lupianez, J.A., Hortelano, P., Sanchez-Medina, F., Sachez-Pogo, A., MacFarlane-Anderson, N., Burnswell, J. and Alleyne, G.A.O. (1981) FEBS Lett. **128**, 361–363
86. Lowry, M. and Ross, B.D. (1980) Biochem. J. **190**, 771–780
87. Vinay, P., Allignet, E., Pichette, C., Watford, M., Lemieux, G. and Gougoux, A. (1980) Kidney Int. **17**, 312–325
88. Schoolwerth, A.C. and LaNoue, K.F. (1983) Am. J. Physiol. **244**, F399–F408
89. Tannen, R.L. and Sastrasinh, S. (1984) Kidney Int. **25**, 1–10
90. Simpson, D.P. and Adams, W. (1975) J. Biol. Chem. **250**, 8148–8158
91. Schoolwerth, A.C. and LaNoue, K.F. (1980) J. Biol. Chem. **255**, 3403–3411
92. Tannen, R.L. and Kunin, A.S. (1981) Am. J. Physiol. **240**, F120–F126
93. Tannen, R.L. and Kunin, A.S. (1982) Kidney Int. **22**, 280–285
94. Yu, H.L., Giammarco, R., Goldstein, M.B., Stinebaugh, B.J. and Halperin, M.L. (1976) J. Clin. Invest. **58**, 557–564
95. Chobanian, M.C. and Julin, C.M. (1991) Am. J. Physiol. **260**, F19–F26
96. Chobanian, M.C. and Hammerman, M.R. (1988) Am. J. Physiol. **255**, F847–F852
97. Chobanian, M.C. and Hammerman, M.R. (1987) Am. J. Physiol. **253**, F1171–F1177
98. Gesek, F.A., Mishkind, M.T. and Schoolwerth, A.C. (1991) Contrib. Nephrol. **92**, 141–148
99. Drewnowska, K. and Schoolwerth, A.C. (1994) Am. J. Physiol. **276**, F153–F159
100. Denton, R.M. and McCormack, J.G. (1985) Am. J. Physiol. **249**, E543–E554

13

A new concept for control of glycolysis

Judit Ovádi* and Ferenc Orosz

Institute of Enzymology, Biological Research Center, Hungarian Academy of Sciences, P.O. Box 7, Budapest H-1518, Hungary

Introduction

Metabolism is defined as the operation of integrated enzyme-catalysed chemical reactions that contribute to the maintenance of the cells in which they occur. Glycolysis is an energy production pathway in cytoplasm that occurs in organisms from microbial cells to human beings. The sequence of the enzymic reactions of the glycolytic pathway is well known; however, their regulation and spatial organization are not completely understood. In intact cells the rate of ATP production is tightly coupled to the rate of ATP consumption. In cell types that rely primarily on oxidative metabolism, this tight coupling implies that the rate of oxygen consumption by mitochondria is highly regulated by cytoplasmic processes [1]. However, the biochemical signals that regulate and relate the rates of ATP synthesis and utilization are unclear. It has been suggested that the ATP/ADP ratio or phosphorylation potential might be responsible for the regulation. There are a number of suggested concepts for control of respiration and ATP synthesis, some compatible and complementary, some incompatible and contradictory, which are reviewed in a recent excellent article [2].

The classical concept of the glycolytic pathway is a system of freely soluble components in the cytoplasmic compartment of the cell where glycolytic enzymes, depending on the cell type, are regulated by allosteric effectors, for example adenine nucleotides, fructose 2,6-bisphosphate and ribose 1,5-bisphosphate predominantly by their actions on hexokinase, phosphofructokinase and pyruvate kinase. However, the sensitivity of these 'rate-limiting' enzymes to allosteric effectors alters with physiological conditions. For example, at high phosphofructokinase concentration [3,4] or under conditions when phosphofructokinase associates with actin filaments in muscle cells [5] or with the cell membrane in erythrocytes [6] the allosteric inhibition of this enzyme by ATP is suspended. Since this feedback control mechanism apparently does not, at least not exclusively, function in certain cases, additional mechanisms have been suggested for the control of glyco-

To whom correspondence should be addressed.

lysis. The physical basis of these concepts is that the glycolytic enzymes do not distribute homogeneously in the cytoplasm, but that they associate with subcellular components of the cells or with each other in ways that can alter their catalytic and regulatory properties. These new aspects will be reviewed in this chapter, with the emphasis on metabolite channelling and micro-compartmentation as special consequences of dynamic enzyme associations occurring within the highly organized cytomatrix.

Diffusion in the cytomatrix versus enzymic conversion

Living cells have 'aqueous compartments' which represent about 75% of the volume and mass of most cells [7]. Glycolysis in living cells occurs in the aqueous cytoplasm, which requires at least 0.1 g of water/g dry mass of cells [8]. The characteristics of the aqueous phase of the cytoplasm as well as cellular viscosity influence a number of intracellular dynamic processes, including small-molecule and macromolecular transport and diffusion-limited enzyme kinetics [9]. A number of special techniques have been developed to assess the motion of metabolite-sized molecules and proteins within the cell. For example, proton NMR studies indicated that proton relaxation times are considerably shorter in living cells than in bulk water. Other studies showed that the viscosity values obtained in the cell after microinjection of small magnetic particles and macromolecules were higher than the fluid-phase cytoplasmic viscosity [10]. The picosecond rotational motion of small probes directly related to the fluid-phase viscosity was analysed by time-resolved fluorescence anisotropy. Since the rotation correlation times of the unbound probe were 20–40% longer than those in water, it was concluded that the fluid-phase cytoplasm is only 1.2–1.4 times as viscous as water [9]. These measurements also indicated that the diffusion coefficients of metabolite-sized particles were identical with those in water only if the short-range transport within the spatial domain of a single interstitial void is considered [9].

Recently, a sophisticated fluorescence method has been developed that measures solvent viscosity more directly [11] by utilizing simultaneously two related indocyanine dyes. The fluorescence quantum yield of one of the dyes depends on solvent viscosity, while the quantum yield of the other is viscosity-insensitive. When the two dyes were covalently coupled to Ficoll 70 (an inert fluorescent tracer particle) and microinjected into living cells, the fluorescence ratio imaging showed that the solvent viscosity of the cytoplasm of living adherent tissue culture cells is not significantly different from that of water. However, the limited spatial resolution of the ratio imaging approach does not allow one to exclude the possibility of a small layer of more or less structured water immediately adjacent to proteins and membrane surfaces.

When the rotational correlation time of a fluorescent probe in the cytoplasmic layer was measured within 50–200 nm of the plasma membrane [12] the value obtained was similar to that measured deeper in the cytoplasm and was not significantly different from that in bulk water. Additional techniques, for example electron spin resonance, fluorescent recovery after photobleaching or time-resolved fluorescence anisotropy, also have methodological uncertainties and limitations. These techniques involve exogenous probes; thus they can only report on compartments to which they have access, and the diffusion coefficient should be sensitive to distance only in a region that is comparable with the obstacle (protein) spacing [13]. Nevertheless, these data make it possible to draw general conclusions as to the constraints on self-diffusion in the cytoplasm of living cells [14–17].

The diffusion of molecules of all sizes is affected by the solvent viscosity of the cytoplasm and by macromolecular crowding (see also Chapters 2 and 3 in the current volume). Because the solvent viscosity of cytoplasm is not substantially different from that of water, the times taken for reactants to encounter each other in the cytoplasm are not much different from those in dilute aqueous solution. The effects of crowding on translational diffusion depend on the size of the diffusing molecules. Ions and other small molecules diffuse nearly as fast as in dilute solution unless they are immobilized by binding. For macromolecular complexes, much larger than the background macromolecules, the crowded solution approximates to a continuum. The free diffusion of a protein monomer with a particle radius of 3.5 nm may be at least 3–4 times slower in cytoplasm than in dilute aqueous solution. As the size of the diffusing molecule increases, the obstruction by the cytoskeletal network becomes increasingly important. The diffusion coefficient for macromolecules is 10–100-fold smaller than for free water [14,16]. Tracer particles greater than 13 nm in radius are excluded from some domains of the peripheral cytoplasm, apparently by a dense network of filaments; tracer particles larger than 26 nm are non-diffusible and require active transport to their targets [17]. Since most macromolecular components of the cell are involved in transient macromolecular associations, the intrinsic macromolecular density is relatively low within the interstitial voids and thus only a small fraction of the total macromolecular content undergoes random thermal motion in cells. Macromolecules in general may undergo much slower transport at rates that are determined by dissociation from cytoskeletal and membraneous binding elements [18]. It may be, then, that a significant fraction of the intracellular macromolecular transport is confined to the active transport of organelles in which they are enclosed or to diffusion along subcellular components.

A pertinent question for enzymic reactions is, however, not only what is the time taken for collision between the reactant molecules, but also what is the time required to manoeuvre into the 'reactive configuration'?. The total reaction time (τ) is the sum of two components: the diffusional transient (transit) time and the reaction transient time. Factors influencing the whole reaction time are well understood, although the calculations are uncertain because uncertain assumptions are included. For example, electrostatic rate enhancements for macromolecular reactions also occur that can increase reaction rates above the expected diffusional limit and extend well beyond the surface of the macromolecule [19]. These fields then guide approaching reactants to the (appropriately charged) active site and thus increase the frequency of successful collisions. In addition, the interactions of macromolecules in solution have special features that can increase the apparent bimolecular association rate [19]. This is because the collision of macromolecules is not elastic, due to their 'stickiness' once they collide, and they tend to drift apart only slowly. Many reiterated minicollisions occur, while the macromolecules undergo appreciable relative rotational arrangements and thus can overcome the limitations of interaction geometry. These rotational rearrangements can overcome the steric factors and thus these actions appear to proceed at essentially diffusion-controlled rates.

The rates of many biological processes can be enhanced by diffusion within reduced dimensions [20]. An excellent example is the movement of myosin molecules along actin filaments in muscle contraction [21]. One-dimensional diffusion may also be involved in the assembly of microtubules or any other cellular processes where proteins or organelles may migrate along microfilaments [22,23]. Also, the rates of protein associations into pores could be greatly enhanced if these ligands could diffuse in two dimensions in the membrane. Therefore planar or linear diffusion as opposed to three-dimensional diffusion results in significant changes in efficiency of transport from source to target [20]. Therefore it is very likely that there are arrangements within the living cell which overcome these diffusional limitations, making successful metabolism possible.

Superstructure of the cytoskeletal network

Prokaryotes and eukaryotes represent two types of structural organization of cells. While eukaryotic cells are larger, with an exceptional variety of subcellular organization, prokaryotic cells do not contain membrane-bound organelles. Eukaryotic cells possess a developed cytoskeleton which can ensure spatial separation of biochemical processes. In prokaryotic cells glycolysis occurs in a minute volume with minimal cellular architectural detail. The absence of membrane-bound organelles suggests that reactions are likely to be organized by direct macromolecular interactions [24], apart from reactions localized in or near the cell membrane. A tendency for spatial organization of cytoplasmic and membraneous proteins can be traced: some of the molecules of the total cell pool of a particular enzyme enter into a dynamic interaction with other enzymes and proteins, forming assemblies with a finite lifetime [25]. The cell cytoplasm of eukaryotic cells is composed of complex networks of the cytoskeletal filament system, which is a dense array of the cytoskeletal elements, i.e. microtubules, microfilaments and intermediate filaments. The concentration of actin in cells in tissue culture is 5–7 mg/ml [17] and in most cells about half of the actin is assembled into filaments. Assuming that all cellular actin is in cytoplasm and that the nucleus occupies not more than half the volume of the cell, the average concentration of F-actin in the cytoplasm corresponds to a volume fraction of 0.015. There are only about 150 microtubules in a cultured mammalian cell. Assuming an average length per microtubule of 50 μm and an average volume for a single cell of 3×10^{-9} ml, the contribution of microtubules to the filament volume fraction is only 0.0012. The content of intermediate filaments varies with the type of cell and with the class of intermediate filament proteins. Assuming that this network in mammalian cells occupies a volume fraction roughly equivalent to that of actin, the total volume occupied by cytoskeletal filaments would still be only 0.03 [17]. However, high-voltage electron microscopy revealed a more complex and richly diverse particulate ultra-structure in eukaryotic cells.

An extreme view is that of Porter and his colleagues [26] who claim that the cytoplasmic organization of macromolecules is essentially complete in the form of the microtrabecular lattice and that the various cytoskeletal elements are interlocked by an ephemeral network [27]. Porter's proposition is that the cell is divided into 'protein-rich and water-rich phases' [26] and that the protein-rich phase is the microtrabecular lattice. This finding was supported by microviscosity studies on intact cells [28]. Furthermore, spatially averaged fluorescence anisotropy (r) with an image analysis system revealed two distinct regions of r in the whole volume of cultured cells [29]: one from the cytoplasm ($r = 0.144$), and a second from the interstitial region ($r = 0.08$). The 'soluble enzymes' are apparently integral parts of this cyto-matrix, the whole constituting a unit system. The aqueous domain of the cytoplasm that occupies the space between the cytoskeletal network contains macromolecules and small organic and inorganic solutes. According to the quantitative data, distances within the intratrabecular space are about 1000 Å [30], much greater than the diameter of BSA (bovine serum albumin). This lattice structure has been also demonstrated by *in situ* diffusion probes [31] (see also below). Therefore the microtrabecular lattice should not retard cytoplasmic diffusion by steric effects [30]. Virtually all cytoplasmic proteins have non-diffusing forms, and many do not diffuse at all on a time scale of hours [32]. Although several criticisms of Porter's views have been made [33], the weight of evidence compels us to accept the existence *in vivo* of a complex highly organized cytoskeletal network.

There are multiple cross-linking proteins in the cytoplasmic actin gel-like structures, the physiological function of which is difficult to demon-strate by mutation or even gene disruption [34]. Consequently, most of our knowledge about the cytoplasmic actin gel is from *in vitro* reconstitution with actin and purified individual cross-linkers such as α-actinin. Quantitative rheological analysis revealed that the cross-linker increases the viscosity and rigidity of the actin filament network. The actin filaments in these bundles are tightly packed in some areas whereas in others they are more disperse [35]. For example, in the presence of phosphofructokinase a distinct cross-striation of F-actin paracrystals was detected by electron microscopy [36]. Also, electron microscopic studies demonstrated that aldolase could bundle actin filaments [37]. Since aldolase is associated with the solid phase of the cell cytoplasm, the effect of aldolase on the organization of actin filaments is probably relevant physiologically. Using fluorescence analogue cytochemistry, digital-imaging microscopy and fluorescence redistribution after photobleaching, Pagliaro and Taylor [31] found that aldolase which bound to and gelled F-actin at physiological concentrations *in vitro* was relatively concentrated in a microdomain around stress fibres *in vivo*. In contrast, enolase has no actin-binding or gelling activity *in vitro* and does not bind to stress fibres *in vivo* [38].

Whereas actin polymerization in muscle is considered relatively static, the microtubule system involved in several essential functions of the cell [39] is much more dynamic in many tissues. Microtubules are ubiquitous cellular structures. The basic building block of microtubules is a tubulin dimer made of α and β subunits. The assembly and functions of microtubules are regulated by microtubule-associated proteins, the major classes of which are the microtubule-associated motors (e.g. kinesin, etc.) and the structural microtubule-associated proteins (MAPs) (e.g. tau, MAP1 and 2, etc.) which modulate the stability and spatial arrangement of the tubules. In addition, a variety of other proteins can interact with microtubules and enhance the formation of bundles [40,41]. There are some reports of cross-linking and bundling of microtubules by the glycolytic enzymes, glyceraldehyde-3-phosphate dehydrogenase and phosphofructokinase [42–46]. Electron microscopic studies show the periodical formation of cross-bridges of microtubules by phosphofructokinase. Three to four closely aligned tubules are connected by rows of highly periodic lateral arms about 13 nm long and 12 nm wide. The centre-to-centre distance between adjacent arms is about 21 nm. The cross-linked area extends over a stretch of about 400–500 nm containing 20–24 arms in a row [46].

A comparable situation occurs in skeletal muscle, where immuno-histochemical data with anti-(ribosomal subunit) antibodies have shown ribosomes to be present in an organized and repetitive fashion along the myofibrils and associated with the myosin-containing A bands [47]. A study combining high-resolution electron microscopy with *in situ* hybridization [48] showed that mRNA species coding for actin, tubulin and vimentin appear to be clustered around filamentous structures in the non-ionic-detergent-insoluble matrix. The extent of the interaction of ribosomes/polysomes and cytoskeleton (microfilaments or myofibrils) varies with different physiological conditions; more mRNAs and polysomes are associated with the cytoskeleton during increased protein synthesis. The association of mRNAs with the cytoskeleton might be important for the transport of mRNA from nucleus to cytoplasm [49]. Polynucleotides associate with some glycolytic enzymes as well, e.g. glyceraldehyde-3-phosphate dehydrogenase forms loose dynamic complexes with polyribosomes [50]. Although this association is relatively weak at physiological ionic strength, a considerable amount of the enzyme could be adsorbed on to the ribosomes in the cell, where the concentrations of both glycolytic enzymes and ribosomes are very high.

Specific associations of glycolytic enzymes

As discussed above, the association of glycolytic enzymes with the cytoskeletal network contributes significantly to the formation of the superstructure of the cytomatrix. The enzymes are partitioned *in vivo* with high concentrations along the I band, as indicated by histochemical and fluorescent antibody staining [51]. Most of the glycolytic enzymes will sediment with F-actin as shown by *in vitro* studies when muscle homogenates are centrifuged [52–54]. Tropomyosin/troponin enhances this interaction [55]. Indeed, in muscle one of the major components that interacts with glycolytic enzymes is actin, whereas creatine kinase and adenylate kinase present in large amounts are not adsorbed. The evidence *in vitro* for the associations of various glycolytic enzymes with F-actin, as well as with other elements of the cytoskeletal network, is abundant and is given in Table 1, and reviews in the literature [5, 56–59] and in several chapters in [60].

Binding sites are located at different interfaces by antigenic probes for aldolase, phosphofructokinase and glyceraldehyde-3-phosphate dehydrogenase on actin monomers in thin filaments [61]. Distinct binding sites for phosphofructokinase and glyceraldehyde-3-phosphate dehydrogenase have been revealed by means of proteolysis [62]. Triosephosphate isomerase, however, apparently binds indirectly via aldolase and glyceraldehyde-3-phosphate dehydrogenase to myofibrils [63].

Mathematical modelling based upon quantitative *in vitro* binding data suggested that a large amount of the enzymes would either be associated with each other in the cytoplasm or associated with F-actin [64]. The existence in muscle cytoplasm of a large multi-enzyme complex, as suggested by Kurganov [66], is not supported by theoretical calculations [64] in agreement with the experimental results [65]. Alternatively, *in vivo* the glycolytic pathway may have different segments, each consisting of not more than four enzymes. These segments may be specifically mobilized at several locations within the cytoplasmic compartment, and often act independently [67].

It was also demonstrated by combining indirect immunofluorescence and cell-permeabilization techniques that there is microcompartmentation of aldose and glyceraldehyde-3-phosphate dehydrogenase in cultured cell types (3T3 normal and transformed cells, fibroblasts, embryocardiomyocytes) [59]. The fraction of aldolase that is bound is also released from F-actin *in*

Table I   **Enzyme associations in glycolysis**

Enzymes involved	K_d (μM)	Consequences	Modulators	Effects of modulators	References
Glucose-phosphate isomerase/PFK (erythrocyte)		Channelling			154
PFK/aldolase (muscle)	2.0–2.5	Shift of oligomeric states			72,155
		PFK activity decreases			72,155
			Calmodulin, ATP	Shift of oligomeric states	155
PFK/aldolase (yeast)	0.1				156
PFK/aldolase (plant)					157
PFK/FBPase (muscle)		Mutual kinetic influence (PFK up, FBPase down)			158
Aldolase/FBPase (liver)					159
Aldolase/triosephosphate isomerase (muscle)	1.2	Aldolase activity decreases			161,162
		Mutual protection against denaturation			160
Aldolase/triosephosphate isomerase (chloroplast)					163
Aldolase/GAPD (muscle)	0.3	Increased K_m for aldolase			80,84
		Channelling			113,164,165
		No channelling			119
			Fru-1,6-P_2	Lower K_d	84
			Fru-1,6-P_2	Higher K_d	156
			NAD$^+$	Higher K_d	166
Aldolase/GAPD (yeast)	0.2	Shift of oligomeric states			156
			Fru-1,6-P_2	Higher K_d	156
Aldolase/glycerol-phosphate dehydrogenase (muscle)	0.2	Shift of oligomeric states			167,168
		Channelling			118,148
			Fru-1,6-P_2	Lower K_d	85
			Fru-2,6-P_2	Lower K_d	85
Triosephosphate isomerase/GAPD (muscle)		Piggy-back binding to F-actin			63,169
GAPD/phosphoglycerate kinase (muscle)	0.3	Channelling			148,170
		No channelling			171,172
			NAD$^+$, ATP, 3-PG	Higher K_d	170

Table 1 (contc.)

Enzymes involved	K_d (μM)	Consequences	Modulators	Effects of modulators	References
GAPD/lactate dehydrogenase (muscle)	5.0	Channelling			148,173
Glycerol-phosphate dehydrogenase/	0.8	Channelling			148,173,174
lactate dehydrogenase (muscle)			NADH	K_d changes	175
Enolase/phosphoglycerate mutase (muscle)	1	Enolase activity decreases			176
Enolase/phosphoglycerate mutase (brain)	10	Enolase activity decreases	2,3-DPG	Reverses activity decrease	177
Mitochondrial membrane/hexokinase		Activation			178
(brain, muscle, liver)		Lower K_m for ATP			179
			Glu-6-P, ATP	Solubilizes	178,180
			Li$^+$	Solubilizes	103
			2-Deoxyglucose	Solubilizes	89
			Mg$^+$, P$_i$	Enhanced binding	181,182
F-actin (muscle) with:					
Glucose-phosphate isomerase					53,183
PFK	0.2	Activation			99,184
		Liberation from ATP-inhibition			99
		Actin cross-linking			36
			Fru-6-P	Enhanced binding	99
			Fru-1,6-P_2	Enhanced binding	185
			Insulin, EGF	Enhanced binding	103
			Ca^{2+}, calmodulin	Enhanced binding	103
			High Ca^{2+}	Solubilizes	104
			5-HT, PLA$_2$	Solubilizes	104
			Li$^+$	Solubilizes	103
Aldolase	0.8				186
		V_{max} increased			187,188
		No change in V_{max}			189
		K_m increased			187–189
		Actin bundling			37,55
			Fru-1,6-P_2	Solubilizes	187–189
			Glu-1,6-P_2, PEP, P$_i$	Solubilizes	187

Table 1 (contd.)

Enzymes involved	K_d (μM)	Consequences	Modulators	Effects of modulators	References
			DHAP, ATP, ADP	Solubilizes	187
			3-PG, 2,3-DPG	Solubilizes	187
			Cytochalasin D	Solubilizes	68
			Ca^{2+}, calmodulin	Enhanced binding	103
			Insulin, EGF	Enhanced binding	103
Triosephosphate isomerase	10	None			186
GAPD	0.6	No activity change			186
		V_{max}, K_m decrease			190
		Actin bundling			191
			GAP, Fru-1,6-P_2	Solubilizes	186,187
			3-PG, 2,3-DPG,	Solubilizes	187
			PEP, ATP, P_i	Solubilizes	187
Phosphoglycerate kinase	10.8	None			186
Pyruvate kinase	1.0, 0.13	Inactivation			186,192
		Actin bundling			191
			Fru-1,6-P_2	Enhanced binding	185
Lactate dehydrogenase	2.1	Inactivation			186
			NADH	Solubilizes	193
Tubulin/microtubules (brain) with:					
Glucose-phosphate isomerase					194
PFK	0.2–0.3	Inactivation			45
		Microtubule bundling			46
			ADP, ATP	Solubilizes	46
			Fru-1,6-P_2	Solubilizes	46
			Fru-2,6-P_2	Solubilizes	46
			Aldolase	Competition	46
			Calmodulin	Competition	102
Aldolase					102,195
		Competitive inhibition			71,102
		Inhibition			70

Table 1 (contd.)

Enzymes involved	K_d (μM)	Consequences	Modulators	Effects of modulators	References
			Fru-1,6-P_2	Solubilizes	102
			PFK	Competition	46
GAPD	1.7				194
	0.76, 0.0064				105
		Inactivation			43,105
		Microtubule bundling			42,44
			ATP	Solubilizes	43
			NAD$^+$, arsenate	Solubilizes	105
Phosphoglycerate kinase					194
Pyruvate kinase	2.2				194
Lactate dehydrogenase (muscle type)	1.0	Inactivation			77
			NADH	Solubilizes	77,194

Sources of enzymes are muscle unless given in parentheses. Abbreviations: PFK, phosphofructokinase; FBPase, fructose-bisphosphatase; GAPD, glyceraldehyde-3-phosphate dehydrogenase; Glu-6-P, glucose 6-phosphate; GAP, glyceraldehyde 3-phosphate; Fru-6-P, fructose 6-phosphate; Fru-1,6-P_2, fructose 1,6-bisphosphate; Fru-2,6-P_2, fructose 2,6-bisphosphate; 3-PG, D-glycerate 3-phosphate; 2,3-DPG, D-glycerate 2,3-bisphosphate; EGF, epidermal growth factor; PLA$_2$, phospholipase A$_2$; PEP, phosphoenolpyruvate; DHAP, dihydroxyacetone phosphate; 5-HT, 5-hydroxytryptamine (serotonin); Glu-1,6-P_2, glucose 1,6-bisphosphate.

vitro when fructose-1,6-bisphosphate is added to a gelled aldolase/F-actin mixture demonstrating specificity and reversibility for its gelling activity. In cultured cells the binding of aldolase is affected by specific inhibitors: $\sim21\%$ of bound aldolase in the perinuclear region of 3T3 cells was released by an inhibitor of glycolysis, 2-deoxyglucose [68]. Therefore, the hypothesis that *in vivo*, aldolase and glyceraldehyde-3-phosphate dehydrogenase exist both as soluble and structure-associated forms is favoured experimentally. The reversible release of the bound fraction of aldolase by cytochalasin D suggests that the distribution of this enzyme is determined by the diverse forms in these cells of the organization of the actin cytoskeleton.

There are much fewer data available about the binding of glycolytic enzymes to microtubules, and those studies were carried out with purified tubulin or MAP-free microtubules. Recent data showed that aldolase [69–71] and probably glyceraldehyde-3-phosphate dehydrogenase [70] bind the acidic C-terminal tail of the α subunit of tubulin. Aldolase and phosphofructokinase may mutually hinder each other in microtubule binding [46]; this might be attributed to competition for microtubule binding. Alternatively, since phosphofructokinase and aldolase interact with each other [72], the formation of a heterologous complex may impede the binding of the enzymes to microtubules. Nevertheless, these observations suggest the possibility that some glycolytic enzymes bind to the same or related domains of microtubules.

The C-terminal binding domain of α tubulin and the N-terminal binding domain of human erythrocyte band 3 membrane protein share many properties, including sequence identity [57]. Steck and his co-workers have shown that glycolytic enzymes bind specifically to the acidic N-terminal region of human erythrocyte band 3 protein [73,74]. Aldolase and glyceraldehyde-3-phosphate dehydrogenase effectively compete with phosphofructokinase for binding to band 3 protein and release the bound phosphofructokinase [75]. This binding site appears to be specific for glycolytic enzymes, as haemoglobin, which is known to bind to band 3, does not release the bound phosphofructokinase. Therefore it has been proposed that these glycolytic enzymes bind to the same or related domains of band 3 [76]. Interestingly, the binding of these glycolytic enzymes to the tubulin/microtubule system or to band 3 protein produces similar functional consequences that will be discussed later.

The association of glycolytic enzymes with the tubulin/microtubulin system is modulated by substrates and allosteric effectors. For example, the binding of phosphofructokinase to microtubules is inhibited by ATP and fructose bisphosphate, but not by some other allosteric effectors, including citrate and NH_4^+ [46]. The binding of glyceraldehyde-3-phosphate dehydrogenase to microtubules is also decreased by ATP [43]. It appears that in many cases substrates release the glycolytic enzymes from the cytoskeletal network by different molecular mechanisms; for example by competition or a ligand-induced shift of the equilibrium of oligomeric forms with different

Fig. 1   **Schematic representation of metabolite-modulated associations of glycolytic enzymes with subcellular elements**

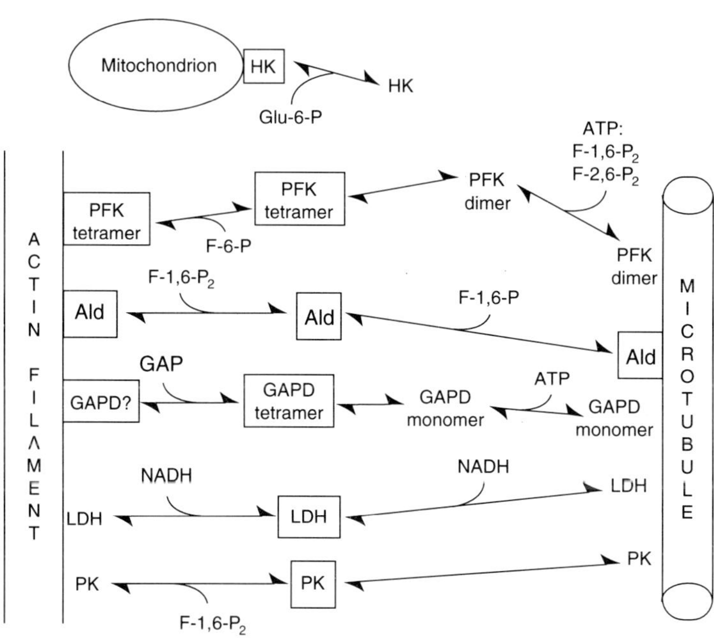

Species in boxes are the more active forms. Abbreviations: HK, hexokinase; PFK, phosphofructokinase; Ald, aldolase; GAPD, glyceraldehyde-3-phosphate dehydrogenase, LDH, lactate dehydrogenase; PK, pyruvate kinase; Glu-6-P, glucose 6-phosphate; F-6-P, fructose 6-phosphate; GAP, glyceraldehyde 3-phosphate; F-1,6-P₂, fructose 1,6-bisphosphate; F-2,6-P₂, fructose 2,6-bisphosphate.

binding properties (Fig. 1). Since in most cases the bound enzymes are less active compared with the free ones (Table 1) the substrate-induced dissociation of enzymes enhances their catalytic activity. As an exception, fructose 6 phosphate strengthens the interaction of active tetrameric phosphofructokinase with actin filaments; however, this effect also increases the overall enzyme activity. These interactions seem to be highly specific, since the well defined conformer(s) of the enzymes recognize the target domain on the cytoskeleton.

Specific binding of isoenzymes as well as its modulation by specific metabolites was also observed. For example, it was found that the muscle-type lactate dehydrogenase, but not the heart-type enzyme, was inhibited by tubulin and that the magnitude of inhibition depended on the NADH concentration, the pH and the buffer medium [77]. Therefore it can be hypothesized that the specific interactions of glycolytic enzymes, and their ability to select targets, could ensure an innovative control mechanism for energy production via glycolysis.

A considerable body of evidence indicates that many glycolytic enzymes are associated with each other in solution at physiological or even lower concentrations (Table 1 and Fig. 1). Several factors are likely to promote the associations of glycolytic enzymes *in vivo* beyond those observed *in vitro*. Firstly, the concentrations of most enzymes in the cell are several orders of magnitude higher than those generally used in kinetic studies *in vitro*. Also, the very high concentrations *in vivo* of proteins other than the interacting species could enhance the association of enzymes due to size-exclusion effects [78] (see also Chapters 2 and 3 in the current volume). However, macromolecular crowding itself cannot promote specific enzyme interactions since it does not provide biorecognition of enzymes. The biorecognition must result from surface complementarity of proteins rather than from higher protein concentrations [79]. As a result of these specific macromolecular associations the kinetic, regulatory or thermodynamic properties of the enzymes are altered compared with their free forms. Specificity is an important criterion in assessing the physiological relevance of enzyme interactions.

In vitro experimental data demonstrate that muscle aldolase (a stable tetrameric enzyme) selectively interacts with dimeric forms of other functionally related muscle enzymes, i.e. phosphofructokinase [72], glyceraldehyde-3-phosphate dehydrogenase [80] and glycerol-phosphate dehydrogenase [81]. The enzyme forms which interact with aldolase are the dimers in the case of all three enzymes, irrespective of whether these are the more active or less active form of the kinase or dehydrogenases. Because the different oligomeric forms have different specific activities, the overall activities of the individual enzymes are altered by these heterologous interactions [82].

Specific ligands can induce changes in the tertiary and quaternary structures of some enzymes and enhance the formation of specific enzyme associations (Table 1). The effects of ligands on heterologous macromolecular interactions are understandable if the 'form-specific' enzyme associations are considered [83]. There are, however, additional mechanisms which may be responsible for the ligand-induced effects. Relatively small, even local, conformational alterations induced by a specific ligand can result in association/dissociation of the heterologous enzyme complexes. For example, co-operative effects of fructose 1,6-bisphosphate on the binding of both glyceraldehyde-3-phosphate dehydrogenase and glycerol-phosphate dehydrogenase to aldolase were found [84,85]. The presence of the key glycolytic metabolite fructose bisphosphate increased specifically the affinity of aldolase for both dehydrogenases.

Hexokinase was identified more than a decade ago as an ambiquitous enzyme that occurs both as a soluble form and bound to mitochondria. Ambiquitous enzymes were originally defined by Wilson in relation to the behaviour of hexokinase [86,87] as having kinetically distinct subsets that partition between soluble and membrane-bound forms in cells. Later, evidence for hexokinase *in vivo* partitioning between soluble and bound forms was presented [88]. Hexokinase is released from mitochondria by glucose 6-phosphate and 2-deoxyglucose [89]. The effect of 2-deoxyglucose is indirect: it increases the level of glucose 6-phosphate, which indirectly inhibits the activity of the free enzyme more effectively than that of the bound form. Therefore the rapidly changeable distribution of hexokinase is important for the control of glycolysis. Recent evidence from Wilson's laboratory shows that hexokinase is released to different extents from brain mitochondria prepared from different species (rat or bovine). It was not possible to distinguish these hexokinases by their isoelectric focusing patterns, kinetic properties or by their molecular masses [90]. Differences in the binding domains of rat and bovine mitochondria were postulated to explain the differences in the extent of solubilization by glucose 6-phosphate.

Isoenzyme-specific interactions probably have a role in the regulation of glycolysis. The involvement of isoenzymes in separating intermediates from competing reactions is well documented [91], e.g. the conversion of glucose 6-phosphate into pyruvate or glycogen via glycolytic or synthetic pathways. The fate of an individual glucose 6-phosphate molecule is specified by the hexokinase isoenzyme responsible for its production [92]. Different pathways utilizing isoenzymes may operate in different compartments [93]. Indeed, the presence of isoenzymes in several metabolic steps can maintain multiple pools of intermediates by isoenzyme–isoenzyme associations. This kind of specific association, e.g. of hexokinase isoenzymes, resulting in functional compartmentation in carbohydrate metabolism, may prevent the shuttling of common intermediates between opposing pathways [92].

The multiple macromolecular interactions present *in vivo* might be expected to stabilize enzyme associations not observed in systems *in vitro* which contain much fewer as well as more dilute macromolecular components. The macromolecular interactions of glycolytic enzymes, however, appear even in the cell to be loose and sensitive to changes in pH and metabolites [94] (Table 1). Hence their intracellular distribution may vary with the metabolic status of the cell [84,95]. Therefore in many cases the intracellular distribution of enzymes is not an invariant property. Whereas the static complexes which are strongly self-associating or covalently linked require no energy to maintain structure and function, dynamic interactions are absolutely dependent on constant energy dissipation [96]. Nevertheless, the terms 'static' and 'dynamic' are phenomenological descriptions of the enzyme associations, and in the nature there is continuous transition between the two extreme association states.

Functional consequences of enzyme associations

The associations of glycolytic enzymes result in mutual effects, termed 'functional duality', that modify not only the ultrastructure and dynamics of the cytoskeleton but also the catalytic and regulatory properties of the enzymes. In these cases the reversible associations with the cytoskeletal network could ensure an effective control mechanism for glycolysis.

An excellent example is the multimodulated muscle phosphofructokinase. The activity of this kinase is regulated by changing the self-association state of the enzyme as well as by macromolecular interactions. At physiological ionic strengths the active tetrameric form of phosphofructokinase is stabilized by binding to F-actin (for review see [97]). This virtually abolishes the allosteric regulation by fructose 1,6-bisphosphate and glucose 1,6-bisphosphate, increases the K_i for ATP and decreases the $K_{0.5}$ for fructose 6-phosphate [98]. The inhibition of phosphofructokinase by high [ATP] is reversed by F-actin at low ionic strengths which increases the apparent affinity of the enzyme for fructose 6-phosphate and there is a small increment in V_{max} [99]. The binding of aldolase and phosphofructokinase to F-actin is increased by both epidermal growth factor and insulin [100]. It was suggested that calmodulin decreases the overall activities of aldolase and phosphofructokinase [101,102]. The binding of these enzymes to the cytoskeleton is increased by both Ca^{2+} and calmodulin [103], while by contrast, high pathological $[Ca^{2+}]$ has opposite effects [104]. The mechanism of any coupling which occurs between these macromolecular complexes has not, however, been elucidated.

Recent data indicated that the inactive dimer forms of muscle phosphofructokinase bind to microtubules, decreasing the overall kinase activity [45]. The kinase periodically cross-links tubules via dimer–dimer interactions; however, these 'artificial' tetramers are not enzymically active, illustrating that the biological activity of the kinase requires not only tetrameric structure but also a highly specific arrangement of monomers. However, these data do not explain why the active tetrameric and the inactive dimeric forms of phosphofructokinase are those which specifically associate with actin and microtubules, respectively. Moreover, fructose bisphosphates have opposite effects on phosphofructokinase–F-actin and phosphofructokinase–microtubule interactions (Table 1 and Fig. 1); they facilitate the binding of the enzyme to F-actin but impede its interaction with microtubules, probably because the tetrameric form of the kinase is stabilized by these metabolites.

In very few cases have the functional consequences of the association of enzymes with tubules been investigated, and these studies were mainly with MAP-free microtubules *in vitro*. The overall activity of glyceraldehyde 3-phosphate dehydrogenase was decreased by interaction with microtubules because of preferential binding of the less active dissociated enzyme molecules [43] (Fig. 1). It was shown recently however, that the tetrameric enzyme was also inhibited by purified tubulin dimers [105]. Two classes of binding sites on tetrameric glyceraldehyde 3-phosphate dehydrogenase for the tubulin dimer have been demonstrated by binding and kinetic data [105]. The catalytic activity of the enzyme is unchanged by tubulin binding to the low-affinity site, although the enzyme is inhibited by tubulin binding to the high-affinity site.

Erythrocyte glyceraldehyde-3-phosphate dehydrogenase activity is inhibited by band 3 protein. Substrates inhibit both dehydrogenase–microtubule and dehydrogenase–(band 3 protein) interactions, and the inhibition is competitive with NAD^+ and arsenate [76,105]. Associations of aldolase with microtubule or band 3 protein were also observed; the enzyme was competitively inhibited by microtubules [102], tubulin [70,102] and band 3 protein [71,74]. Homologous binding peptides of α tubulin from *Plasmodium falciparum* and human band 3 protein were identified, and these were competitive inhibitors of *Plasmodium falciparum* aldolase [71].

Direct evidence for the control of glycolysis in erythrocytes by binding of some enzymes to the cytoplasmic extension of the anion transporter band 3 protein *in vivo* was provided after the development of rigorous tests. By changing the availability of binding sites for glycolytic enzymes at the extreme N-terminus of band 3 the glycolytic flux could be varied over 30-fold [106]. The rate of lactate formation was increased by approx. 3-fold by anti-peptide antibodies raised against residues 1–15 of band 3 which blocked these inhibitory sites. The rate of lactate formation was decreased by more than 10-fold by enrichment of cytoplasm of erythrocytes with the band 3 peptide (the antibodies described above were raised against this). Hexokinase may be one of the enzymes effected by binding to band 3 during antibody treatment, as indicated by analysis of changes in the concentrations of glycolytic intermediates. The cell, therefore, can regulate its glycolytic flux over a wide range by controlling the extent of occupation of the enzyme-binding site at the N-terminus of the anion transporter. The reversible covalent blockade of an inhibitory membrane binding site provides the basis for this type of metabolic control [106]. The regulation of enzyme interactions with the band 3 peptide may be an auxiliary pathway to increase or decrease energy production, although the classical regulatory mechanisms appear to predominate in metabolic control in erythrocytes [106].

Possible significance of channelling in glycolysis

Not only can the properties of the individual enzyme be modified as a result of enzyme associations, but these associations may provide advantages for catalysis by arranging enzymes of a pathway next to each other. Such an organization of metabolic sequences may permit 'substrate channelling' and the resulting microcompartmentation of metabolites that might ensure physiologically significant consequences. These consequences can be fulfilled via different molecular mechanisms that require specific enzyme associations, for example interactions between sequential enzymes or associations of sequential enzymes on the actin filament close to each other. In fact, such a sequential arrangement of phosphofructokinase, aldolase and glyceraldehyde-

3-phosphate dehydrogenase on actin filaments was demonstrated by using antigenic probes [61]. This spatial arrangement of active sites can ensure that the intermediate binds to the next enzyme with a high probability instead of leaving the complex [107]. Thus the catalytic efficiency of the overall process is increased without an alteration of the intrinsic catalytic activities of the components. However, the sequential arrangement of metabolically linked enzymes may alter not only the local properties of the enzymes but also the system (glycolysis) properties. These and related issues are extensively reviewed elsewhere [56,58,65,108,109] and discussed in other chapters of this book.

Lag-time analysis is a simple and powerful tool for analysis of metabolic channelling [107,110–113]. The transient time is the most physiologically realistic temporal response during which a metabolic system undergoes a transition from one steady state to another after a perturbation (e.g. through variation in the rate of substrate supply or in the presence of external effector substances) [114]. The (total) transient (lag) time, τ, is composed of the diffusional transient time, τ_d, and reaction transient time, τ_r (see the Introduction). The reciprocal values, $1/\tau_d$ and $1/\tau_r$, are the pseudo-first-order rate constants for the velocity at which a substrate molecule encounters the 'recognition volume' of the enzyme active site and for formation of the enzyme–substrate complex, respectively. In the cases of multi-step reactions the overall transition time for a whole metabolic pathway is the sum of the τ values for all its component enzyme reactions, and it is given by the ratio of steady-state intermediate concentrations to steady-state flux [114–117].

For non-interacting systems the transient times can be estimated from the kinetic constants of the individual enzymes [110]. If we consider simple two-step irreversible consecutive reactions catalysed by enzymes E_1 and E_2 under conditions whereby the first reaction proceeds at constant velocity and the concentration of intermediate, [I], is low enough for the second reaction to be first order, then the progress curve of product formation for a non-interacting bulk system can be described as follows:

$$P(t) = v\tau - v\tau(1 - e^{-t/\tau})$$

where v is the steady-state velocity of the overall reaction catalysed by the two-enzyme sequence. In a non-interacting system v is just the activity of free E_1 ($v = v_{E1}$) and τ is inversely proportional to the concentration of E_2 ($\tau = K_m/V_{max}$) [110].

However, channelling may be indicated if the transient time in a coupled reaction is less than predicted. Kinetic approaches have been developed to detect metabolic channelling and to identify the mechanism of intermediate transfer. Many of these kinetic methods are based upon measuring the steady-state flux in consecutive reactions catalysed by functionally related enzymes as well as determining the time required to attain the steady-state flux. One possibility is to compare the kinetic behaviour of interacting and non-interacting systems by determining the transient times and steady-state velocities of coupled reactions (i) at given enzyme concentrations under interacting conditions and analysing the deviation from a non-interacting system calculated from the parameters of the individual enzymes; (ii) at various enzyme concentrations and analysing the deviations as a function of enzyme concentration, keeping the ratios of the enzymes constant; and (iii) under non-interacting (i.e. high ionic strength, low enzyme concentrations) and interacting (i.e. crowding agents, preincubation, high enzyme concentrations) conditions at given enzyme concentrations.

However, these analyses have to include the determination of the kinetic parameters of the individual enzyme reactions in the presence of the other enzyme(s), since the interactions of enzymes may induce alterations in their tertiary and quaternary structure which alter transient time and/or steady-state velocity values due to the 'kinetically significant' interaction of enzymes, even if the free diffusion mechanism holds [112]. These effects are considered in our simple kinetic approach, which is based upon the identification of the relationship among macroscopic kinetic parameters [112,113]. The time courses of coupled and individual reactions catalysed by aldolase and glycerol-3-phosphate dehydrogenase as a typical example are presented in Fig. 2 [118]. The relationship between the transient time (τ_{app}) for the coupled reactions catalysed by the complexed and uncomplexed enzyme species and the pseudo-first-order rate constants (dehydrogenase reaction) measured in the absence (k_{E2}) and presence ($k_{E2,E1}$) of E_1 (aldolase) are indicative of the mechanism in the interacting enzyme system. If the interaction of the two enzymes induces alterations in the kinetic properties of the complexed enzymes without producing channelling of the intermediate, the following relationships hold: $v_{E1} \leq \geq v_{E1,E2}$ and $k_{E2} \leq \geq k_{E2,E1}$. If the intermediate produced endogenously by the $E_1 \cdot E_2$ complex is channelled between the two enzymes, the transient time is reduced with respect to that measured in a non-interacting system. This relationship may result either from steric hindrance, which impedes the diffusion of intermediate into the bulk solution, or simply from the juxtaposition of active sites of the enzymes in complexed form. The former case is represented by the aldolase/glycerol-3-phosphate dehydrogenase system, where the following relationship between kinetic parameters holds:

$$1/\tau > k_{app}[\text{dehydrogenase}] > k_{app}[\text{dehydrogenase} + \text{aldolase}]$$

which means that aldolase impedes the binding of exogeneous intermediate to the dehydrogenase via steric hindrance.

The latter case, which can be considered as a special one, we defined as a 'leaky' channel. A leaky channel mechanism for the intermediate was identified when the aldolase/glyceraldehyde-3-phosphate dehydrogenase system was used [113]. Conflicting results were obtained for this system [119] that have been reviewed elsewhere [58,83,120]. However, it is important to emphasize that at high E_2 concentrations the transient time for a non-interacting system reaches that measured for an interacting one, since both the free and channelled pools are minimized [107,121]. Thus with a large excess of second enzyme the free diffusion and channelled mechanisms cannot be distinguished. This is especially important for workers who re-examine 'channelling mechanisms' at high excess of second enzyme and draw incorrect conclusions regarding the mechanism of intermediate transfer [119].

The leaky channelling mechanism for triosephosphate transfer from aldolase to glyceraldehyde-3-phosphate dehydrogenase was also demonstrated using an isotope dilution technique [113]. This mechanism means that the exogenous intermediate binds to the complexed dehydrogenase with the same probability as to the free one. This finding indicates that the active site of the dehydrogenase in its complexed form may not be blocked completely by aldolase. In fact, this is the situation which is expected for enzymes involved in non-processive metabolic pathways such as glycolysis. Recently, the compartmentalized glycolytic sequence consisting of aldolase, triosephosphate isomerase, glyceraldehyde-3-phosphate dehydrogenase and phosphoglycerate kinase was reported for isolated skeletal muscle triads [122].

Fig. 2   **Time courses of coupled and individual reactions catalysed by aldolase and glycerol-3-phosphate dehydrogenase**

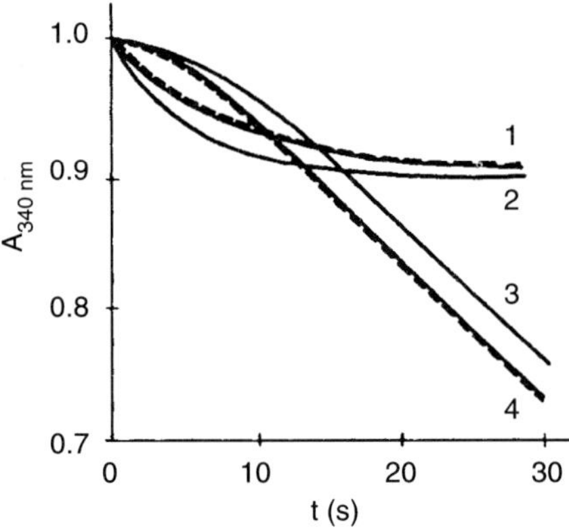

Curves 1 and 2, conversion of exogenous dihydroxyacetone phosphate catalysed by dehydrogenase in the presence of aldolase but in the absence of fructose 1,6-bisphosphate. Curves 3 and 4, progress curves of NADH oxidation catalysed by aldolase and dehydrogenase. Broken lines are experimental curves. The continuous curves were computed by assuming $k_{E2} = 0.11\ s^{-1}$ (curve 1) and $0.18\ s^{-1}$ (curve 2) for the individual reactions, and $1/\tau = 0.11\ s^{-1}$ (curve 3) and $0.18\ s^{-1}$ (curve 4) for the coupled reactions. The steady-state velocity of the coupled reaction was $0.011\,\Delta A_{340}/s$. The enzyme concentrations were $0.15\ \mu M$ and $2.0\ \mu M$ for dehydrogenase and aldolase, respectively. The initial concentrations of fructose 1,6-bisphosphate and dihydroxyacetone phosphate, if present, were $1.0\ mM$ and $0.016\ mM$, respectively. Reproduced with permission from [118].

Although this kinetic analysis displays limitations, since it assumes zero-order and pseudo-first order kinetic behaviour of E_1 and E_2, respectively and irreversible conversions, the advantages are significant: (i) knowledge of the catalytic mechanisms of enzymes is not required; (ii) the mechanism of intermediate transfer can be identified; (iii) the identification does not require knowledge of the dissociation constant of the enzyme complex, since the kinetic parameters of the consecutive and the individual reactions are determined at the same E_1 and E_2 concentrations in both sets of experiments; and (iv) if the dissociation constant is known from independent measurements then the efficiency of the channel can be deduced.

The second and third points are especially important for recent studies. The second point allows the possibility to differentiate between 'kinetically significant' and 'channelling' enzyme complexes that makes this approach unique among kinetic analyses, including Metabolic Control Analysis. The validity of the third point renders it possible to analyse complex (e.g. *in situ*) biological systems for the existence of metabolite channelling. In fact, the channelling of carbamoyl phosphate, the intermediate of the reactions catalysed by aspartate transcarbamoylase and carbamoyl-phosphate synthase, was analysed in permeabilized cells using our kinetic approach [123]. The data showed that within this multifunctional enzyme the intermediate is partially channelled; thus it could leak and diffuse outside the complex.

Microcompartmentation in the glycolytic pathway

Multiple pools may occur in the cell as a result of metabolite segregation or enzyme associations. An intermediate pool within enzyme complexes can be formed due to the juxtaposition of the active site of the relevant enzymes or if the diffusion of the intermediate into the bulk solution is impeded by steric hindrance [96,124,125]. These 'internal pools' are smaller than in the situation where the enzymes and intermediates diffuse freely; thus the next enzyme in the sequence meets a higher concentration of the localized metabolites and this might serve to maintain a high local concentration of intermediates for efficient functioning of an enzyme. There are additional advantages of the existence of separate intermediate pools depending on physiological need. Studies of metabolite compartmentation of glycolytic intermediates have been carried out with a number of cell types using a wide variety of methodologies. In this section we attempt to give a representative view of these *in situ* and *in vitro* experiments.

Clegg and colleagues have developed a permeabilization technique using dextran sulphate to study channelling of glycolysis in mouse fibroblasts (L-292 cells) [126–128]. Although these cells are permeable to high molecular mass proteins (up to 400 kDa), they nevertheless maintain a high rate of glycolysis when incubated in a medium of appropriate composition. The glycolytic rate is higher than in intact cells, presumably because of the constraints in the intact cells resulting from compartmentation. When the dextran-permeabilized cells were incubated with ^{14}C-glucose the dilution by exogenous intermediates of the ^{14}C-lactate formed was not what would have been expected if there were complete mixing of the intermediates with the 'bulk' phase in the incubation medium. When the oxidation of glucose to $^{14}CO_2$ was determined in the dextran-permeabilized cells it was shown that various unlabelled glycolytic intermediates diluted the ^{14}C-label. Exogenous pyruvate, however, had remarkably little effect on isotope dilution, indicating that pyruvate derived from glucose does not equilibrate with the bulk phase during entry into mitochondria. Furthermore, exogenous pyruvate had little effect on stimulation of respiration in the permeabilized cells despite oxidation of pyruvate derived from glucose. These data were interpreted as indicating that pyruvate formed from glucose does not mix with the pyruvate pool that is derived from exogenous lactate or pyruvate.

Evidence for more than one pyruvate pool has also been obtained from studies on the isolated rat heart perfused by the Langendorff technique [129,130]. The perfused heart was studied in steady-state conditions using various labelled substrates, including [3,4-^{14}C]glucose and [1-^{14}C]pyruvate or [1-^{14}C]lactate and the incorporation of label into pyruvate, lactate and alanine were determined. Two pyruvate pools were demonstrated. Further evidence for compartmentation of pyruvate was obtained using dichloroacetate, a potent activator of pyruvate dehydrogenase via inhibition of the protein kinase [130]. It was suggested that multiple pools result from close functional interactions between cytoplasmic pyruvate kinase and the mitochondrial pyruvate dehydrogenase complex.

An aggregate or complex consisting of four sequential glycolytic enzymes (aldolase, triosephosphate isomerase, glyceraldehyde-3-phosphate dehydrogenase and phosphoglycerate kinase) has been demonstrated in the skeletal muscle triad at the site of excitation contraction coupling [122]. There is evidence that the ATP formed via phosphoglycerate kinase cannot be used by an exogenous ATP-consuming system involving hexokinase and 2-deoxyglucose. The implication is that the ATP generated in the muscle triads is utilized at the site of production by coupling to an ATP-requiring system and/or that there is restricted diffusion of ATP from this microcompartment. These and other observations suggest that ATP production and utilization are not in equilibrium with a 'bulk' myoplasmic ATP pool.

Various studies have provided evidence for interactions between the integrity of the cytoskeleton and ATP metabolism [131]. Actin-containing bundles differ in their sensitivity to ATP [132] and accordingly the ATP formed via glycolysis determines the organization of the filament structure. NMR has been used in studies on the perfused heart to investigate the interaction between aerobic glycolysis and ischaemic contraction [133]. Although the cause of the ischaemic contraction remains controversial, there is evidence that during ischaemia the ATP-deficient myosin cross-bridge

binds to actin [134]. While it is generally accepted that in the normal heart ischaemic contraction is caused by rigor bond formation because of a lowering of ATP availability in the myofibrils, there is evidence that the onset of contraction is induced by the rate of ATP production *per se*, rather than by the overall ATP concentration. It is possible that the phosphocreatine/creatine kinase system enables the transfer of ATP (and likewise removal of ADP) to the cross-bridge rather than diffusion of ATP and ADP between the cross-bridge and the bulk phase. A possible implication from such a model is that compartmentation of intermediates or channelling of adenine nucleotides might delay the onset of ischaemic contractions [133].

Vascular smooth muscle cells have been used by Paul and colleagues to study the control of glycolysis and oxidative phosphorylation, because these cells maintain a high rate of lactate production in well-oxygenated conditions [135]. Using porcine carotid artery, which comprises mainly tonic vascular smooth muscle, they showed that lactate production and oxidative phosphorylation change independently [136] and suggested that ATP formed via oxidative phosphorylation is utilized for muscle contraction while ATP derived via glycolysis in a microcompartment associated with the plasma membrane is used for the Na/K-ATPase and Ca^{2+}-ATPase [137,138].

Isolated hepatocytes have been used by Berry and colleagues to study the balance of glucose metabolism between glycolysis and gluconeogenesis [139]. During incubation with various glucose concentrations, the rate of lactate formation from glucose is not linear with time but gradually declines and reaches a steady state. This decline in lactate production is not due to conversion to pyruvate and uptake into mitochondria but to a decline in the rate of glycolytic flux. The actual steady-state concentration of extracellular lactate when there is no further net glycolysis is a function of the extracellular glucose concentration. The concentrations of intermediary metabolites that are known to modulate phosphofructokinase activity such as citrate, fructose 1,6-bisphosphate and adenine nucleotides do not change. Thus the decline in flux cannot be attributed to changes in the elasticity coefficients of phosphofructokinase. At steady state when there is no net glycolytic flux, the system is very far removed from thermodynamic equilibrium ([lactate]/[glucose] $> 10^6$). The conclusion drawn from these studies was that the free energy of glycolysis is balanced by intracellular forces. It was hypothesized that the complexity of intracellular organization maintains the compartmentation of glycolytic intermediates in the hepatocytes [140,141].

The question of whether exogenous glucose and endogenous glycogen are metabolized by separate or distinct glycolytic routes has been studied by Hardin and colleagues in smooth muscle using ^{13}C NMR [142]. By following the position of the ^{13}C label it was shown that the label from exogenous glucose was recovered in lactate, whereas that from endogenous glycogen was metabolized intramitochondrially. Furthermore, the glycolytic intermediates of the two pathways did not mix completely, despite simultaneous net metabolism of glucose and catabolism of glycogen, suggesting that either or both pathways may be in part channelled.

In other studies Hardin and colleagues used exogenous ^{13}C-labelled fructose 1,6-bisphosphate to study compartmentation of glycolysis in vascular smooth muscle [143,144] (Fig. 3). The metabolism of exogeneously added ^{13}C-labelled fructose 1,6-bisphosphate and of [2-^{13}C]glucose in well-oxygenated and well-superfused hog carotid artery segments was examined [143]. When [1,6-^{13}C]fructose 1,6-bisphosphate or [1-^{13}C]fructose 1,6-bisphosphate was utilized individually, gluconeogenic flux occurred without metabolism through aldolase and triosephosphate isomerase, resulting in the formation of [1,6-^{13}C]glucose and [1-^{13}C]glucose, respectively. When [2-^{13}C]glucose was the sole exogenous substrate, it was utilized and participated exclusively in glycolytic flux, with production of [2-^{13}C]lactate and no gluconeogenic flux from the trioses to [5-^{13}C]glucose. When both glucose and fructose bisphosphate were provided together as

Fig. 3   **Schematic representation of label positions derived from [2-^{13}C]glucose, [1,6-^{13}C]fructose 1,6-bisphosphate and [1-^{13}C]fructose 1,6-bisphosphate**

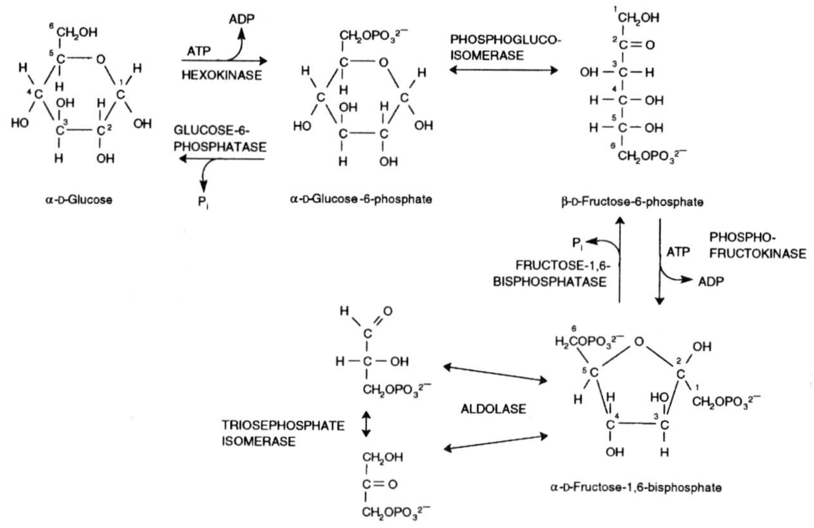

If gluconeogenesis from [1-^{13}C]fructose 1,6-bisphosphate occurs without reaction through aldolase and triosephosphate isomerase, the glucose formed will be labelled in the same positions as the starting fructose 1,6-bisphosphate ([1-^{13}C]glucose). However, if isomerization occurs then both [1-^{13}C]glucose and [6-^{13}C]glucose will be observed. Similarly, if glucose catabolism proceeds beyond the aldolase step and the resulting trioses participate in gluconeogenesis, then resonances from [5-^{13}C]glucose and [2-^{13}C]glucose will be observed. Reproduced with permission from [144].

exogenous substrates, glucose still participated exclusively in glycolytic flux, with no trioses participating in gluconeogenesis, whereas fructose bisphosphate partly participated in glycolytic flux, with production of [3-^{13}C]lactate. It was concluded that the intermediates of glucose utilization and catabolism to lactate do not appear to mix with the intermediates of exogenous fructose 1,6-bisphosphate metabolism. Therefore the existence of simultaneous yet separable fluxes of glycolysis and gluconeogenesis indicates a structural organization of carbohydrate metabolism in vascular smooth muscle.

Discussion

Ultrastructural evidence for the association of glycolytic enzymes with the contractile apparatus of muscle was reported 30 years ago [145]. Compelling evidence now exists for the structural organization of glycolytic enzymes in *in vivo*, *in situ* and *in vitro* systems. These associations are relatively weak, frequently transient, and their association states depend on the experimental or cellular conditions, and most importantly on cell type.

Molecular models based upon dynamic enzyme associations have been suggested with special features. For example, Masters and colleagues [67] proposed that glycolysis exists *in vivo* as a number of segments consisting of four enzymes or less. Characteristically these are capable of being mobilized at several locations within the cytoplasmic compartment, and often act independently of other segments. Metabolite-modulated bienzyme associations of sequential glycolytic enzymes were postulated as a control mechanism of glycolysis with special consideration of oligomer-form specific interactions [83]. The possibility that intermediates might be involved in enzyme distribution by adsorption–desorption mechanisms has been also discussed by Ryazanov and co-workers [146]. The enzyme associations coupled with the polymerization–depolymerization of actin and microtubular systems have been suggested to function as intracellular mechanisms which synchronize local and global processes [147]. These models as potential control mechanisms have to be taken into account as well as or instead of the classic mechanisms of feedback inhibition/activation or covalent modification of the key glycolytic enzymes in order to understand the complex energy production of living cells.

Enzyme complex formation, therefore (even if no metabolite channelling occurs), can increase glycolytic flux through selected enzyme forms and decrease flux through others, resulting in effective metabolic regulation [64,67,83]. This kind of enzyme association may provide a new regulatory mechanism for glycolysis. For example, actin filaments activate phosphofructokinase [149] whereas microtubules inactivate it [45]. These phenomena are based upon different multiple equilibria of actin–phosphofructokinase and microtubule–phosphofructokinase systems. Different oligomeric forms of the enzyme are stabilized upon binding: the active tetramer is stabilized by F-actin whereas the inactive dimers preferentially associate with microtubules. In addition, the modulating effects of metabolites on these associations are opposite (Table 1). Because of limited data it is difficult to speculate about the physiological relevance of these phenomena. Nevertheless, the bound enzymes may serve other non-enzymic functions under some metabolic conditions [35]. For example, the inactive oligomeric forms of phosphofructokinase periodically cross-link microtubules [46], altering their stability and resistance to effectors.

Several functional consequences (advantages) of metabolite channelling due to the association of glycolytic enzymes have been postulated [150]: (i) it prevents or impedes loss of intermediates by diffusion; (ii) it decreases the transit time required for intermediates to reach the active site of the next enzyme; (iii) the transient time for the system to reach a new steady state is reduced; (iv) it protects chemically labile intermediates, e.g. the glyceraldehyde 3-phosphate; (v) it circumvents unfavourable equilibria, e.g. aldolase-catalysed reactions; and (vi) it segregates the intermediates of competing chemical and enzymic reaction. These consequences probably confer advantages for glycolysis. For instance, in muscle glycolysis metabolic channelling facilitates a 1000-fold increase in flux, without a significant lag phase, which is accomplished in less than 1 s in response to external stimuli [79].

Glycolysis is an example of an amphibolic pathway, since the intermediates are also used in many pathways in the cells. In enzyme complexes, in which several enzymes are permanently associated and catalyse the conversion of intermediates via several steps, the space where these reactions occur obviously cannot be completely closed off from the medium. Rather, this space must be open to let in the first metabolite and to let out the final metabolite (product) of the complex. Since glycolytic intermediates have multiple reaction fates, there has to be leakiness in the channelling process in order that the intermediates (e.g. triosephosphates) are shared among metabolic pathways (e.g. glycolysis and lipid synthesis). This co-ordinate effect can determine the direction of sugar phosphate conversion within the enzyme complexes. This may be achievable via modulation of weak pair-wise enzyme–enzyme interactions at metabolic branch-points by key regulatory substrates [84,95,148]. In addition, the intermediates can be kept in a limited microenvironment, and competition with other pathways can be minimized. Therefore the co-ordinate effect of channelling mechanisms could act elegantly in dynamically associated enzyme systems where the channelling process is a system- and time-dependent phenomenon. Particularly in the case of actin-filament-associated enzymes, the vectorial motion of specific metabolites might ensure catalytic advantages for glycolysis. Accordingly, the triose- and hexose-phosphates could be compartmentalized in a highly specific fashion *in vivo*.

In any textbook of biochemistry written during the last two decades very little change can be found in the discussion of the principles of regulation of glycolysis. As Srere [151] pointed out, the problem is that the metabolic pathways are treated as sequential, isolated events, the control of which exists as the sum of properties of individual enzymes, and there are 'rate-limiting' enzymes that control glycolysis. Now it is clear that glycolysis is a more complex process. In a recent study glycolytic flux and the work performed by rat heart were measured under conditions where the hearts were perfused with glucose, glucose plus insulin, glucose plus ketone bodies or glucose, insulin and ketone bodies [152]. These data indicated that control of glucose utilization does not reside at a single step, and control by different steps varied as conditions were varied. Recent NMR data with overexpressed phosphofructokinase showed that the overexpression had no effect on glycolytic flux under anaerobic conditions, but under aerobic conditions it increased glycolytic flux up to anaerobic rates [153]. The enzymes share the control of glycolysis, and their contributions to this control depend on the metabolic conditions. Therefore, the classic metabolic concept has been replaced by new ones which consider the complexity of metabolic regulation. With regard to glycolysis, dynamic enzyme associations are complicated by the diversity of interactions and microenvironmental factors which affect these associations, as well as by the diverse types of energy requirement from glycolysis in a variety of physiological situations.

This work was supported by grants from the Hungarian National Science Foundation (OTKA T-5412, T-6349 and T-17830) to J.O.

References

1. From, A.H.L., Zimmer, S.D., Michurski, S.P., Mohanakrishnan, P., Ulstad, V.K., Thoma, W.J. and Ugurbil, K. (1990) Biochemistry **29**, 3731–3743
2. Brown, G.C. (1992) Biochem. J. **284**, 1–13
3. Aragon, J.J. and Sánchez, V. (1985) Biochem. Biophys. Res. Commun. **131**, 849–855
4. Aragon, J.J. and Sols, A. (1991) FASEB J. **5**, 2945–2950
5. Masters, C. (1984) J. Cell Biol. **99**, 222S–225S
6. Uyeda, K. (1979) Adv. Enzymol. **48**, 193–244
7. Clegg, J.S. (1987) in Molecular Mechanisms in the Regulation of Cell Behavior (Waymouth, C., ed.), pp. 151–156, A.R. Liss, New York
8. Clegg, J.S. (1986) in Membranes, Metabolism and Dry Organisms (Leopold, A.C., ed.), pp. 169–187, Cornell University Press, New York
9. Fushimi, K. and Verkman, A.S. (1991) J. Cell Biol. **112**, 719–725
10. Valberg, P.A. and Albertini, D.F. (1985) J. Cell Biol. **101**, 130–140
11. Luby-Phelps, K., Mujumdar, S., Mujumdar, R., Ernst, L., Galbraith, W. and Waggoner, A. (1993) Biophys. J. **65**, 236–242
12. Bicknese, N., Periasamy, N., Shohet, S.B. and Verkman, A.S. (1993) Biophys. J. **65**, 1272–1282
13. Scalettar, B.A. and Abney, J.R. (1991) Comments Mol. Cell. Biophys. **7**, 79–107
14. Mastro, A.M. and Hurley, D.J. (1986) in Organization of Cell Metabolism (Welch, G.R. and Clegg, J.S., eds.), pp. 57–74, Plenum Press, New York
15. Kao, H.P., Abney, J.R. and Verkman, A.S. (1993) J. Cell Biol. **120**, 175–184
16. Luby-Phelps, K., Lanni, F. and Taylor, D.L. (1988) Annu. Rev. Biophys. Chem **17**, 369–396

17. Luby-Phelps, K. (1994) Comments Mol. Cell. Biophys. **8**, 199–216
18. Jacobson, K. and Wojcieszyn, J. (1984) Proc. Natl. Acad. Sci. U.S.A. **81**, 6747–6751
19. von Hippel, P.H. and Berg, O.G. (1989) J. Biol. Chem. **264**, 675–678
20. Adam, G. and Delbrück, M. (1968) in Structural Chemistry and Molecular Biology (Rich, A. and Davidson, N., eds.), pp. 198–215, W.H. Freeman, San Francisco
21. Northrup, S.H., Boles, J.O. and Reynolds, J.C.L. (1988) Science **241**, 67–70
22. Katchalski-Katzir, E., Rishpon, J., Sahar, E. and Lamed, R. (1985) Biopolymers **24**, 257–277
23. Berg, O.G. (1985) Biophys. J. **47**, 1–14
24. Moses, V. (1986) in Organization of Cell Metabolism (Welch, G.R. and Clegg, J.S., eds.), pp. 121–129, Plenum Press, New York
25. Kaprelyants, A.S. (1988) Trends Biochem. Sci. **13**, 43–46
26. Porter, K.R. (1986) in Organization of Cell Metabolism (Welch, G.R. and Clegg, J.S., eds.), pp. 9–25, Plenum Press, New York
27. Porter, K.R. (1984) J. Cell Biol. **99**, 3S–12S
28. Mastro, A.M., Babich, M.A., Taylor, W.D. and Keith, A.D. (1984) Proc. Natl. Acad. Sci. U.S.A. **81**, 3414–3418
29. Dix, J. and Verkman, A.S. (1990) Biophys. J. **57**, 231–240
30. Gershon, N.D., Porter, K.R. and Trus, B.L. (1985) Proc. Natl. Acad. Sci. U.S.A. **82**, 5030–5034
31. Pagliaro, L. and Taylor, D.L. (1988) J. Cell Biol. **107**, 981–991
32. Fulton, A.B. (1982) Cell **30**, 345–347
33. Small, J.V. (1988) Electron Microsc. Rev. **1**, 155–174
34. Wallraff, E., Schleicher, M., Modersitzki, M., Rieger, D., Isenberg, G. and Gerisch, G. (1986) EMBO J. **5**, 61–67
35. Maciver, S.K., Wachsstock, D.H., Schwarz, W.H. and Pollard, T.D. (1991) J. Cell Biol. **115**, 1621–1628
36. Roberts, S.J. and Somero, G.N. (1987) Biochemistry **26**, 3437–3442
37. Morton, D.G., Clarke, F.M. and Masters, C.J. (1977) J. Cell Biol. **74**, 1016–1023
38. Pagliaro, L., Kerr, K. and Taylor, D.L. (1989) J. Cell Sci. **94**, 333–342
39. Bershadsky, A.D. and Vasiliev, J.M. (1988) Cytoskeleton, Plenum Press, New York
40. MacRae, T.H. (1992) Biochim. Biophys. Acta **1160**, 145–155
41. Bennett, A.F. and Baines, A.J. (1992) Eur. J. Biochem. **206**, 783–792
42. Somers, M., Engelborghs, Y. and Baert, J. (1990) Eur. J. Biochem. **193**, 437–444
43. Durrieu, C., Bernier-Valentin, F. and Rousset, B. (1987) Arch. Biochem. Biophys. **252**, 32–40
44. Huitorel, P. and Pantaloni, D. (1985) Eur. J. Biochem. **150**, 265–269
45. Lehotzky, A., Telegdi, M., Liliom, K. and Ovádi, J. (1993) J. Biol. Chem. **268**, 10888–10894
46. Lehotzky, A., Pálfia, Z., Kovács, J., Molnár, A. and Ovádi, J. (1994) Biochem. Biophys. Res. Commun. **204**, 585–591
47. Horne, Z. and Hesketh, J.E. (1990) Biochem. J. **268**, 231–236
48. Singer, R.H., Langevin, G.L. and Lawrence, J.B. (1989) J. Cell Biol. **108**, 2343–2353
49. Agutter, P.S. (1990) Between Nucleus and Cytoplasm, Chapman and Hall, London
50. Ryazanov, A.G. (1985) FEBS Lett. **192**, 131–134
51. Dolken, G., Leisner, E. and Pette, D. (1975) Histochemistry **43**, 113–121
52. Arnold, H. and Pette, D. (1968) Eur. J. Biochem. **6**, 163–171
53. Clarke, F.M. and Masters, C.J. (1975) Biochim. Biophys. Acta **381**, 37–46
54. Clarke, F.M. and Masters, C.J. (1976) Int. J. Biochem. **7**, 359–365
55. Stewart, M., Morton, D.J. and Clarke, F.M. (1980) Biochem. J. **186**, 99–104
56. Clarke, F., Stephan, P., Morton, D. and Weidemann, J. (1985) Regulation of Carbohydrate Metabolism (Beitner, R., ed.), vol. 2, pp. 1–31, CRC Press, Boca Raton, FL
57. Knull, H.R. and Walsh, J.L. (1992) Curr. Top. Cell. Regul. **33**, 15–30
58. Keleti, T., Ovádi, J. and Batke, J. (1989) Prog. Biophys. Mol. Biol. **53**, 105–152
59. Minaschek, G., Stewart, U.G., Blum, S. and Bereiter-Hahn, J. (1992) Eur. J. Cell Biol. **58**, 418–428
60. Cornish-Bowden, A. and Cardenas, M.L. (eds.) (1990) Control of Metabolic Processes, Plenum Press, New York

61. Méjean, C., Pons, F., Benyamin, Y. and Roustan, C. (1989) Biochem. J. **264**, 671–677
62. Humphreys, L., Reid, S. and Masters, C.J. (1986) Int. J. Biochem. **18**, 445–451
63. Stephan, P., Clarke, F. and Morton, D. (1986) Biochim. Biophys. Acta **873**, 127–135
64. Brooks, S.P.J. and Storey, K.B. (1991) FEBS Lett. **278**, 135–138
65. Masters, C. (1989) Trends Biochem. Sci. **14**, 361
66. Kurganov, B.I. (1986) J. Theor. Biol. **119**, 445–452
67. Masters, C., Reid, S. and Don, M. (1987) Mol. Cell. Biochem. **76**, 3–14
68. Pagliaro, L. and Taylor, D.L. (1992) J. Cell Biol. **118**, 859–863
69. Carr, D. and Knull, H. (1993) Biochem. Biophys. Res. Commun. **195**, 289–293
70. Volker, K.W. and Knull, H.R. (1993) J. Mol. Recognit. **6**, 167–177
71. Itin, C., Burki, Y., Certa, U. and Dobeli, H. (1993) Mol. Biochem. Parasitol. **58**, 135–143
72. Orosz, F., Christova, T.Y. and Ovádi, J. (1987) Biochem. Biophys. Res. Commun. **147**, 1121–1128
73. Tsai, I., Murthy, S.N.P. and Steck, T.L. (1982) J. Biol. Chem. **257**, 1438–1442
74. Jenkins, J.D., Kezdy, F.J. and Steck, T.L. (1985) J. Biol. Chem. **260**, 10426–10433
75. Higashi, T., Richards, C.S. and Uyeda, K. (1979) J. Biol. Chem. **254**, 9542–9550
76. Uyeda, K. (1992) Curr. Top. Cell. Regul. **33**, 31–46
77. Marmillot, P., Keith, T., Srivastava, D.K. and Knull, H.R. (1994) Arch. Biochem. Biophys. **315**, 467–472
78. Minton, A.P. (1983) Mol. Cell. Biochem. **55**, 119–140
79. Srivastava, D.K. (1991) J. Theor. Biol. **152**, 93–101
80. Ovádi, J., Salerno, C., Keleti, T. and Fasella, P. (1978) Eur. J. Biochem. **90**, 499–503
81. Ovádi, J., Mohamed Osman, I.R. and Batke, J. (1983) Eur. J. Biochem. **133**, 433–437
82. Ovádi, J. (1989) Acta Biochim. Biophys. Hung. **24**, 41–59
83. Ovádi, J. (1988) Trends Biochem. Sci. **13**, 486–490
84. Neuzil, J., Danielson, H., Welch, G.R. and Ovádi, J. (1990) Biochim. Biophys. Acta **1037**, 307–312
85. Vértessy, G.B., Orosz, F. and Ovádi, J. (1991) Biochim. Biophys. Acta **1078**, 236–242
86. Wilson, J.E. (1978) Trends Biochem. Sci. **3**, 124–125
87. Wilson, J.E. (1980) Curr. Top. Cell. Regul. **16**, 1–54
88. Laursen, S.E., Belknap, J.K., Sampson, K.E. and Knull, H.R. (1990) Biochim. Biophys. Acta **1034**, 118–121
89. Lynch, R.M., Fogarty, K.E. and Fay, F.S. (1991) J. Cell Biol. **112**, 385–395
90. Kabir, F. and Wilson, J.E. (1993) Arch. Biochem. Biophys. **300**, 641–650
91. Ureta, T. (1978) Curr. Top. Cell. Regul. **13**, 233–251
92. Ureta, T. (1991) J. Theor. Biol. **152**, 81–84
93. Lynch, R.M. and Paul, R.J. (1983) Science **222**, 1344–1346
94. Shearwin, K. and Masters, C. (1990) Biochem. Int. **22**, 735–740
95. Tompa, P., Batke, J., Ovádi, J., Welch, G.R. and Srere, P.A. (1987) J. Biol. Chem. **262**, 6089–6092
96. Welch, G.R. (1977) Prog. Biophys. Mol. Biol. **32**, 103–191
97. Somero, G.N. and Hand, S.C. (1990) Physiol. Zool. **63**, 443–471
98. Beitner, R. (1990) Int. J. Biochem. **22**, 553–557
99. Liou, R.-S. and Anderson, S. (1980) Biochemistry **19**, 2684–2688
100. Chen-Zion, M., Livnat, T., Morgenstern, H. and Beitner, R. (1992) Isr. J. Med. Sci. **28**, 764–771
101. Mayr, G.W. (1984) Eur. J. Biochem. **143**, 513–520
102. Ovádi, J. and Orosz, F. (1992) Curr. Top. Cell Regul. **33**, 105–126
103. Beitner, R. (1993) Int. J. Biochem. **25**, 297–305
104. Lilling, G. and Beitner, R. (1990) Int. J. Biochem. **22**, 857–863
105. Muronetz, V.I., Wang, Z.-X., Keith, T.J., Knull, H.R. and Srivastava, D.K. (1994) Arch. Biochem. Biophys. **313**, 253–260
106. Low, P.S., Rathinavelu, P. and Harrison, M.L. (1993) J. Biol. Chem. **268**, 14627–14631
107. Tompa, P., Batke, J. and Ovádi, J. (1987) FEBS Lett. **214**, 244–248
108. Knull, J.R. (1990) UCLA Symp. Mol. Cell. Biol. **133**, 215–228
109. Ovádi, J. (1991) J. Theor. Biol. **152**, 1–22

110. Hess, B. and Wurster, B. (1970) FEBS Lett. **9**, 73–77
111. Easterby, J.S. (1973) Biochim. Biophys. Acta **293**, 552–558
112. Ovádi, J., Tompa, P., Vértessy, B., Orosz, F., Keleti, T. and Welch, G.R. (1989) Biochem. J. **57**, 187–190
113. Orosz, F. and Ovádi, J. (1987) Biochim. Biophys. Acta **915**, 53–59
114. Easterby, J.S. (1981) Biochem. J. **199**, 155–161
115. Walsh, T.D., Masters, C.J., Morton, D.J. and Clarke, F.M. (1981) Biochim. Biophys. Acta **675**, 29–30
116. Westerhoff, H.V. and Welch, G.R. (1992) Curr. Top. Cell. Regul. **33**, 361–390
117. Welch, G.R. and Easterby, J.S. (1994) Trends Biochem. Sci. **19**, 193–197
118. Vértessy, B. and Ovádi, J. (1987) Eur. J. Biochem. **164**, 655–659
119. Kvassman, J.M., Pettersson, G. and Ryde-Pettersson, U. (1988) Eur. J. Biochem. **172**, 427–431
120. Srere, P.A. and Ovádi, J. (1990) FEBS Lett. **268**, 360–367
121. Easterby, J.S. (1989) Biochem. J. **264**, 605–607
122. Han, J.W., Thieleczek, R., Varsányi, M. and Heilmeyer, L.M.G., Jr. (1992) Biochemistry **31**, 377–384
123. Penverne, B., Belkaid, M. and Hervé, G. (1994) Arch. Biochem. Biophys. **309**, 85–93
124. Friedrich, P. (1985) in Organized Multienzyme Systems: Catalytic Properties (Welch, G.R., ed.), pp. 141–176, Academic Press, Orlando and London
125. Keleti, T. and Ovádi, J. (1988) Curr. Top. Cell. Regul. **29**, 1–33
126. Clegg, J.S. and Jackson, S.A. (1988) Biochem. J. **255**, 335–344
127. Clegg, J.S. and Jackson, S.A. (1989) Biochem. Biophys. Res. Commun. **160**, 1409–1414
128. Clegg, J.S. and Jackson, S.A. (1990) Arch. Biochem. Biophys. **278**, 452–460
129. Peuhkurinen, K.J., Hiltunen, J.K. and Hassinan, I.E. (1983) Biochem. J. **210**, 193–198
130. Schadewaldt, P., Münch, U. and Staib, W. (1983) Biochem. J. **216**, 761–764
131. Bershadsky, A.D. and Gelfand, V.I. (1983) Cell Biol. Int. Rep. **7**, 173–187
132. Bereiter-Hahn, J., Tillmann, U. and Voth, M. (1984) Cell Tissue Res. **238**, 129–134
133. Kingsley, P.B., Sako, E.Y., Yang, M.Q., Zimmer, S.D., Ugurbil, K., Foker, J.E. and From, A.H.L. (1991) Am. J. Physiol. **261**, H469–H478
134. Bremel, R.D. and Weber, A. (1972) Nature (London) **238**, 97–101
135. Paul, R.J. (1981) in Handbook of Physiology, Sect. 2: The Cardiovascular System, Vol. 2 (Bohr, D.F., Somlyo, A.P. and Sparks, H., eds.), pp. 201–235, Williams and Wilkins, Baltimore
136. Paul, R.J. (1983) Am. J. Physiol. **244**, C399–C409
137. Champbell, J.D. and Paul, R.J. (1992) J. Physiol. (London) **447**, 67–82
138. Hardin, C.D., Raeymaekers, L. and Paul, R.J. (1992) J. Gen. Physiol. **99**, 21–40
139. Berry, M.N., Gregory, R.B., Grivell, A.R., Henly, D.C., Philips, J.W., Wallace, P.G. and Welch, G.R. (1990) in Control of Metabolic Processes (Cornish-Bowden, A. and Cardenas, M.L., eds.), pp. 343–350, Plenum Press, New York
140. Berry, M.N., Gregory, R.B., Grivell, A.R., Henly, D.C., Philips, J.W., Wallace, P.G. and Welch, G.R. (1987) FEBS Lett. **224**, 201–207
141. Berry, M.N., Gregory, R.B., Grivell, A.R., Henly, D.C., Nobes, C.D., Philips, J.W. and Wallace, P.G. (1988) Biochim. Biophys. Acta **936**, 294–306
142. Hardin, C.D. and Kushmerick, M.J. (1994) J. Mol. Cell. Cardiol. **26**, 1197–1210
143. Hardin, C.H. and Roberts, T.M. (1994) Am. J. Physiol. **267**, H2325–H2332
144. Hardin, C.D. and Robers, T.M. (1995) Biochemistry **34**, 1323–1331
145. Amberson, W.R., Roisen, F.J. and Bauer, A.C. (1965) J. Cell. Comp. Physiol. **66**, 71–90
146. Ryazanov, A.G., Ashmarina, L.I. and Muronetz, V.I. (1988) Eur. J. Biochem. **171**, 301–305
147. Cortassa, S. and Aon, M.A. (1994) Cell Biol. Int. **18**, 687–713
148. Srivastava, D.K. and Bernhard, S.A. (1986) Curr. Top. Cell. Regul. **28**, 1–68
149. Luther, M.A., Cai, G.-Z. and Lee, J.C. (1986) Biochemistry **25**, 7931–7937
150. Ovádi, J. (1995) Cell Architecture and Metabolite Channelling, R.G. Landes Co., Austin and Springer Verlag, Heidelberg

151. Srere, P.A. (1994) Trends Biochem. Sci. **19**, 519–520
152. Kashiwaya, Y., Sato, K., Tsuchiya, N., Thomas, S., Fell, D.A., Veech, R.L. and Passonneau, J.V. (1994) J. Biol. Chem. **269**, 25502–25514
153. Davies, S.E.C. and Brindle, K.M. (1992) Biochemistry **31**, 4729–4735
154. Zahner, D. and Malaisse, W.J. (1993) Int. J. Biochem. **25**, 1303–1307
155. Orosz, F., Christova, T.Y. and Ovádi, J. (1988) Biochim. Biophys. Acta **957**, 293–300
156. Tompa, P., Bar, J. and Batke, J. (1986) Eur. J. Biochem. **159**, 117–124
157. Moorhead., G.B.G. and Plaxton, W.C. (1992) FEBS Lett. **313**, 277–280
158. Ovádi, J., Aragon, J.J. and Sols, A. (1986) Biochem. Biophys. Res. Commun. **135**, 852–856
159. MacGregor, J.S., Singh, V.N., Davoust, S., Melloni, E., Pontremolli, S. and Horecker, B.L. (1980) Proc. Natl. Acad. Sci. U.S.A. **77**, 3889–3892
160. Salerno, C. and Ovádi, J. (1982) FEBS Lett. **138**, 270–272
161. Orosz, F., Nuridsány, M. and Ovádi, J. (1986) J. Biochem. Biophys. Methods **13**, 325–332
162. Orosz, F. and Ovádi, J. (1986) Eur. J. Biochem. **160**, 615–619
163. Xiang, M. and Anderson, L.E. (1992) Plant Physiol. **99**, S334
164. Ovádi, J. and Keleti, T. (1978) Eur. J. Biochem. **85**, 157–161
165. Patthy, L. and Vas, M. (1978) Nature (London) **276**, 94–95
166. Kálmán, M. and Boross, L. (1982) Biochim. Biophys. Acta **704**, 272–277
167. Ovádi, J., Mátrai, G., Bartha, F. and Batke, J. (1985) Biochem. J. **229**, 57–62
168. Batke, J., Asbóth, G., Lakatos, S., Schmitt, B. and Cohen, R. (1980) Eur. J. Biochem. **107**, 389–394
169. Beeckmans, S., Van Driessche, E. and Kanarek, L. (1990) J. Cell. Biochem. **43**, 297–306
170. Sukhodolets, M.V., Muronetz, V.I. and Nagradova, N.K. (1989) Biochem. Biophys. Res. Commun. **161**, 187–196
171. Vas, M. and Batke, J. (1981) Biochim. Biophys. Acta **660**, 193–198
172. Kvassman, J. and Pettersson, G. (1989) Eur. J. Biochem. **186**, 265–272
173. Batke, J. (1989) FEBS Lett. **251**, 13–16
174. Srivastava, D.K., Smolen, P., Betts, G.F., Fukushima, T., Spivey, O.H. and Bernhard, S.A. (1989) Proc. Natl. Acad. Sci. U.S.A. **86**, 6464–6468
175. Yong, H., Thomas, G.A. and Peticolas, W.L. (1993) Biochemistry **32**, 11124–11131
176. Nazaryan, K.B., Climent, F., Simonian, S., Tompa, P. and Batke, J. (1992) Arch. Biochem. Biophys. **296**, 650–653
177. Batke, J., Nazaryan, K.B. and Karapetian, N.H. (1988) Arch. Biochem. Biophys. **264**, 510–518
178. Gots, R.E., Gorin, F.A. and Bessman, S.P. (1972) Biochem. Biophys. Res. Commun. **261**, 1753–1759
179. Wilson, J.E. (1988) in Microcompartmentation (Jones, D.P., ed.), pp. 171–190, CRC Press Inc., Boca Raton, FL
180. Wilson, J.E. (1968) J. Biol. Chem. **243**, 3640–3647
181. Craven, P.A. and Basford, R.E. (1972) Biochim. Biophys. Acta **255**, 620–630
182. Purich, D.L. and Fromm, H.J. (1971) J. Biol. Chem. **246**, 3456–3463
183. Walsh, J.L. and Knull, J.R. (1987) Biochim. Biophys. Acta **952**, 83–91
184. Luther, M.A. and Lee, J.C. (1986) J. Biol. Chem. **261**, 1753–1759
185. Nanhua, C., Nancarrow, D. and Masters, C. (1986) Biochem. Int. **13**, 539–546
186. Arnold, H., Henning, R. and Pette, D. (1971) Eur. J. Biochem. **22**, 121–126
187. Arnold, H. and Pette, D. (1970) Eur. J. Biochem. **15**, 360–366
188. Walsh, T.D., Clarke, F.M. and Masters, C.J. (1977) Biochem. J. **165**, 165–167
189. Harris, S.J. and Windsor, D.J. (1987) Biochim. Biophys. Acta **911**, 121–126
190. Dagher, S.M. and Hultin, H.O. (1975) Eur. J. Biochem. **55**, 185–192
191. Clarke, F., Stephan, P., Morton, D. and Weidemann, J. (1983) in Actin: Structure and Function in Muscle and Non-muscle Cells (Barden, J. and Dos Remedios, C., eds.), pp. 249–257, Academic Press, Sydney
192. Chan, L.M., Hickmon, T., Collins, C.J. and Davidson, Y.Y. (1986) Fed. Proc. Fed Am. Soc. Exp. Med. **45**, 1657
193. Ratner, J.H., Nitisewojo, P., Hirway, S. and Hultin, H.O. (1974) Int. J. Biochem. **5**,

     525–533
194. Walsh, J.L., Keith, T.J. and Knull, H.R. (1989) Biochim. Biophys. Acta **999**, 64–70
195. Balaban, N. and Goldman, R. (1990) Exp. Cell Res. **191**, 219–226

14

The role of channelling in glycogen metabolism

Enrique Meléndez-Hevia*‡, Joan J. Guinovart† and Marta Cascante†

*Universidad de La Laguna, Departamento de Bioquímica, Facultad de Biología, 38206 Tenerife, Canary Islands, Spain, and †Universitat de Barcelona, Departament de Bioquímica, Facultat de Química, Martí i Franquès 1, 08028 Barcelona, Catalunya, Spain

General aspects of the metabolic role of glycogen

The main function of skeletal muscle glycogen is as a source of glucose for anaerobic glycolysis. This is not only a means of producing ATP in the absence of an oxygen supply, but represents a very rapid metabolic source of ATP to support rapid macroscopic motion. This is because anaerobic glycolysis is a short pathway for ATP production, and therefore the time taken to reach a steady state is small [1,2]. The amount of glucose used during anaerobic glycolysis (about 11–16 times more than during aerobic metabolism to supply the same amount of ATP) necessitates a very large glucose store situated as close as possible to contractile myofibrils. Despite its poor energy yield, anaerobic glycolysis has an interesting metabolic role as a good energetic support for rapid movement.

Glycogen, as a storage molecule, must have an appropriate design for performing this role. It is a polymer, which is a very efficient way of storing a large amount of cytoplasmic glucose without a significant increase in osmolarity. The total amount of fuel sugar stored in liver cells as glycogen is equivalent to 200–400 mM glucose, while the concentration of glycogen is only 5–10 μM. In the skeletal muscle of a trained runner the concentration of glycogen is about 2 μM, which is equivalent to 80 mM glucose. The branching structure of glycogen supplies many points for phosphorylase attack, allowing the release of many glucose molecules simultaneously. A β-particle of glycogen has a diameter of 40 nm; such a particle contains about 55 000 glucose residues and 2100 non-reducing ends, and has about 20–25 phosphorylase molecules attached.

The kinetic design of glycolysis and glycogen metabolism correlates well with the purpose of the quick release of large amounts of glucose 1-phosphate (Glc 1-P). It has been demonstrated by several groups [3–7] that the availability of phosphorylated glucose is the most critical variable in

‡*To whom correspondence should be addressed.*

controlling the glycolytic flux. Accordingly, the regulatory mechanism that triggers the release of Glc 1-P from glycogen is extremely efficient and rapid [8]. The amplification effect of the cascade is in accordance with the required amounts of enzymes involved. Phosphorylase is enormously abundant in skeletal muscle, accounting for 2% of the total soluble protein [9]; phosphorylase and glycolytic enzymes are much more active in anaerobic (white) muscles than in aerobic (red) muscles [10–12]. Muscle fatigue is the result of an increase in diprotonated phosphate H_2PO_4, phosphocreatine depletion, a fall in pH and the accumulation of P_i or ADP. Vigorous exercise is usually accompanied by a fall in muscle pH due to lactic acidosis and an accumulation of P_i resulting from ATP hydrolysis by myosin. Bertocci et al. [13] have shown that all these effects are a consequence of glycogen depletion after anaerobic exercise. Aerobic exercise does not use muscle glycogen and so does not produce fatigue.

Liver glycogen plays a different role, as it is the main source of blood glucose, but this does not mean that its target in evolutionary optimization should be different. There are, in fact, no important differences in the structure of glycogen in these two organs and, although for different reasons, the release of glucose from liver glycogen into the blood also has to be quick. The fact that liver cells also show the cascade regulatory mechanism supports this reasoning. Liver cell size seems to be a critical feature conditioning glycogen content; cell size decreases during fasting and increases during refeeding, and glycogen content changes in parallel. Accordingly, Agius and co-workers have proposed that the increase in cell volume promoted by insulin is the cause, rather than the consequence, of glycogen deposition [14].

Optimization of glycogen structure

The efficiency of the features of animal macroscopic behaviour related to glycogen metabolism depends on good design of the glycogen molecule. This must maximize the capacity for storing a very large amount of glucose in the least possible volume. In addition, when under attack by the appropriate enzymes, as much glucose as possible must be released quickly. The design of such a molecule depends on the values of certain parameters, such as the degree of branching and the chain length. The question which arises here is: are the values of these parameters developed by cells throughout evolution the most appropriate for the optimized design of the glycogen molecule? The mathematical modelling approach presented here allows us to answer this question. Let us first discuss the general features of glycogen structure.

Glycogen structure

Whelan's model [15,16], derived from glycogen enzymic degradation data, is generally accepted for describing glycogen structure [17–19]. According to this model, the main features of glycogen structure can be described as

Fig. I   **Structure of glycogen**

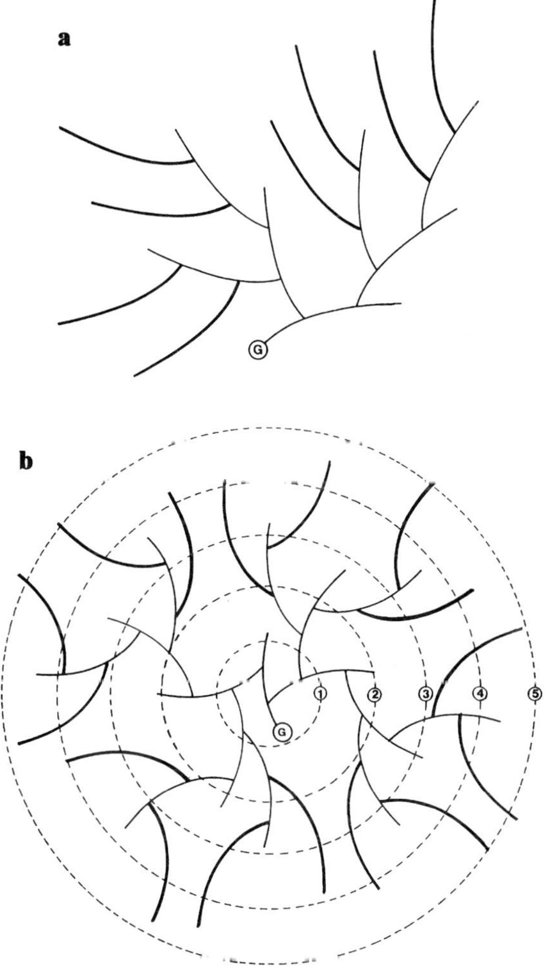

Scheme showing the structure of the glycogen molecule. (a) Extended structure to show the branching structure; (b) a more realistic drawing showing the disposition of the successive branches forming concentric tiers (numbered circles). Both schemes show a simplified molecule, with only four tiers in (a) and five in (b). A-chains (in the external tier) are emboldened.

follows (see Fig. 1). The glycogen molecule is formed by two different kinds of chains: B-chains, which are branched, and A-chains, which are not. The branching of the B-chains is uniformly distributed (degree of branching = 2), so that every B-chain has two branches on it, creating further A- or B-chains. There are four glucose residues between branches and a tail after the second branch in the B-chains. Both A- and B-chains have a uniform length, which is the same for both kinds of chains; this length has a mean value of 13 glucose residues. Phosphorylase can only act on A-chains, since the tail of the B-chains is too short (about four glucose residues, which is at the limit of phosphorylase action). The glycogen molecule is spherical and formed by concentric tiers; each tier has the same thickness (1.9 nm). There are 12 tiers in a β-particle, giving a total radius of 21 nm. All A-chains are in the most external tier. As a consequence of the degree of branching ($r = 2$; every B-chain gives two chains), the number of chains in any tier is twice that in the previous one, and the same as the total number of chains in all other previous tiers. From these data it can be calculated that there is the same number of A-chains (all in the external tier) as B-chains, and that the amount of glucose directly available to be released by phosphorylase is 34.6% of the total molecule.

Assuming an organization of glycogen as described above, changes in the values of certain parameters of the design can result in glycogen molecules with different structural features whose properties condition different functional possibilities. These parameters are: the chain length (g_c), the degree of branching (r) and the number of tiers (t). Any value for these parameters different from those of cellular glycogen would give a molecule with a similar shape but different properties. Meléndez-Hevia et al. [19] analysed these questions using a mathematical model describing glycogen structure, in order to calculate the values of the three parameters mentioned above, for obtaining a molecular design giving maximization of all stored glucose, glucose available to phosphorylase and the number of A-chains (points of attack for phosphorylase), and minimization of the molecular volume. These results were then compared with the values of these parameters in cellular glycogen.

Mathematical model

The model is obtained using a set of hypotheses according to the general features of Whelan's model [15–19]. The structure of the glycogen molecule can be described by the following set of equations. Let r be the degree of branching (number of branch points on each B-chain), and thus the factor which, when multiplied by the number of chains in a tier, gives the number of chains in the next tier. Let t be the number of tiers in the molecule. The number of chains of glucose residues doubles in each tier of the glycogen molecule, since $r = 2$. The total number of chains, C_T, may be represented by the series for t tiers:

$$C_T = r^0 + r^1 + r^2 + r^3 + \ldots + r^{(t-1)} = 1 + r + r^2 + r^3 + \ldots + r^{(t-1)}$$

Since this is a series of the form $1 + x + x^2 + x^3 + \ldots + x^n$ whose sum is $(1 - x^{n+1})/(1 - x)$, it follows that the total number of chains, C_T, is given by:

$$C_T = \sum_{i=1}^{t} r^{(i-1)} = \frac{1 - r^t}{1 - r} \tag{1}$$

and the number of chains in a given tier (C_{t_i}) is:

$$C_{t_i} = r^{(t_i-1)} \tag{2}$$

All A-chains are in the most external tier. Thus eqn. (2) gives us the number of A-chains (C_A):

$$C_A = r^{(t-1)} \tag{3}$$

Let g_c be the number of glucose residues in any A-chain. Not all of these units can be released by phosphorylase; a physical limit, empirically determined, of four residues exists in the ability of phosphorylase to digest any A-chain. The number of glucose residues available for phosphorylase in each A-chain (G_{PC}), therefore, is:

$$G_{PC} = g_c - 4 \tag{4}$$

The total amount of glucose available for phosphorylase in the whole molecule (G_{PT}) is written as:

$$G_{PT} = C_A \cdot G_{PC} = C_A \cdot (g_c - 4) \tag{5}$$

and the total glucose in the whole molecule (G_T) is given by:

$$G_T = C_T \cdot g_c \tag{6}$$

which by eqn. (1) gives:

$$G_T = g_c \cdot \sum_{i=1}^{t} r^{(i-1)} = g_c \cdot \frac{1 - r^t}{1 - r} \tag{7}$$

Structural analysis [17] shows that, on average, a branch starts half-way up a chain, gaining 0.35 nm in the $(1 \rightarrow 6)$ bond; the length per glucose in a chain is 0.24 nm. This gives an effective thickness per tier (L_t) of:

$$L_t = 0.12g_c + 0.35 \text{ nm} \tag{8}$$

The molecule has a spherical shape; this is consistent with Whelan's model and experimental data, including electron micrographs. The radius of a sphere with t tiers (R_S) is:

$$R_S = L_t \cdot t$$

which, by applying eqn. (8), gives:

$$R_S = t \cdot (0.12g_c + 0.35) \text{ nm}$$

and the volume of the sphere (V_S) is:

$$V_S = (4/3)\pi \cdot t^3 \cdot (0.12g_c + 0.35)^3 \text{ nm}^3 \tag{9}$$

Thus our mathematical model described in eqns. (3), (5), (7) and (9) will allow us to calculate any of the variables of the glycogen molecule mentioned above as a function of the parameters r, t and g_c. We shall use these equations to obtain the values for these parameters that optimize the variables.

Number of tiers

The cellular glycogen molecule contains 12 tiers [17]. The volume of a hypothetical 13th tier in a glycogen molecule (according to these structural features) would be $10\,000\ nm^3$, and there would be about 55000 glucose residues in such a tier. Assuming a van der Waals volume of $0.113\ nm^3$ for the glucose molecule, this would give a total volume for glucose of $6215\ nm^3$, which means that in this tier 62% of the space would be occupied by glucose, leaving practically no space for phosphorylase or glycogen-synthesizing enzymes. This is a very efficient way of controlling molecule size. Thus the physical limit to the size of the glycogen molecule at 12 tiers is not only empirically known; the sizes of the enzymes involved in glycogen metabolism can explain it. It is interesting to note that in glycogen storage disease type II (Pompe's disease), in which a lack of lysosomal amylo($1 \rightarrow 4$)glucosidase occurs, there is a significant increase in the amount of glycogen in liver and muscle cells. However, this is because of a large increase in the number of glycogen particles accumulated in lysosomal vacuoles, not because of a larger molecule [20].

Degree of branching

The degree of branching in the glycogen molecule can not be very high, because it would give an extremely dense molecule which would be useless for glucose storage and phosphorylase action (see Fig. 2). Calculations using the mathematical model explained earlier demonstrate that if the degree of branching were $r = 3$, then a molecule with the same density as cellular glycogen (the maximum allowed density, see earlier) could only have seven tiers, and it would be much less efficient than cellular glycogen: its capacity for storing glucose is 27% and glucose is available to phosphorylase only 36% of the cellular glycogen. These values decrease dramatically for larger values of r: for $r = 4$, a molecule with a similar density would have five tiers, 8% stored glucose and 13% of glucose available to phosphorylase cellular glycogen. It is thus concluded that a degree of branching of $r = 2$ (as in cellular glycogen) is optimal.

Chain length in the glycogen molecule

Fig. 3 shows two glycogen molecules containing the same amount of stored glucose but with different designs. The chain length is the only difference; chains are short in Fig 3(a) and long in Fig. 3(b). A number of properties are derived from the value of this parameter; for example, for a given total amount of glucose stored, the design in Fig. 3(a) occupies less space and

Fig. 2   Degree of branching in the glycogen structure

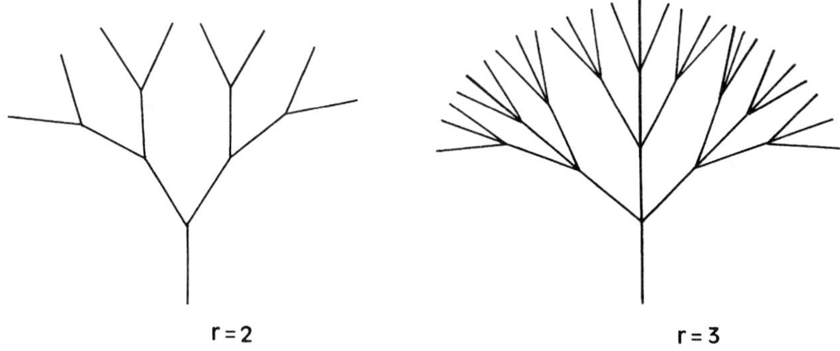

A very simplified scheme for the structure of glycogen, showing the properties which derive from the degree of branching. Left, r = 2, as in cellular glycogen; right, r = 3. Larger values of r give an extremely dense molecule with a poor capacity for storing glucose, since it will contain few tiers.

contains more A-chains (more tiers). However, the chains are longer in Fig. 3(b) and there are more glucose units available for phosphorylase. The four properties which an optimized molecule should have are: (a) maximum number of points for phosphorylase attack; (b) maximum amount of stored glucose; (c) maximum number of glucose residues directly available for phosphorylase with no previous debranching; and (d) minimum molecule volume. All of these properties must be optimized, so this is a case of multi-objective optimization.

Fig. 3   Chain length in glycogen structure

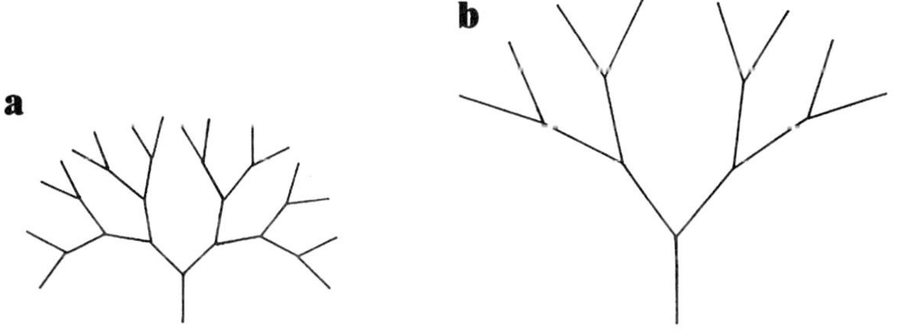

Scheme illustrating the problem of optimization for determining the most appropriate chain length of the glycogen molecule. The different properties of two glycogen designs, both with the same degree of branching (r = 2) but with different chain lengths, are shown as (a) and (b). Design (a) has short chains and design (b) has long chains. The diagrams depict two glycogens containing the same amount of stored glucose (the same amount of ink was used for each one).

Each of these properties can be expressed by a given variable, all of them being related by the equations of the model described. In effect, A-chains (C_A) are the points for phosphorylase attack, G_T is the total stored glucose in the molecule, G_{PT} is the total glucose available for phosphorylase, and V_S is the volume of the molecule. The relationships among these variables are given by eqns. (3), (5), (7) and (9). They describe the properties of the glycogen molecule whose variables have to be optimized. In accordance with the previous reasoning, the aim now is to find the values of t and g_c which maximize C_A, G_T and G_{PT} and which minimize V_S. This purpose is achieved by maximizing the function:

$$f = G_T \cdot C_A \cdot G_{PT}/V_S \tag{10}$$

C_A, G_T, G_{PT} and V_S are related by eqns. (3), (5), (7) and (9). According to the results of the previous section, $r = 2$. Therefore eqn. (10) can be written as:

$$f = K \cdot \frac{g_c \cdot (g_c - 4)}{(0.12 g_c + 0.35)^3} \tag{11}$$

with:

$$K = \frac{(6C_A - 3) \cdot C_A^2}{4\pi t^3} = \frac{[6 \cdot 2^{(3t-3)}] - [3 \cdot 2^{(2t-2)}]}{4\pi t^3} \tag{12}$$

The value of g_c that maximizes f from the root of $df/dg_c = 0$ is 12.93. The optimization function is plotted in Fig. 4; $g_c = 13$ is, therefore, the value of the chain length that optimizes the structure of glycogen. Empirical data obtained by several groups are in good agreement with this theoretical result, as Table 1 shows. The optimization function shown in Fig. 4 demonstrates that the small ranges around the value of 13 do not indicate a significant deviation from the optimum, and allows us to conclude that living cells have achieved a well optimized chain length for their glycogen structure.

Optimization principles have been used to study several aspects of cellular organization [28–32]. The results reported here represent a special case, i.e. the optimization of molecular structure, and indicate a close structure/function relationship in a biological molecule. Glycogen is a material for which the aim of design optimization is to maximize the rapid and substantial activity of phosphorylase for fuel supply in anaerobic glycolysis; this is in good agreement with the regulatory paraphernalia of this enzyme, and with the specific design of anaerobic glycolysis (see distribution of lactate dehydrogenase isoenzymes in [33]).

How did the cell evolve a glycogen molecule with these optimized features? The specificity of the enzymes which build glycogen obviously determines the value of certain parameters, such as the minimum distance between branches; however, more than enzyme specificity is involved. The results reported by Smith [34] suggest that the ratio between glycogen synthase and the branching enzyme plays an important role in achieving the optimized design of glycogen: in a system of glycogen synthesis by chain elongation and branching, variation in the ratio of these enzymes leads to different degrees of branching in the molecule. Another example is glycogen storage disease type IV (Andersen's disease); low activity of the branching enzyme promotes a glycogen molecule with very long outer branches. Furthermore, some 'abnormal' physiological situations such as glucose or fructose infusion in rabbit liver result in glycogen molecules with longer chains ($g_c = 16$–17) [21].

The latest results in the research of glycogen optimization (R. Meléndez, E. Meléndez-Hevia and M. Cascante, unpublished work) have demonstrated analytically that the degree of branching ($r = 2$) is also optimized, and that each tier of a glycogen molecule has its structure optimized. A glycogen molecule with $r = 2$ (the minimum possible, since $r = 1$ means no branching) is distributed in small spheres, which maximizes the surface and allows the simultaneous attack of more phosphorylase molecules.

The design of the starch molecule seems to pursue different purposes. In general, this reasoning only applies to animal glycogen, where a quick response is of vital importance. The mechanisms which account for this

---

Fig. 4   Plot of the optimization function for the glycogen molecule

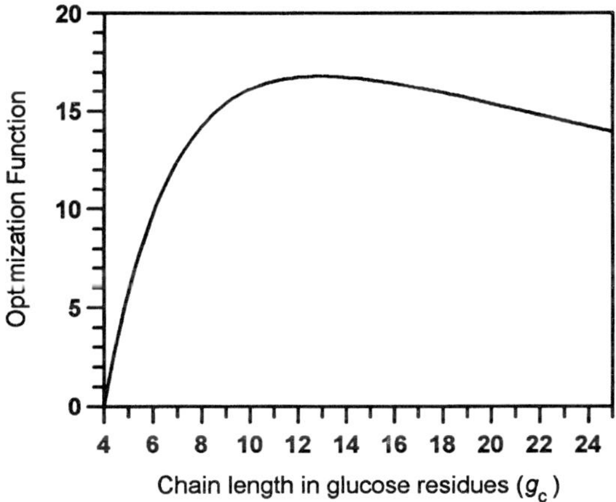

Optimization of the chain length (g_c) in the glycogen molecule in order to maximize the capacity for storing glucose in the least possible volume, the total amount of glucose which can be released by phosphorylase before any debranching occurs, and the points of attack for the enzyme. Glycogen has its structure optimized with a chain length of 13 glucose residues The optimization function has dimensions of glucose available for phosphorylase multiplied by density, and it represents the maximum available glucose stored in a molecule which has the maximum possible density.

fast metabolism have not been seen in plants. Potato phosphorylase is not phosphorylated or stimulated by AMP, and lacks the regulatory and allosteric properties characteristic of muscle phosphorylase [35]. The design of amylopectin is rather different from that of glycogen, with chain lengths of between 22 and 25 glucose residues. It is likely that chain length in amylopectin has also been optimized, but the target there seems to have been different than in animal glycogen; it is probably only storage capacity, which would explain the longer chains.

Channelling in glycogen metabolism

Our knowledge on channelling is quite different with respect to different pathways of metabolism. With glycogen metabolism there is perhaps no direct experimental evidence for channelling, such as, for instance, that

Table 1   Chain lengths of glycogen molecules from different sources

Glycogen source	Chain length (g_c)	Refs.
12 different species	10.8–15.4	21
Fetal guinea pig liver	13.0	21
62 glycogens analysed	11.0–13.0	22
Rat liver	13.0	21,23
Rabbit muscle	13.0	16,23,24
Rabbit muscle	14.0	25
Cat liver	12.5	21
Cat liver	13.0	22
Cat liver	14.0	16
Human muscle	11.5	16
Skate liver	12.0	16
Ascaris lumbricoides	12.5	16
Trichomonas foetus	14.5	16
Horse diaphragm	15.0	16
White-rabbit liver	12.0–14.0	18
Mouse muscle	12.8	24
Hen liver	15.0	25
Pig liver	15.0–16.0	25
Pig muscle	11.0–16.0	25
Mouse liver	14.0	25
Human placenta	11.6	26
Most glycogens analysed	12.0–14.0	27

Glycogen molecules were analysed by several groups, using different analytical techniques.

provided by the elegant experiments of Raijman's group on the urea cycle (see Chapter 10), and by Ovádi on glycolysis (see Chapter 13), but there are many data strongly suggesting that such channelling may exist. Such data concern a close coupling between gluconeogenesis and glycogen synthesis in liver, and so we will discuss this here. Liver glycogen metabolism is involved in three metabolic pathways: (a) glycogenesis, the net conversion of glucose into glycogen; (b) gluconeogenesis, the conversion of C_3 precursors, such as lactate or alanine, into glucose; and (c) glycogenolysis, the release of glucose from glycogen. Muscle gluconeogenesis has no relevant role, and glycogenolysis in this tissue is closely coupled with anaerobic glycolysis, with a net conversion of glycogen into lactate. In the liver a close relationship between glycogen synthesis and gluconeogenesis seems to exist, resulting in a long pathway from lactate (or eventually from other pyruvate precursors such as alanine) to glycogen. A number of experimental results strongly suggest that glucose 6-phosphate (Glc 6-P), Glc 1-P and other intermediates are channelled, not allowing their escape to other pathways or their incorporation from other processes. We will present here a brief summary of the main data in support of this assertion, and the theoretical basis that can explain it.

Thermodynamics: channelling would be very convenient

It is necessary to look at the thermodynamic features of glycolysis and gluconeogenesis in order to understand the organization of glycogen metabolism. Good design of a metabolic pathway involves having a high global equilibrium constant capable of accounting for a large net exergonism under a broad variety of environmental conditions. The chemical affinity of the reaction, defined as the global exergonism ($-\Delta G$), is related to the reaction rate by the equation:

$$v = k \cdot S \cdot (1 - e^{\Delta G/RT}) \tag{13}$$

where v is the reaction velocity, k is the rate constant and S is the substrate concentration. Eqn. (13) applies to any chemical reaction, and shows that the greater the chemical affinity, the faster the reaction, assuming that other variables are constant. It can be also written as:

$$v = \frac{k \cdot E_T \cdot (S \cdot K_{eq} - P)}{1 + K_{eq}} \tag{14}$$

where k is a specific catalytic constant, E_T is the total amount of enzyme, K_{eq} is the equilibrium constant of the reaction, and S and P are the concentrations of the substrate and product respectively [36]. In addition, we have found recently (R. Heinrich, F. Montero, E. Klipp, T.G. Waddell and E. Meléndez-Hevia, unpublished work) that the specific distribution of local exergonisms has a dramatic influence on the kinetic yield of the pathway: the optimum design must have the highly exergonic steps concentrated at the beginning of the pathway, and the lesser ones at the end. This ideal design is, however, strongly constrained by the chemical possibilities for the reactions, and it may be that in some cases the best design of a chemical reaction mechanism is still very far from a good thermodynamic design, leading to an end-point state that evolution cannot improve.

The thermodynamic design of a metabolic pathway is defined as its standard free energy change ($\Delta G^{\circ\prime}$) profile (Fig. 5). Cell metabolism occurs, of course, under non-standard conditions, but the concept of thermodynamic design is based on standard values, since they give the same information as equilibrium constants, by the relationship:

$$\Delta G^{\circ\prime} = RT \cdot \ln K_{eq} \tag{15}$$

A scale of standard free energy is thus a logarithmic scale of equilibrium constants. Thermodynamic design is the thermodynamic basis of a pathway; i.e. the thermodynamic background on which metabolism can work. A comparison of the standard free energies of hydrolysis of ATP and of glycerol phosphate illustrates this point. ATP is often described as having a 'high-energy phosphate bond' because its equilibrium constant of hydrolysis is large (its *standard* free energy is very negative; $\Delta G^{\circ\prime} = -30.4$ kJ/mol). Hydrolysis of an ester phosphate bond, such as glycerol phosphate $R–CH_2–O–PO_3H^{2-}$, i.e.:

$$R–CH_2–O–PO_3H^{2-} + H_2O \rightarrow R–CH_2–OH + R'–COOH$$

has a low equilibrium constant, which gives $\Delta G^{\circ\prime} = -9.2$ kJ/mol. However, this reaction might be able to drive energy traffic under appropriate conditions. If, for example, the following concentrations occur: [glycerol phosphate] $= 20$ mM, [glycerol] $= 0.5$ mM and $[P_i] = 0.5$ mM, then $\Delta G = -37.15$ kJ/mol; this demands a large difference in concentrations which is non-physiological. ATP has the advantage that its high equilibrium constant allows it to work well under reasonably high P_i concentrations, e.g. 3 mM in the cytosol, making easier other reactions where phosphate traffic is also involved to, for example, supply leaving groups for transfer of chemical groups. (In fact, under cellular conditions such as 3 mM ATP, 0.3 mM ADP and 3 mM P_i in the cytosol, ATP hydrolysis has an actual free energy value of $\Delta G = -50.48$ kJ/mol.) So, with regard to the structure of ATP and its hydrolysis reaction, we can state that cellular energy metabolism based on it is *well designed*. Life with energy traffic based on glycerol phosphate is of course possible, but it would be poorly designed!

Every metabolic pathway, in order to work, requires a high net exergonism ($\Delta G \ll 0$) as the necessary chemical affinity; this is easy to achieve if the equilibrium constant is high. However, in cases where equilibrium constants are low, cellular evolution has had to achieve high exergonism by the use of dramatic differences in the concentrations of reactants. Therefore, because the evolutionary target (from the thermodynamic point of view) is the same for every metabolic pathway, the chemical affinities of

Fig. 5   Thermodynamic designs of glycolysis and gluconeogenesis

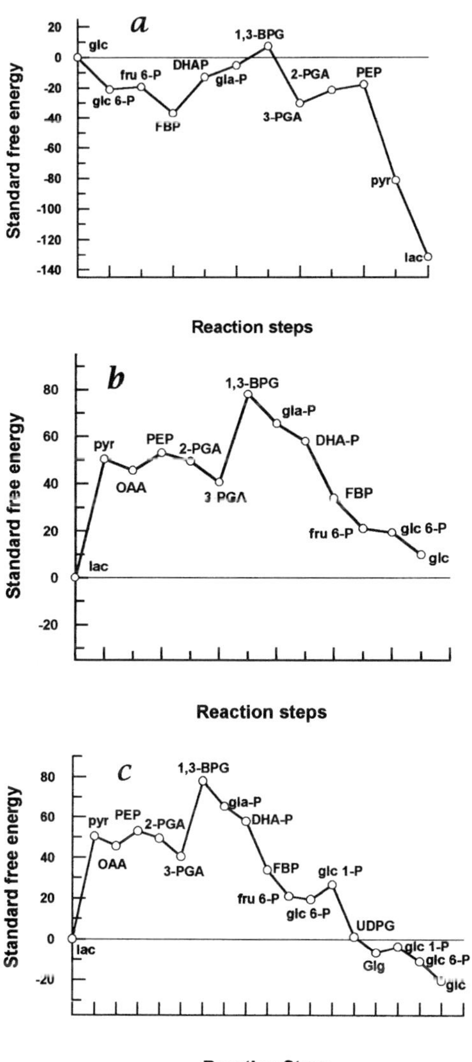

Thermodynamic profiles of these pathways, plotted as standard free energy change of each step of the pathway; this is equivalent to a logarithmic scale of the equilibrium constants. (a) Glycolysis; (b) gluconeogenesis by the direct route from lactate to glucose; (c) possible channelled gluconeogenesis passing through glycogen synthesis and degradation. Free energy under standard conditions is given in kJ/mol of glucose converted or produced. Abbreviations: glc, glucose; glc 1-P, glucose 1-phosphate; glc 6-P, glucose 6-phosphate; fru 6-P, fructose 6-phosphate; FBP, fructose 1,6-bisphosphate; DHA-P, dihydroxyacetone phosphate; gla-P, glyceraldehyde 3-phosphate; 1,3-BPG, 1,3-bisphosphoglycerate; 3-PGA, 3-phosphoglycerate; 2-PGA, 2-phosphoglycerate; PEP, phosphoenolpyruvate; pyr, pyruvate; lac, lactate; OAA, oxaloacetate; UDPG, uridine diphosphate glucose; Glg, glycogen.

pathways of the same length are expected to be similar. This reasoning also demonstrates that we must use *standard* free energy values (or equilibrium constants), and not the actual ones, to analyse the *thermodynamic design* of a pathway. The actual free energy values are also very interesting, but they give quite different information and must be used for other purposes.

A pathway with good thermodynamic design must have a high global equilibrium constant to allow the pathway to work without a dependence on the mass action ratio, and thus well designed metabolism should allow the functioning of antagonistic pathways under minimally changing substrate concentrations. The glycolysis/gluconeogenesis system should have an appropriate thermodynamic design which allows the separate functioning of these pathways with the same substrate concentrations. Thus the activity of each pathway should be a response to regulatory mechanisms and not the consequence of a change in the mass action ratio.

Fig. 5 shows the thermodynamic design of glycolysis and gluconeogenesis. The profile for glycolysis is good, with a global standard free energy of $\Delta G^{o\prime} = -131.47$ kJ/mol of glucose for the whole conversion:

$$\text{Glucose} + 2\text{ADP} + 2\text{P}_i \rightarrow 2\text{lactate} + 2\text{ATP} \quad (K_{eq} = 1.13 \times 10^{23})$$

However, that for gluconeogenesis is not: the global conversion of lactate (the most frequent gluconeogeneic substrate) into glucose has $\Delta G^{o\prime} = +9.87$ kJ/mol of glucose ($K_{eq} = 0.018$). It is obvious that gluconeogenesis has a serious problem of thermodynamic design.

This large difference in equilibrium constants, or thermodynamic support, between glycolysis and gluconeogenesis could determine important differences in the metabolic possibilities for the cell with regard to these pathways, and could also be the origin of regulation problems. From these data we can deduce, in principle, that glycolysis works well under a broad set of environmental conditions (extensive range of lactate, glucose or ATP concentrations), while the possibilities for gluconeogenesis would be much more restricted. This thermodynamic problem in gluconeogenesis design is probably inevitable for reasons of chemical bio-organic mechanisms, as there is no obvious step in the pathway where more ATP could be consumed to increase the global exergonism. However, this problem could be solved in part if channelling occurs, forcing the route to pass through glycogen synthesis and degradation. This would then involve the consumption of one extra ATP for each glucose produced, which adds $\Delta G^{o\prime} = -30.4$ kJ/mol per glucose produced. This changes the global standard free energy value of gluconeogenesis to $\Delta G^{o\prime} = -20.53$ kJ/mol, a value of standard exergonism still much lower than that of glycolysis, but somewhat better than in the absence of channelling. Such channelling would be a way to separate the two Glc 6-P pools in order to guarantee the consumption of this extra ATP which chemical mechanisms do not allow elsewhere along the pathway. Table 2 shows the standard free energy values of several possible pathways of glycolysis, gluconeogenesis and glycogen metabolism.

Table 2   Global thermodynamics of glycolysis, gluconeogenesis and glycogenesis

	$\Delta G^{\circ\prime}$ (kJ/mol)	ATP consumed (mol/mol of glucose)
Glycolysis		
Glucose → lactate	− 131.47	− 2
Glycogen → lactate	− 114.41	− 3
Gluconeogenesis		
Lactate → glucose (direct)	+ 9.87	4
Alanine → glucose (direct)	− 39.53	4
Lactate → glycogen	− 6.72	5
Alanine → glycogen	− 58.12	5
Lactate → glycogen → glucose	− 20.53	5
Alanine → glycogen → glucose	− 69.93	5
Fructose → glucose (direct, through C_3)	− 61.57	2
Fructose → (C_3) → glycogen → glucose	− 91.97	3
Glycogenesis		
Glucose → glycogen (direct)	− 46.99	2
Glucose → glycogen (through C_3)	− 77.39	3
Fructose → glycogen (direct, through C_3)	− 78.16	3

Free energy under standard conditions is given in kJ per mol of glucose. Several possible starting substrates and end-products are considered.

Regulation: strong indications for channelling

Co-ordinated activation of gluconeogenesis and glycogen synthesis

It has been well known since the classical work by Cori's group [37] that gluconeogenesis is, under a number of physiological conditions, closely coupled with glycogen synthesis. Glucocorticoid hormones activate gluconeogenesis and glycogen synthesis simultaneously. Direct stimulation of gluconeogenesis by glucocorticoids has been related to their ability to induce the synthesis of phosphoenolpyruvate carboxykinase (PEPCK). In contrast, direct effects of glucocorticoids on glycogen metabolism are much less well established. The direct effects of dexamethasone on glycogen synthase and phosphorylase, and on glycogen content, have been investigated in primary cultured rat hepatocytes (S. Baqué, A. Roca, J.J. Guinovart and A. Gómez-Foix, unpublished work); these results indicate that dexamethasone induces the activation of both glycogen synthase and phosphorylase, driving the metabolic flux through a route equivalent to a futile cycle. Such simultaneous activation of PEPCK and glycogen synthase emphasizes that the long pathway formed by closely coupled gluconeogenesis and glycogen synthesis would be driven by two 'regulatory pumps': a 'propellent' pump at PEPCK and a 'suction' pump at glycogen synthase. Finally, the coupling of this with phosphorylase activation leads to depletion of hepatocyte glycogen. There is much evidence that the phosphorylase and synthase can be activated simultaneously (see also [38,39]); this has been observed in the presence of glutamine and adenosine [40], and is also promoted by fructose, a very effective gluconeogeneic substrate [41,42]. Epidermal growth factor has been reported to be an activator of both glycogen synthase [43] and phosphorylase [44,45]. These facts strongly suggest a close coupling between gluconeogenesis and glycogen synthesis, whereby the Glc 6-P produced is not able to escape from the synthetic pathway but is obliged to form glycogen, in turn yielding free glucose.

The activation of both the synthase and the phosphorylase by fructose [41,42] is also consistent with this conclusion. Fructose is metabolized in the liver via the pathway:

fructose → fructose 1-phosphate

    → dihydroxyacetone phosphate + glyceraldehyde

    → 2 glyceraldehyde 3-phosphate

Thus the net conversion of fructose into glucose must involve at least the last steps of gluconeogenesis. According to the hypothesis of a close coupling between gluconeogenesis and glycogen synthesis, the synthase and phosphorylase should therefore be activated to convert fructose into glucose (see Figs. 5 and 6).

The effects of glucagon on the regulation of glycogen metabolism are complex, and perhaps not fully understood. Glucagon activates gluconeogenesis by promoting PEPCK synthesis, activates glycogen degradation by means of the covalent cascade on phosphorylase, and inactivates the synthase through activation of protein kinase A, which increases the phosphorylation of this enzyme. These facts have been interpreted for a long time as reflecting the co-ordinated action of glucagon in releasing glucose by two different routes (gluconeogenesis and glycogenolysis), and could be the consequence of glucagon dissipating channelling under acute conditions. However, the extension of this effect could only account for a fraction of the synthase activity. Re-activation of phosphorylated glycogen synthase in muscle has been reported at physiological Glc 6-P concentrations [46]. If this effect also occurs in liver, then it could account for the re-activation of synthase previously inactivated by glucagon, forcing a certain fraction of the gluconeogenic flux towards glucose via glycogen. In this case the channelling coupling gluconeogenesis and glycogen synthesis (see Fig. 6) would not have been totally lost.

A 'futile cycle' in glycogen metabolism

A futile cycle occurs when two antagonistic pathways (e.g. glucokinase/glucose-6-phosphatase; phosphofructokinase/fructose-1,6-bisphosphatase; pyruvate kinase/pyruvate kinase, PEPCK; etc.) are working simultaneously. The reason why futile cycles exist in cellular metabolism has been discussed, with suggestions that they have some role in metabolic regulation, as highly sensitive points of control [47,48], as well as in thermogenesis. However, these are surely cases where evolutionary opportunism has taken advantage of this feature, utilizing something that already existed. The initial, real reason

Fig. 6   Possible scheme for liver glycogen metabolism with channelling connecting gluconeogenesis and glycogen synthesis

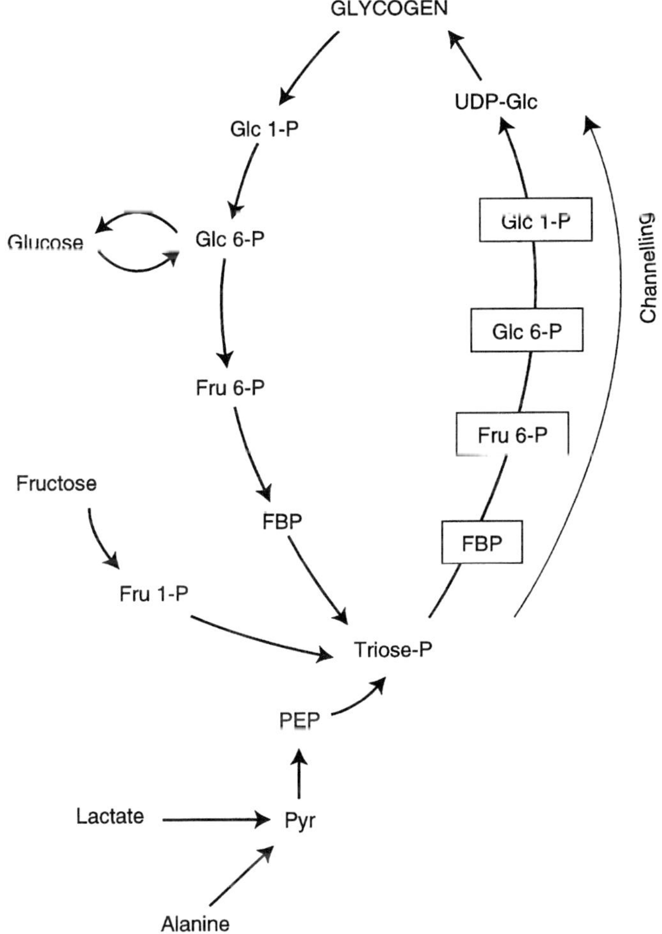

Channelling between gluconeogenesis and glycogen synthesis separates Glc 6-P, Glc 1-P and other intermediates (boxed) of this route from the soluble pools involved in glycolysis, glycogenolysis and other pathways. This scheme can explain many experimental data which are difficult to reconcile with the presence of only a common freely interchangeable pool of Glc 6-P. Abbreviations: Fru, fructose; FBP, fructose 1,6-bisphosphate; PEP, phosphoenolpyruvate.

for the existence of metabolic futile cycles is that they could not be avoided. Futile cycles are inevitable unless each enzyme in the cycle has a very efficient mechanism of regulation which inhibits fully its activity when the antagonistic enzyme is activated [48]. Allosterism (usually with a Hill coefficient of between 2 and 3) is a good mechanism for regulating enzyme activity, but over the physiological range of the modulator the enzyme activity cannot be completely inhibited, with inhibition to below 15% of the maximal possible activity being rare. Thus a futile cycle cannot be avoided.

In glycogen metabolism, the regulatory mechanisms of the activities of glycogen synthase and phosphorylase are both based on covalent modifications of the enzyme structure; this is very effective as a regulatory mechanism, and indeed is the only one capable of completely activating/inactivating one enzyme [8]. Thus one would expect that a well defined antagonistic regulatory mechanism exists between the synthesis and degradation of glycogen, ensuring that a futile cycle does not occur. It is therefore surprising to observe that, as discussed above, in a number of physiological situations both the synthase and the phosphorylase are active, apparently forming a futile cycle. There is, however, a singularity here: a futile cycle usually exists because allosterism or other regulatory mechanisms cannot fully inactivate an enzyme; however, in glycogen metabolism the futile cycle occurs, despite the cascade which can operate as a switch, because the effector which activates one enzyme also activates the other. The futile cycle of phosphofructokinase is thus *inevitable*, while that involving glycogen is *intentional*. In a typical futile cycle the stimulus that activates one enzyme usually inactivates the antagonistic one (e.g. AMP and fructose 2,6-bisphosphate are activators of phosphofructokinase and inhibitors of fructose-2,6-bisphosphatase), or there are different modulators for each enzyme of the cycle, but with an antagonistic metabolic effect (e.g. alanine, a typical precursor of gluconeogenesis, inhibits pyruvate kinase, a glycolytic enzyme). This feature also seems to occur in glycogen metabolism under certain conditions, as glucagon activates the phosphorylase and inactivates the synthase; however, in this case the regulatory effects mentioned above, which simultaneously activate both the synthesis and the degradation of glycogen, produce a futile cycle effect deliberately. Now regarding the role that channelling can play here, we see that the simultaneous activation of both the synthesis and the degradation of glycogen does not really produce a futile cycle, but rather a longer route. Channelling connecting gluconeogenesis with glycogen synthesis does not promote a proper futile cycle, since the metabolite is not really recycled. Rather, the pathway (Glc 6-P)$_a$ → glycogen → (Glc 6-P)$_b$ is a means of separating the two Glc 6-P pools. The reason for this pathway lengthening, i.e. to allow consumption of extra ATP (as UTP), has been discussed above.

Metabolic fluxes: difficult to explain without channelling

Thermodynamic data based on equilibrium constants suggest that the design of gluconeogenesis could be greatly improved if the path from lactate to glucose passes through glycogen by means of channelling to avoid the escape of Glc 6-P. Thermodynamic data are therefore in good agreement with channelling in glycogen metabolism, but they cannot prove it. Data from studies of metabolic regulation described above demonstrate that such coupling really exists, i.e. they confirm the thermodynamic predictions. These data suggest more strongly the existence of channelling as the mechanism of coupling; however, again this is only a suggestion since, although difficult, any of these effects can be explained without invoking the existence of channelling. Finally, however, data on metabolic fluxes seem impossible to explain if channelling does not occur.

Some experimental results suggest that substrates entering the gluconeogenic pathway at the level of trioses or lactate are better precursors than glucose for glycogen synthesis. This fact, widely observed and discussed by several groups, is what Katz has called 'the glucose paradox' [49,50]. Hepatocytes encounter very high glucose concentrations and they have the full complement of enzymes required to convert this substrate into glycogen. However, glucose is poorly utilized for this purpose in the liver; instead, other compounds, such as lactate, fructose and alanine, are the main metabolic substrates for glycogen synthesis in this organ. How can a long route be more efficient than a short one?

On the other hand, there is much experimental evidence to suggest that gluconeogenesis is closely coupled with glycogen synthesis under certain physiological conditions, so that glucose output comes from glycogen rather than directly from the gluconeogenic Glc 6-P pool. A number of results [51] led to the conclusion that a major fraction of rat liver glycogen deposited in response to exogenous carbohydrate is formed by a pathway involving the prior conversion of glucose into a C_3 compound. This also suggests that the last steps of gluconeogenesis and its connection with the glycogen synthesis pathway might be channelled. Katz's group have measured the fluxes from glucose to glycogen in rats infused with ^{13}C-enriched glucose [52,53]. This isotopomer approach makes it possible to evaluate whether glucose is directly converted into glycogen (the direct pathway), or if it is first broken down to give C_3 compounds. In the former case the labelling of glucose into glycogen is the same as in the substrate used, and thus only two species of glucose will be found, of molecular mass 180 kDa (non-labelled) and 186 kDa (all carbons labelled). On the other hand, if the indirect pathway is occurring then there will be a random mixture of labelled and non-labelled trioses or pyruvate, giving glucose of molecular mass 183 kDa; interactions with other metabolic processes will result in glucose with different labelling, with molecular masses of 181, 182, 184 and/or 185 kDa. Therefore the analysis by mass spectrometry of the molecular mass of glucose obtained from isolated liver glycogen gives a measure of the partitioning of the pathways operating in liver for the conversion of glucose into glycogen. The results vary according to physiological state (fasting, glucagon administration), and demonstrate that the contribution of the indirect pathway is between 25 and 65% of the total. These results suggest again the occurrence of channelling, illustrating the limited availability of the glycolytic Glc 6-P pool for use in glycogen synthesis. They also give information on the extent of such channelling, suggesting that it can be of varying importance depending on physiological conditions.

More direct evidence of channelling

The existence of two separate pools of glycolytic and gluconeogenic intermediates in hepatocytes has been suggested since the late 1960s [54]. This separation was supported by the slow exchange of radioactivity, not compatible with the existence of a general pool of each intermediate. This separate compartmentation of glycolytic and gluconeogenic substrates could be extended from phosphoenolpyruvate to UDP-glucose, i.e. practically the whole of gluconeogenesis plus glycogen synthesis, in good accordance with Fig. 6. More recently, Christ and Jungerman [55], using ^{14}C-labelled Glc 6-P and ^{14}C-prelabelled glycogen in permeabilized hepatocytes, showed that [^{14}C]glucose production from prelabelled glycogen was not altered by the addition of 5 mM Glc 6-P to the incubation medium; they concluded that at least two separate, mutually non-accessible, Glc 6-P pools exist in rat hepatocytes, linked to glycolysis and gluconeogenesis respectively. Srere [56], reviewing the data on the regulation and kinetic behaviour of the enzymes of glycolysis and gluconeogenesis, also arrived at the conclusion that such results can be most easily interpreted if two separate systems exist in the cytosol for glycolysis and gluconeogenesis.

Many of the results discussed above, and particularly those concerned with the direct (C_6) and indirect (C_3) pathways, have been interpreted in terms of liver zonation (for a review, see [57]). According to such a hypothesis, some liver cells convert glucose into lactate (or some other C_3 metabolite), which is then transferred to cells in another part of the liver, where it is metabolized as a glycogen precursor. There is in fact much experimental evidence for differences in the metabolic roles of different liver hepatocyte populations; it can be concluded that the periportal zone is more gluconeogenic, whereas the perivenous zone is more glycolytic [57]. Glycogen metabolism has also been shown to be different in periportal and perivenous hepatocytes: Agius and her colleagues have shown that synthesis of glycogen from lactate was between 2- and 4-fold greater in periportal than in perivenous hepatocytes, whereas glycogen synthesis from glucose was similar [58]. The different metabolic roles of the periportal and perivenous zones of the liver thus have been well demonstrated experimentally. However, it is unlikely that liver zonation by itself can explain the data discussed above, since they imply intracellular, rather than extracellular, compartmentation. In fact, the two types of hepatocyte show the same response to hormonal stimuli [58,59]. It is interesting to note that the simple model presented here (Fig. 6), with the compartmentation of these pathways in the same cell, can account for all data discussed.

Conclusions

In Fig. 6 we present a plausible metabolic scheme for liver carbon traffic involving the synthesis and degradation of glycogen, with channelling involving Glc 6-P and Glc 1-P for coupling between gluconeogenesis and glycogen synthesis. According to this model, the three pathways involved in glycogen metabolism in the liver are as follows. (a) Glycogenesis (conversion of glucose into glycogen) would pass through the glycolytic pathway until some intermediate between pyruvate and triosephosphate, and the carbon flux would continue from there to glycogen through the gluconeogenesis and glycogen synthesis pathways. (b) Gluconeogenesis (conversion of lactate or other C_3 compound, or even fructose, into glucose) would pass through glycogen synthesis and degradation. (c) Glycogenolysis (release of glucose from glycogen) is a direct pathway. Soluble pools of Glc 1-P, Glc 6-P, fructose 6-phosphate and fructose bisphosphate would be involved in glycogenolysis, glycolysis and the pentose cycle, etc. Channelled pools of these intermediates are boxed in Fig. 6. The channelling must also involve fructose 6-phosphate and fructose 1,6-bisphosphate (and perhaps some C_3 intermediate) in order to explain the incorporation of glucose into glycogen via C_3 metabolites [51–53]. The variable proportions of the direct and indirect pathways for glycogenesis seem to suggest that this might be dynamic channelling, with a variable degree of mixing of the different pools of intermediates. It is noteworthy that in the model of channelling presented in Fig. 6 there is no opportunity for futile cycles, as glycolytic and gluconeogenic pools are separate; but our model could also explain the experimental results on glucose and fructose 6-P recycling, previously reported as evidence for futile cycles in gluconeogenesis. Whether channelling occurs at the C3 intermediate level between triosephosphate and pyruvate is not known.

The model shown can explain the conflicting results described in this chapter, and this type of metabolic organization would give a general solution to the problems reviewed: it is a means of rearranging the thermodynamic constraints more favourably, an explanation of apparent contradictions in regulation, and also a way to explain the carbon fluxes seen in metabolism, including futile cycles. It is interesting to note that all data on liver carbohydrate metabolism that are difficult to explain, including Katz's glucose paradox, are based on the assumption of a free interchange and circulation of Glc 6-P. If the new ideas on channelled metabolism apply, they would account for the close coupling between gluconeogenesis and glycogen synthesis, limiting the availability of the Glc-6-P pool. Previous results should be reviewed in the light of this hypothesis, which also suggests new experiments and approaches for further research, as well as new approaches to questions concerning diabetes and obesity.

Channelling has usually been considered as a mechanism that can improve cellular metabolic design by decreasing the concentrations of metabolic pools, enhancing fluxes and reducing transition times [60–63], and its selective value in metabolic evolution has been based on these features [63,64]. The analysis of the thermodynamics of gluconeogenesis and glycogen synthesis presented here leads us to acknowledge another interesting property of metabolite channelling, i.e. as a more efficient mechanism for the thermodynamic coupling of metabolic processes. The selective value of this feature could be critical in the evolution of some metabolic designs.

This work, as well as the work of the authors quoted, was supported by grants from Dirección General de Investigación Científica y Técnica, Ministerio de Educación y Ciencia (Spain) (PB90–0846, PB91–0276, PB92–0852 and PB94–0593); Consejería de Educación del Gobierno de Canarias (Spain) (91/10); and CIRIT, Generalitat de Catalunya (Spain) (QFN94–4683-E). We thank Professor F. Montero and Professor J. Corzo the critical reading of the manuscript.

References

1. Easterby, J.S. (1981) Biochem. J. **199**, 155–161
2. Torres, N.V., Sicilia, J. and Meléndez-Hevia, E. (1991) Biochem. J. **276**, 231–236
3. Aragón, J.J., Tornheim, K. and Lowensteim, J.M. (1980) FEBS Lett. **117** (Suppl.), K56–K64
4. Helmreich, E. and Cori, C.F. (1965) Adv. Enzyme Regul. **3**, 91–107
5. Torres, N.V., Mateo, F., Meléndez-Hevia, E. and Kacser, H. (1986) Biochem. J. **234**, 169–174
6. Torres, N.V., Mateo, F. and Meléndez-Hevia, E. (1988) FEBS Lett. **233**, 83–86
7. Rapoport, T.A., Heinrich, R., Jacobasch, G. and Rapoport, S. (1974) Eur. J. Biochem. **42**, 107–120
8. Cárdenas, M.L. and Cornish-Bowden, A. (1989) Biochem. J. **257**, 339–345
9. Ryman, B.E. and Whelan, W.J. (1971) Adv. Enzymol. Relat. Areas Mol. Biol. **34**, 285–433
10. Opie, L.H. and Newsholme, E.A. (1967) Biochem. J. **103**, 391–399
11. Newsholme, E.A. and Start, C. (1973) Regulation in Metabolism, Wiley, London
12. Banks, P., Bartley, W. and Birt, L.M. (1976) in The Biochemistry of the Tissues, 2nd edn., pp. 148–150, Wiley, Chichester
13. Bertocci, L.A., Fleckenstein, J.L. and Antonio, J. (1992) J.Appl. Physiol. **73**, 75–81
14. Agius, L., Peak, M. and Al-Habori, M. (1991) Biochem. J. **276**, 843–845
15. Gunja-Smith, Z., Marshall, J.J., Mercier, C., Smith, E.E. and Whelan, W.J. (1970) FEBS Lett. **12**, 101–104
16. Gunja-Smith, Z., Marshall, J.J. and Smith, E.E. (1971) FEBS Lett. **13**, 309–311
17. Goldsmith, E., Sprang, S. and Fletterick, R. (1982) J. Mol. Biol. **156**, 411–427
18. Bullivant, H.M., Geddes, R. and Wills, P.R. (1983) Biochem. Int. **6**, 497–506
19. Meléndez-Hevia, E., Waddell, T.G. and Shelton, E. (1994) Biochem. J. **295**, 477–483
20. Garancis, J.C. (1968) Am. J. Med. **44**, 289–300

21. Illingworth, B., Larner, J. and Cori, G.T. (1952) J. Biol. Chem. **199**, 631–640
22. Manners, D.J. (1957) Adv. Carbohydr. Chem. **12**, 261–298
23. Manners, D.J. and Wright, A. (1962) J. Chem. Soc. 1597–1602
24. Calder, P.C. (1987) Ph.D. Thesis, University of Auckland, New Zealand
25. Kjolberg, O., Manners, D.J. and Wright, A. (1963) Comp. Biochem. Physiol. **8**, 353–365
26. Blows, J.M.H., Calder, P.C., Geddes, R. and Willis, P.R. (1988) Placenta **9**, 493–500
27. Ryman, B.E. and Wheland, W.J. (1971) Adv. Enzymol. Relat. Areas Mol. Biol. **34**, 285–443
28. Meléndez-Hevia, E. and Isidoro, A. (1985) J. Theor. Biol. **117**, 251–263
29. Meléndez-Hevia, E. (1990) Biomed. Biochim. Acta **49**, 903–916
30. Meléndez-Hevia, E., Waddell, T.G. and Montero, F. (1994) J. Theor. Biol. **166**, 201–220
31. Heinrich, R., Schuster, S. and Holzhntter, H.G. (1991) Eur. J. Biochem. **201**, 1–21
32. Heinrich, R. and Hoffmann, E. (1991) J. Theor. Biol. **151**, 249–283
33. Kaplan, N.O. (1964) Brookhaven Symp. Biol. **17**, 131–153
34. Smith, E.E. (1968) in Control of Glycogen Metabolism (Whelan, W.J., ed.), pp. 203–213, Universitetsforlaget, Oslo, and Academic Press, London
35. ap Rees, T. (1974) MTP Int. Rev. Sci. Plant Biochem. **11**, 89–127
36. Heinrich, R. and Hoffmann, E. (1991) J. Theor. Biol. **151**, 249–283
37. Cori, C.F. (1981) Curr. Top. Cell. Regul. **18**, 377–387
38. Hue, L., Bontemps, F. and Hers, H.G. (1975) Biochem. J. **152**, 105–114
39. Hutson, N.J., Brumley, F.T., Assimacopoulos, F.D., Harper, S.C. and Exton, J.H. (1976) J. Biol. Chem. **251**, 5200–5208
40. Carabaza, A., Ricart, M.D., Mor, A., Guinovart, J.J. and Ciudad, C.J. (1990) J. Biol. Chem. **265**, 2724–2732
41. Ciudad, C.J., Massagué, J. and Guinovart, J.J. (1979) FEBS Lett. **99**, 321–324
42. Katz, J., Golden, S. and Wals, P. (1979) Biochem. J. **180**, 389–402
43. Bosch, F., Bouscarel, B., Slaton, J., Blackmore, P.F. and Exton, J.H. (1986) Biochem. J. **239**, 523–530
44. Hughes, P.B., Crofts, J.N., Auld, A.M., Read, L.C. and Barritt, G.J. (1987) Biochem. J. **249**, 911–918
45. Quintana, I., Grau, M., Moreno, F., Soler,C., Ramírez, I. and Soley, M. (1995) Biochem. J. **308**, 889–894
46. Villar Palasí, C. (1991) Biochim. Biophys. Acta **1095**, 261–267
47. Hue, L. (1982) in Metabolic Compartmentation (Sies, H., ed.), pp. 71–97, Academic Press, London
48. Hers, H.G. and Hue, L. (1983) Annu. Rev. Biochem. **52**, 617–653
49. Katz, J. and McGarry, J.D. (1984) J. Clin. Invest. **74**, 1901–1909
50. Katz, J., Kuwajima, M., Foster, D.W. and Garry, J.D. (1986) Trends Biochem. Sci. **11**, 136–140
51. Newgard, C.B., Hirsch, L.J., Foster, D.W. and McGarry, J.D. (1983) J. Biol. Chem. **258**, 8046–8052
52. Katz, J., Lee, W.N.P., Wals, P.A. and Bergner, E.A. (1989) J. Biol. Chem. **264**, 12994–13001
53. Katz, J., Wals, P.A. and Lee, W.N.P. (1991) Proc. Natl. Acad. Sci. U S A **88**, 2103–2107
54. Threlfall, C.J. and Heath, D.F. (1968) Biochem. J. **110**, 303–312
55. Christ, B. and Jungermann, K. (1987) FEBS Lett. **221**, 375–380
56. Srere, P.A. (1987) Annu. Rev. Biochem. **56**, 89–124
57. Jungerman, K. and Katz, N. (1989) Physiol. Rev. **69**, 708–764
58. Agius, L., Peak, M. and Alberti, G.M.M. (1990) Biochem. J. **266**, 91–102
59. Agius, L., Tosh, D. and Peak, M. (1993) Biochem. J. **289**, 255–262
60. Ovádi, J. (1991) J. Theor. Biol. **152**, 1–22
61. Heinrich, R. and Schuster, S. (1991) J. Theor. Biol. **152**, 57–61
62. Mendes, P., Kell, D.B. and Westerhoff, H.V. (1992) Eur. J. Biochem. **204**, 257–266
63. Meléndez-Hevia, E. and Montero, F. (1991) J. Theor. Biol. **152**, 77–79
64. Cascante, M., Sorribas, A. and Canela, E.I. (1994) Biochem. J. **298**, 313–320

15

Substrate channelling in β-oxidation: myth or reality?

Harald Osmundsen*||, Kim Bartlett†, Morteza Pourfarzam†,
Simon Eaton† and Jowita Sleboda*

*Department of Physiology and Biochemistry, University of Oslo, Oslo,
Norway, and †Department of Child Health, University of Newcastle upon
Tyne, Newcastle upon Tyne, U.K.

Introduction

The pivotal role of the β-oxidation of fatty acids in the energy metabolism of higher organisms is well known. This sequence of reactions enables mammals to utilize the huge store of energy which is found in the fatty acids stored in adipose tissue as triacylglycerol. Whereas mammalian carbohydrate stores may last for 12–48 h during fasting, the triacylglycerol stores can last for weeks.

Fatty acid β-oxidation has two facets, mitochondrial β-oxidation and peroxisomal β-oxidation; the latter is most active in liver, although both types of β-oxidation are thought to occur in most tissues. Mitochondrial β-oxidation represents the major fraction of cellular β-oxidation. In the liver (and kidney cortex) of rodents the activity of peroxisomal β-oxidation is increased some 10–20-fold on treatment with fibrate-type drugs [1], dihydroepiandrosterone [2] or diethylhexylphthalate [3]. These aspects of peroxisomal β-oxidation have been reviewed elsewhere [4–6].

Enzymes of mitochondrial β-oxidation and their organization

The enzymes of mitochondrial β-oxidation are summarized in Table 1. In brief, for each of the constituent steps of the pathway there are multiple enzymes which vary in their chain-length specificity. In the case of acyl-CoA dehydrogenation there are four enzymes: short-chain acyl-CoA dehydrogenase (active with C_4 and C_6), medium-chain acyl-CoA dehydrogenase (active with C_4–C_{12}), long-chain acyl-CoA dehydrogenase (active with C_8–C_{20}) and very-long-chain acyl-CoA dehydrogenase (active with C_{12}–C_{24}). Each of these enzymes catalyses the formation of 2-enoyl-CoA from the corresponding saturated ester. Short-, medium- and long-chain acyl-

||*To whom correspondence should be addressed.*

CoA dehydrogenases are homotetramers located in the matrix. Very-long-chain acyl-CoA dehydrogenase, however, is a homodimer and is located in the mitochondrial inner membrane.

Similarly, it appears that there are three 2-enoyl-CoA hydratases. One, a soluble matrix enzyme, is most active towards short-chain substrates, although it will act on substrates up to C_{16} at a much lower rate and with higher K_m values [7–9]. This was the first enzyme of mammalian mitochondrial β-oxidation to be purified (crotonase; short-chain enoyl-CoA hydratase; EC 4.2.1.17) [10]. The long-chain enzyme (EC 4.2.1.74) is most active with C_6–C_{10} substrates, and virtually inactive with crotonyl-CoA (C_4), the preferred substrate of crotonase [11–13]. Studies of patients with inherited disorders suggested a third, medium-chain-specific, enzyme [14], and this activity has now been partially purified from pig and human liver [14a].

The third step of the pathway, L-3-hydroxyacyl-CoA dehydrogenation, is catalysed by two enzymes with overlapping chain-length specificities. The short-chain-specific enzyme (EC 1.1.1.35) is a soluble matrix enzyme which will act on substrates of chain length C_4–C_{16} although, as with crotonase, the shorter-chain-length substrates are preferred [15–18]. A long-chain 3-hydroxyacyl-CoA dehydrogenase was first demonstrated by El Fakhri and

Table 1 Enzymes of mitochondrial β-oxidation

Enzyme	Structure	Molecular mass (kDa)	References
Very-long-chain acyl-CoA dehydrogenase	Homodimer	150	45
Long-chain acyl-CoA dehydrogenase	Homotetramer	180	82
Medium-chain acyl-CoA dehydrogenase	Homotetramer	180	83
Short-chain acyl-CoA dehydrogenase	Homotetramer	168	84
Long-chain 3-hydroxyacyl-CoA dehydrogenase	Hetero-octomer	460	25
Long-chain 2-enoyl-CoA hydratase			
Long-chain 3-oxoacyl-CoA thiolase			
Short-chain 2-enoyl-CoA hydratase	Homohexamer	164	8
Short-chain 3-oxoacyl-CoA thiolase	Homotetramer	169	85
General 3-oxoacyl-CoA thiolase	Homotetramer	200	24
ETF	Heterodimer	57	84
ETF:ubiquinone oxidoreductase	Monomer	68	86
2,4-Dienoyl-CoA reductase	Homotetramer	124	87
Δ^3,Δ^2-Enoyl-CoA isomerase	Homodimer	70	88,89
$\Delta^{3,5},\Delta^{2,4}$-Dienoyl-CoA isomerase	Homotetramer	126	90

Middleton [19]. This enzyme is firmly associated with the mitochondrial inner membrane and is active with medium- and long-chain substrates, with C_{16} being the preferred substrate.

The final step of the pathway, thiolytic cleavage of 3-oxoacyl-CoA to yield acetyl-CoA and a chain-shortened intermediate, is catalysed by three enzymes. Two soluble activities have been identified. One is specific for acetoacetyl-CoA and 2-methylacetoacetyl-CoA [20–22]. The second thiolase, the 'general' thiolase, is active with all substrates from C_6 to C_{16} to approximately equal extents [23,24]. The third activity is part of a newly described trifunctional enzyme which also comprises, it appears, the long-chain 2-enoyl-CoA hydratase and long-chain 3-hydroxyacyl-CoA dehydrogenase activities described above. This complex, a heterodimer closely associated with the mitochondrial inner membrane, was first described by Uchida and co-workers [25] and rapidly confirmed by others [26,27].

Intriguingly, a complex of activities associated with carnitine palmitoyltransferase II has also been reported by Kerner and Bieber [28]. However, in this study the constituent activities were not characterized with any precision, and it is difficult to know if Bieber's complex also involved the trifunctional enzyme. In any event, there can be no doubt that carnitine palmitoyltransferase II, very-long-chain acyl-CoA dehydrogenase and the trifunctional protein are associated with the mitochondrial inner membrane together with Complex I, electron transfer flavoprotein (ETF):CoQ oxido-reductase and the remainder of the respiratory chain. The medium- and short-chain activities appear to have a matrix localization. In effect this suggests the presence of two mitochondrial β-oxidation systems: one in the matrix and one associated with the inner membrane (Fig. 1). What then are the functional consequence of such an arrangement? This and related questions are discussed below.

Enzymes of peroxisomal β-oxidation

Hepatic peroxisomes are conventionally visualized as spherical vacuoles enclosed by a single bilayer membrane (for review see [29]). The peroxisomal membrane contains a cytochrome b_5 reductase [30–32] and long-chain acyl-CoA synthase activity [33]. It also contains a protein thought to render the membrane freely permeable to all metabolites of molecular mass less than 10 kDa [34]. In this sense the peroxisomal membrane is more like the mitochondrial outer membrane. This situation may therefore also result in peroxisomal β-oxidation operational characteristics which are markedly different from those of mitochondrial β-oxidation.

The chemistry of peroxisomal β-oxidation is identical with that of mitochondrial β-oxidation as far as the fatty acyl-CoA is concerned. The enzymes of peroxisomal β-oxidation are presented in Table 2. It is evident

Table 2   **Enzymes of hepatic peroxisomal β-oxidation**

Enzyme	Substrate	Comment	Reference
Long-chain acyl-CoA oxidase	Straight-chain acyl-CoA		55
Pristanoyl-CoA oxidase	2-Methyl-branched acyl-CoAs		35
Trihydroxycoprostanoyl-CoA oxidase	CoA-esters of bile acid intermediates		35
Δ^2-Enoyl-CoA hydratase	Δ^2-Enoyl-CoA	Part of trifunctional enzyme	49
3-Hydroxyacyl-CoA dehydrogenase	3-Hydroxyacyl-CoA	Part of trifunctional enzyme	49
Δ^3,Δ^2-Enoyl-CoA isomerase	Δ^3-Enoyl-CoA	Part of trifunctional enzyme	36
Thiolase	3-Oxoacyl-CoA		91
Four additional 3-hydroxyacyl-CoA dehydrogenases	3-Hydroxyacyl-CoA?	Function unknown	39

All enzymes of peroxisomal β-oxidation are most active with long-chain substrates. In vitro, optimal activity is usually found with acyl-CoA esters of carbon chain lengths of 12–16 carbon atoms.

Fig. I   Organization of mitochondrial β-oxidation and its relationship with the respiratory chain

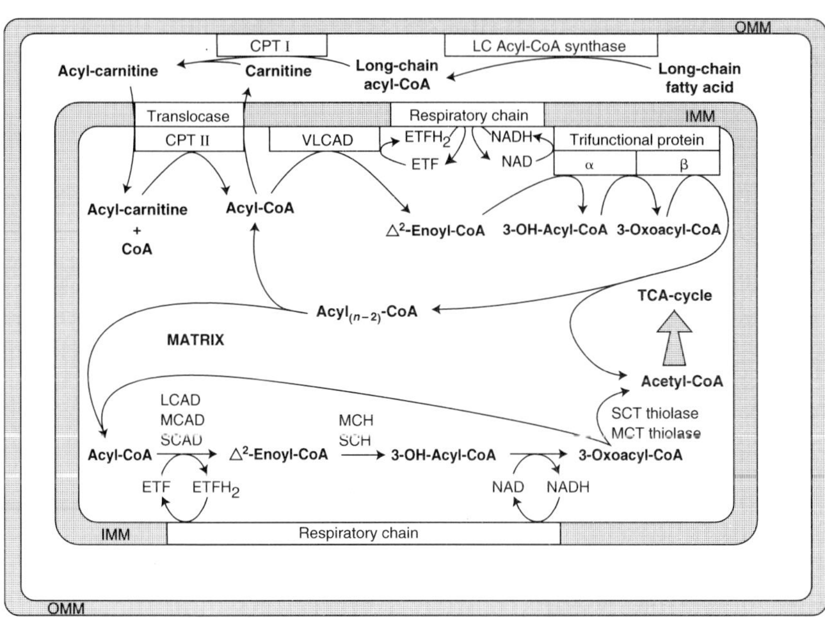

The following abbreviations have been used: LC, long chain; MCT, medium chain; SCT, short chain; VLCAD, very-long-chain acyl-CoA dehydrogenase; LCAD, long-chain acyl-CoA dehydrogenase; MCAD, medium-chain acyl-CoA dehydrogenase; SCAD, short-chain acyl-CoA dehydrogenase; MCH, medium-chain acyl-CoA hydratase; SCH, short-chain acyl-CoA dehydrogenase; CPT, carnitine palmitoyltransferase; TCA-cycle, tricarboxylic acid cycle; OMM, mitochondrial outer membrane; IMM, mitochondrial inner membrane.

that the multiplicity of enzymes found in mitochondrial β-oxidation is, as yet, not thought to be present in peroxisomes. Although peroxisomes contain three different acyl-CoA oxidases, these are characterized by differences in substrate specificity (not primarily related to carbon chain length) [35]. Peroxisomes are known to contain one enoyl-CoA hydratase and one 3-hydroxyacyl-CoA dehydrogenase activity, both of which reside on a trifunctional enzyme together with Δ^3,Δ^2-enoyl-CoA isomerase [36]. Also, only one peroxisomal thiolase has been described [37], as well as a medium-chain-length carnitine acyltransferase which is also active with, for example, hexadecanoyl-CoA [38]. All peroxisomal enzymes are generally optimally active with long-chain-length substrates. Recently evidence of four additional 3-hydroxyacyl-CoA dehydrogenases was presented [39]. Their function is as yet unknown. This finding demonstrates that our knowledge of the enzymology of peroxisomal β-oxidation remains incomplete.

Is there a rationale for channelling of β-oxidation intermediates?

Several authors have pointed out that, at the concentration of protein which must exist in the mitochondrial matrix (about 500 mg/ml [40]), the matrix will possess a gel-like consistency. In this environment rates of diffusion of both macromolecules and low-molecular-mass metabolites will probably be smaller than those found in free solution. On the other hand, dense packing of proteins means that the diffusion distance from one enzyme to the next in the sequence may be decreased, hence counteracting decreased rates of diffusion. In an environment with diminished molecular mobility this may be of little value, however, unless the active sites of enzymes are juxtapositioned so as to make optimal use of the proximity effect. This is of course the idea behind the metabolon concept [41]. The concept is ideally suited for β-oxidation, as these intermediates have no other known metabolic function. With peroxisomal β-oxidation this may not be true, because chain-shortened (i.e. partially β-oxidized) fatty acids may be regarded as a metabolic product [5,42].

Furthermore, the amount of CoA in the mitochondrial matrix is finite, and it is almost completely acylated during the β-oxidation of, for example, hexadecanoylcarnitine, most of it accumulating as hexadecanoyl-CoA and acetyl-CoA [43]. Any further accumulation of intermediates would represent an undesirable drain on the CoA pool and would be likely to diminish rates of β-oxidation. As 29 intermediates are involved in the β-oxidation of hexadecanoate, their accumulation can be regarded as undesirable. In addition, their solvation would require water molecules, already much in demand due to the high concentration of proteins in the matrix.

In mitochondria, at least, there are therefore several good reasons why channelling could be beneficial. With peroxisomal β-oxidation the situation is less clear because of the permeability of the peroxisomal membrane.

Studies of three enzymes of mitochondrial β-oxidation have demonstrated their binding to the mitochondrial inner membrane with a high degree of specificity [44]. Using preparations from pig heart it was shown that short-chain crotonase, thiolase and β-hydroxyacyl-CoA dehydrogenase were bound to the matrix surface of mitochondrial inner membrane fractions, but not to liposomes. In contrast, succinyl-CoA:acetoacetate CoA-transferase, a mitochondrial matrix enzyme, did not bind to this membrane fraction. The interpretation of this was that enzymes of β-oxidation can form a complex with the mitochondrial inner membrane. This suggestion is made more realistic by the findings that the very-long-chain acyl-CoA dehydrogenase [45] and the trifunctional enzyme [25] are associated with the mitochondrial inner membrane. The physical verification of such a complex has yet to be achieved.

The enzymes of peroxisomal β-oxidation have been shown to differ with respect to their degree of solubilization [46]. The peroxisomal thiolase was shown to readily leak out of peroxisomes, much like catalase. The trifunctional enzyme and long-chain acyl-CoA synthase remained particulate, while about 50% of the acyl-CoA oxidase activity was solubilized by freezing–thawing or by ultrasonication [46]. The peroxisomal long-chain acyl-CoA synthase is an established membrane protein [33,47]. Alexson et al. [46] suggested that the poor solubility of the trifunctional enzyme may be caused by the protein associating with other matrix or membrane proteins. None of these enzymes were found to be associated with the dense cores (i.e. crystalline urate oxidase). These data therefore hint at a possible protein complex involving some enzymes of peroxisomal β-oxidation.

Multifunctional enzymes in β-oxidation

Multifunctional enzymes are prime candidates for substrate transfer between active sites by channelling. Bacterial β-oxidation, at least in *Escherichia coli*, is well recognized to involve a multifunctional enzyme [48]. This is a tetra-functional enzyme having active sites for enoyl-CoA hydratase, 3-hydroxyacyl-CoA dehydrogenase, Δ^3-*cis*,Δ^2-*trans*-enoyl-CoA isomerase and 3-hydroxyacyl-CoA epimerase. Likewise, in peroxisomal β-oxidation enoyl-CoA hydratase and 3-hydroxyacyl-CoA dehydrogenase were found to reside on the same protein (the bifunctional protein [49]). The peroxisomal Δ^3-*cis*,Δ^2-*trans*-enoyl-CoA isomerase activity was subsequently shown also to reside on this same protein, turning the bifunctional protein into a trifunc-tional protein [36]. Similarly, a trifunctional enzyme is also found in yeast peroxisomes [50], with an epimerase activity replacing the isomerase activity found in the rat liver enzyme.

More recently the mitochondrial long-chain 3-hydroxyacyl-CoA dehydrogenase was also shown to be a trifunctional protein, as both long-chain enoyl-CoA hydratase and long-chain 3-oxoacyl-CoA thiolase activities are also associated with this protein as isolated from rat liver mitochondria [25] and pig heart mitochondria [27]. Hence a multifunctional enzyme appears to be a common denominator as regards the enzymes of β-oxidation All these multifunctional enzymes possess enoyl-CoA hydratase and 3-hydroxyacyl-CoA dehydrogenase activities, whereas additional activities vary.

The apparently universal presence of a multifunctional enzyme in the β-oxidation sequence suggests that this type of enzyme must fulfil some essential function. One advantage of a multifunctional enzyme is its potential to transfer the product from one reaction directly to the substrate-binding site of the succeeding reaction. In this way a high local concentration of substrate is achieved, and the reaction products are immediately metabolized further. This can have clear kinetic advantages. Indeed, with the multifunc-tional enzymes from both *E. coli* and rat liver peroxisomes, channelling of β-oxidation intermediates has been demonstrated to occur in the conversion of enoyl-CoA into the corresponding 3-oxoacyl-CoA [51,52]. Available evidence suggests that the reason why channelling has been implemented at this stage of β-oxidation is to circumvent an unfavourable reaction equilibrium. An example is found in the β-oxidation of polyunsaturated fatty acids. Hydration of 2-*trans*,4-*trans*-decadienoyl-CoA into 4-*trans*-3-hydroxyenoyl-CoA occurs with an equilibrium constant estimated to be of the order of 10^{-3} [52]. Effective hydration of this intermediate (which will be formed during β-oxidation of a *trans*-fatty acid) would require a non-physiological (i.e. very high) concentration of substrate, unless the product (4-*trans*-3-hydroxyenoyl-CoA) was very quickly metabolized further. This is achieved by channelling of the 4-*trans*-3-hydroxyenoyl-CoA from the active site of the hydratase to that of the 3-hydroxyacyl-CoA dehydrogenase. The product from the hydratase reaction is thus metabolized as soon as it is formed. A high rate of β-oxidation is maintained because channelling removes an intermediate which otherwise would reverse the enoyl-CoA hydratase reaction and inhibit β-oxidation.

No corresponding channelling has yet been demonstrated for the mitochondrial trifunctional enzyme. This enzyme would also appear to have this potential, but this will have to be verified by future investigators.

Although we have evidence for channelling on multifunctional enzymes of β-oxidation, the full explanation for its presence may still be lacking. The reason for this is the existence of supplementary enzymes required for β-oxidation of polyunsaturated fatty acids, e.g. Δ^2,Δ^4-dienoyl-CoA intermediates using NADPH (for a review see [53]), and hence the problem of their slow hydration. It is, however, possible that nature has built an element of redundancy into β-oxidation to ensure that these intermediates (which must be frequently formed during cellular β-oxidation) will not inhibit β-oxidation.

Available evidence suggests this is a problem emanating from the chemistry of hydration of the Δ^2 double bond when present in the conjugated Δ^2,Δ^4-dienoyl-CoA structure [52,54] produced by chain shortening of polyunsaturated acyl-CoA esters. It is, therefore, a problem which is universal to β-oxidation; hence the need for this problem to be solved whether β-oxidation operates in bacteria, yeast or mammalian cells. We might, therefore, expect to find a multifunctional enzyme of β-oxidation possessing at least enoyl-CoA hydratase and 3-hydroxyacyl-CoA dehydrogenase activity in all organisms possessing a functional β-oxidation sequence. Any additional activities are variable, and probably suited to the physiological demands of the species in which the activity is present.

Is there a case for metabolite channelling in β-oxidation?

Whereas the mitochondrial β-oxidation process is intimately integrated with the respiratory chain, peroxisomal β-oxidation has no direct link to an electron transport chain. Both sequences are catabolic sequences, where there are no known metabolic functions for the intermediates. It is generally considered that this property renders a metabolic sequence likely to exhibit metabolite channelling (for a review see [41]).

As in mitochondrial β-oxidation, acetyl-CoA is also the product of peroxisomal β-oxidation. During unperturbed, ADP-stimulated β-oxidation by rat liver mitochondria acetyl-CoA is the only metabolite derived from the fatty acid carbon chain, while peroxisomal β-oxidation also produces chain-shortened fatty acids [55–57]. It has been tacitly assumed, because of the 'low' concentration of acyl intermediates detected during mitochondrial β-oxidation by early workers [43], that metabolite channelling occurs. However, more recent studies have demonstrated the concentration of C_{16}–C_{14} acyl-CoA intermediates to be in the range 0.5–1.2 nmol/mg of protein in skeletal muscle mitochondria incubated with 60 μM hexadecanoate [58]. The flux under these conditions is approx. 1–5 nmol of acetyl units/min per mg of protein. Incubation of liver mitochondria under the same conditions resulted in fluxes of 10–15 nmol of acetyl units/min per mg of protein and the detection of 0.5–2.5 nmol of C_{16}–C_{14} acyl-CoA intermediates/mg of protein [59]. Shorter-chain-length intermediates, although detectable, are present at much lower concentrations. A typical chromatogram is shown in Fig. 2.

The pattern of acyl-CoA intermediates generated from the oxidation of hexadecanoyl-CoA is quite different in the two pathways. In the case of mitochondrial β-oxidation, although there are species and tissue differences, in general intermediates of chain length C_{16}–C_{10} are present at concentrations which decrease sharply with decreasing chain length, and intermediates of lower chain length are not seen. The precise pattern of intermediates depends on the time of incubation, i.e. at what point during a substrate-limited pulse of β-oxidation a measurement is made. In liver, saturated acyl-CoA esters are prominent, although in skeletal and cardiac muscle there are greater amounts of 3-hydroxyacyl- and 2-enoyl-CoA esters (for further discussion of the significance of this observation, see below). In peroxisomal β-oxidation, in contrast, intermediates of all chain lengths are always observed, in addition to acetyl-CoA, although medium-chain intermediates are present at the lowest concentrations (see below for a more detailed discussion). The amount of intermediates produced exceeds that formed during mitochondrial β-oxidation by a factor of 100. The mode of operation of the peroxisomal pathway is therefore fundamentally different from that of mitochondrial β-oxidation. Superficially this would suggest that substrate channelling does not occur within peroxisomal β-oxidation, while the issue remains open as regards mitochondrial β-oxidation.

Intermediates formed during peroxisomal β-oxidation

During *in vitro* peroxisomal β-oxidation of [U-^{14}C]hexadecanoate, intermediates spanning the entire range of possible saturated intermediates from 14 to 4 carbon atoms are accumulated (Fig. 3). Acetoacetyl-CoA, 3-oxohexadecanoyl-CoA and 3-oxotetradecanoyl-CoA are also observed, being particularly prominent when peroxisomes are exposed to relatively high concentrations of substrate [60,61]. There is therefore no evidence to suggest a 'leaky hose-pipe' model for peroxisomal β-oxidation. In peroxisomes the leaks in the β-oxidation hose-pipe, by analogy, must be substantial compared with the flux through the sequence to acetyl-CoA.

Several phenomena may contribute to the observed pattern, and channelling is not the most likely. The low levels of octanoyl- and decanoyl-CoA may simply be caused by a peroxisomal acyl-CoA hydrolase with particularly high affinity for acyl-CoAs of these chain lengths, or by peroxisomal β-oxidation having a particularly high affinity for octanoyl- and decanoyl-CoA.

With optimized conditions for *in vitro* peroxisomal β-oxidation, 2-enoyl-CoA or 3-hydroxyacyl-CoA esters have never been detected as intermediates of β-oxidation. When, however, an NAD$^+$ regenerator is not

Fig. 2   **Radiochromatogram of the acyl-CoA intermediates generated by the β-oxidation of 60 μM [U-^{14}C]hexadecanoate by intact rat liver mitochondria**

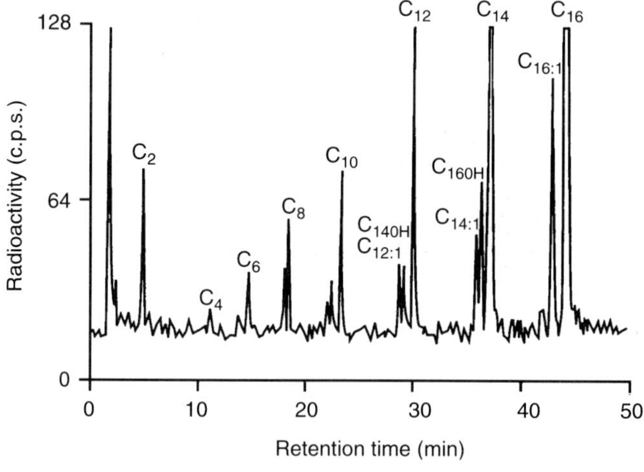

The conditions of incubation and analysis were as described in [59]. The numbers indicate the carbon chain-lengths of the acyl-groups; OH indicates 3-hydroxyderivatives; and :1 indicates Δ^2-enoyl esters.

present in the incubations these intermediates are found [42,60]. This could imply the presence of channelling within a limited segment of β-oxidation which is no longer operational when the NAD^+/NADH ratio becomes too small. At this point during β-oxidation the trifunctional enzyme is involved, which has been shown to carry out channelling between two of its active sites [51,52], as discussed above.

The formation of acetoacetyl-CoA during peroxisomal β-oxidation, and from added acetyl-CoA [62], is unexpected because the equilibrium of the thiolase reaction strongly favours the formation of acetyl-CoA from acetoacetyl-CoA. In addition, the formation of acetoacetyl-CoA disappears when peroxisomes are solubilized by detergent [62]. Conversion of 2 molecules of acetyl-CoA into acetoacetyl-CoA and CoA presumably would require a high concentration of acetyl-CoA and a low concentration of CoA. This suggests the presence of a microenvironment in the non-solubilized peroxisome which somehow fulfils these criteria, facilitating formation of

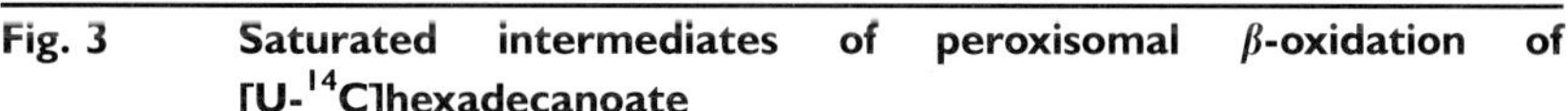

Fig. 3	**Saturated intermediates of peroxisomal β-oxidation of [U-^{14}C]hexadecanoate**

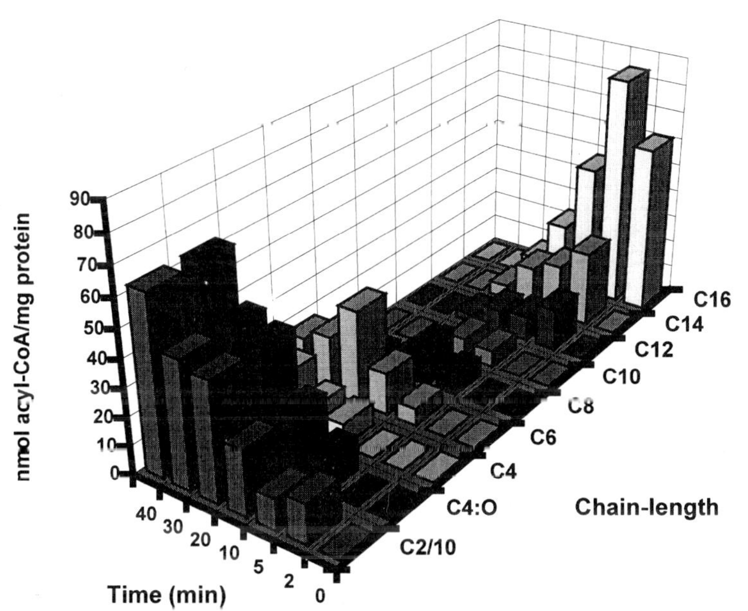

Freshly isolated rat liver peroxisomes were incubated under iso-osmotic conditions as described in [60] in the presence of 20 μM [U-^{14}C]hexadecanoate. At the times indicated, samples were removed for analysis of acyl-CoA esters by radio-HPLC. The following abbreviations have been used: C2, acetyl-CoA; C4:0, 3-oxobutyryl-CoA; C4, butyryl-CoA; C6, hexanoyl-CoA; C8, octanoyl-CoA; C10, decanoyl-CoA; C12, dodecanoyl-CoA; C14, tetradecanoyl-CoA; C16, hexadecanoyl-CoA.

acetoacetyl-CoA from acetyl-CoA. Treatment of isolated peroxisomal fractions with Triton X-100 is known to solubilize virtually all of the peroxisomal thiolase [46]. Any intraperoxisomal microenvironment involving thiolase is therefore certain to be destroyed.

Time course of β-oxidation as an indicator of channelling

In the absence of any channelling, simulation studies of β-oxidation have shown that a plot of acetyl-CoA produced against time should exhibit a short lag phase [63]. Also, when comparing the time course of the appearance of radioactive β-oxidation products (mainly acetyl-CoA, acetoacetate and citrate) a clear lag-phase is expected when an ω-^{14}C-labelled fatty acid is β-oxidized, but not when a 1-^{14}C-labelled fatty acid is the substrate [63]. These phenomena are illustrated by the curves presented in Fig. 4. In a β-oxidation sequence which is 100% channelled, lag phases should not be present because any one fatty acid molecule is oxidized to completion prior to the initiation of β-oxidation of another molecule. There is now no need to build up a pool of intermediates prior to the appearance of acetyl-CoA. Also, for the same reason, the ω-^{14}C label should appear in acetyl-CoA as quickly as the 1-^{14}C label.

Stewart et al. [63] demonstrated that, in a solubilized mitochondrial extract, β-oxidation behaves as expected for a sequence devoid of any detectable channelling. This conclusion was based on the finding that acetyl groups derived from a 1-^{14}C-labelled substrate bring about a more rapid labelling of the acetyl-CoA-pool than acetyl groups derived from β-oxidation of an ω-^{14}C-labelled fatty acid. These authors were, however, unable to detect any deviation from linearity of the β-oxidation time course.

In addition, with intact mitochondria, no lag phase is demonstrable in the time course of the release of acid-soluble radioactivity using [16-^{14}C]hexadecanoylcarnitine [64], or [U-^{14}C]hexadecanoylcarnitine or [1-^{14}C]hexadecanoylcarnitine [65] as substrate. This would be expected in the presence of a significant degree of channelling. Therefore steady-state levels of any intermediates are achieved within seconds of the initiation of β-oxidation. With intact isolated rat liver mitochondria, Stanley and Tubbs [66] observed that the addition of unlabelled hexadecanoylcarnitines during a pulse of oxidation of [16-^{14}C]hexadecanoylcarnitine inhibited the decline in levels of radioactive intermediates observed in the absence of added unlabelled hexadecanoylcarnitine.

This is one key observation which led these authors to formulate the leaky hose-pipe model for β-oxidation. In studies of peroxisomal β-oxidation we have, however, observed a similar phenomenon. When unlabelled tetradecanoyl-CoA was added to peroxisomes during a pulse of oxidation of [U-^{14}C]hexadecanoate a very marked increase in intermediates containing 12 carbon atoms or less was observed (Fig. 5). This was interpreted to indicate that the non-radioactive tetradecanoyl-CoA, and intermediates derived from this substrate, were preferentially β-oxidized. This phenomenon, however, was observed with a β-oxidation system in which extensive accumulation of intermediates occurs. Although the experimental set-up is somewhat different from that used by Stanley and Tubbs [64], the experiments are sufficiently similar to suggest that this phenomenon is not a straightforward indicator for a leaky hose-pipe type of model for β-oxidation [64].

Careful studies of the time course of peroxisomal β-oxidation using freshly prepared non-solubilized peroxisomes demonstrate that a lag phase is apparent when β-oxidation is measured as the release of acid-soluble β-oxidation products from [U-^{14}C]hexadecanoate (Fig. 6). With non-solubilized peroxisomes this lag phase is enhanced in the presence of 20 μM tetradecanoyl-CoA, whereas this has no effect with solubilized peroxisomes (Fig. 6). This lag phase could be due to an initial build-up of a critical concentration of [U-^{14}C]hexadecanoyl-CoA (due to the activity of hexadecanoyl-CoA synthetase) being required before rapid β-oxidation is

---

Fig. 4   **Theoretical simulation of β-oxidation**

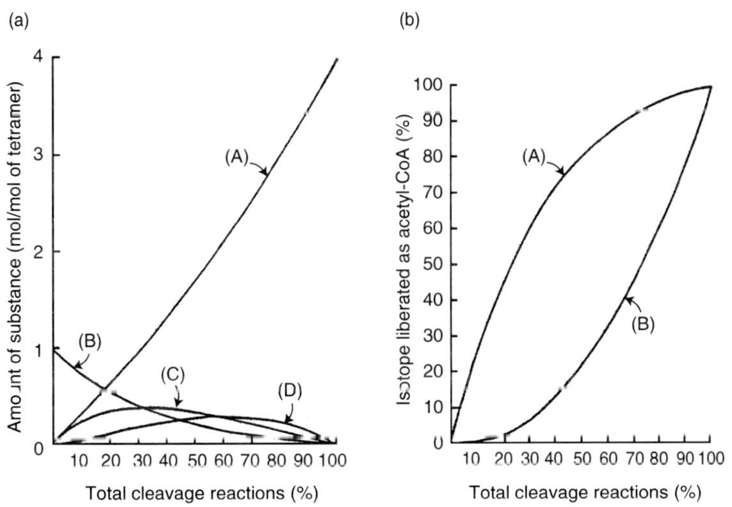

The graphs illustrate depolymerization of a linear tetramer from one end by three equivalent cleavages to form four monomers. This process is similar to complete β-oxidation of octanoyl-CoA to acetyl-CoA, assuming that the probability of each intermediate participating in further cleavage events is proportional to its relative concentration. (a) Disappearance of substrate and appearance of intermediates and final product (i.e. acetyl-CoA). Curve (A), acetyl-CoA production; (B), octanoyl-CoA disappearance; (C) and (D), concentrations of C_6 and C_4 intermediates respectively. (b) Liberation of ^{14}C as a percentage of the total amount of radioactivity in a labelled precursor present in the system of (a). Curve (A), precursor is [1-^{14}C]octanoyl-CoA; (B), precursor is [8-^{14}C]octanoyl-CoA. Reproduced from [63], with permission.

possible. The absence of an effect of tetradecanoyl-CoA with solubilized peroxisomes, however, suggests that this is unlikely to be the complete explanation of this phenomenon.

Intermediates of mitochondrial β-oxidation

Mitochondrial β-oxidation is linked to the respiratory chain at two stages: the 3-hydroxyacyl-CoA dehydrogenase activities to Complex 1 via NAD^+/ NADH, and the acyl-CoA dehydrogenases to ubiquinone via the ETF and its oxidoreductase (ETF-CoQ). Inhibition of respiratory chain activity at the level of Complex 1 leads to diminished β-oxidation flux and the accumulation of 3-hydroxyacyl- and 2-enoyl-CoA and carnitine esters [64,66–70]. This may lead to further inhibition of flux at the level of the acyl-CoA dehydrogenases [71,72]. Similarly, a deficiency of ETF or ETF-CoQ leads to diminished β-oxidation flux and an accumulation of long-chain saturated

---

Fig. 5　　　**Effects of addition of myristoyl-CoA on intermediates of the peroxisomal β-oxidation of [U-^{14}C]hexadecanoate**

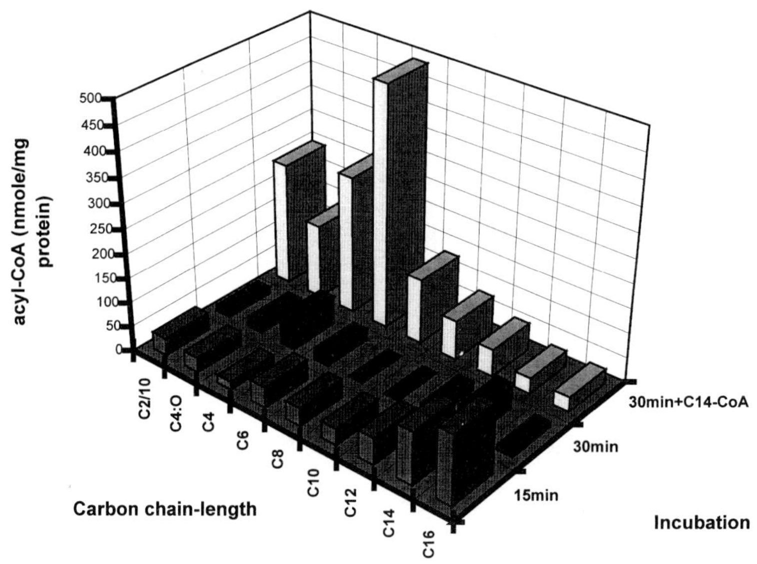

Freshly isolated rat liver peroxisomes were incubated under iso-osmotic conditions as described in the legend to Fig. 3, except that 100 μM [U-^{14}C]hexadecanoate was used. The radioactive acyl-CoA esters found after 15 min of incubation are shown in the first series (15 min). Tetradecanoyl-CoA (20 μM) was added, and radioactive acyl-CoA esters were measured after a further 15 min of incubation (30 min + C14-CoA). Results from a 30 min incubation in the absence of added tetradecanoyl-CoA are also shown (30 min). The following abbreviations have been used: C2, acetyl-CoA; C4:0, 3-oxobutyryl-CoA; C4, butyryl-CoA; C6, hexanoyl-CoA; C8, octanoyl-CoA; C10, decanoyl-CoA; C12, dodecanoyl-CoA; C14, tetradecanoyl-CoA; C16, hexadecanoyl-CoA.

acyl-CoA and acylcarnitine esters [73]. Measurement of the CoA and carnitine esters arising from β-oxidation of [U-^{14}C]hexadecanoate by isolated rat skeletal muscle mitochondria and of NAD$^+$ and NADH has led to the suggestion that there may be tight channelling of a small recycling pool of NAD$^+$ and NADH between Complex 1 of the respiratory chain and the trifunctional protein of β-oxidation ([74]; see also Chapter 4 in the current volume). Thus it is suggested that a major portion of the control of mitochondrial β-oxidation flux resides in the properties of the trifunctional protein and its relationship with other components of the mitochondrial inner membrane such as Complex 1. Such a model could explain our observation of the accumulation of 3-hydroxyacyl-CoA and 2-enoyl-CoA esters in

---

Fig. 6   **Time course of peroxisomal β-oxidation**

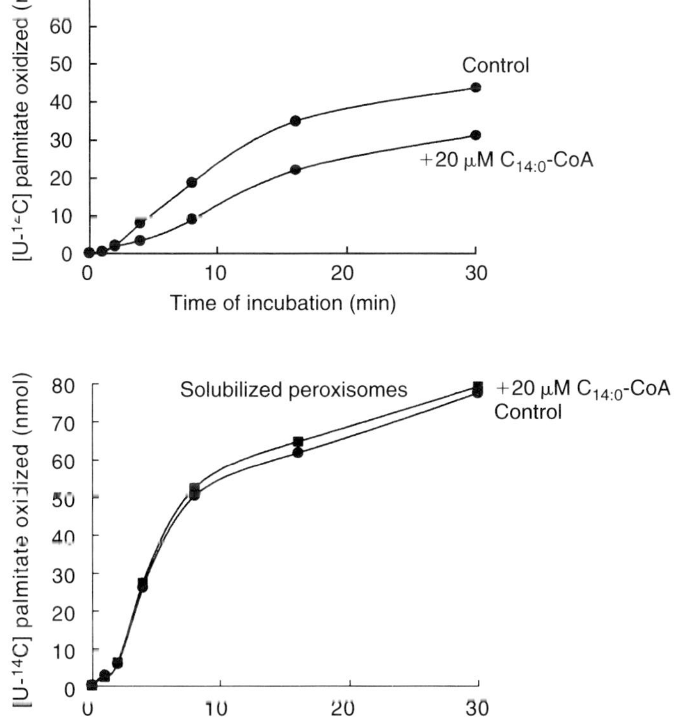

Freshly isolated peroxisomes were incubated as described in legend to Fig. 3 in the presence of 100 µM [U-^{14}C]hexadecanoate, in the absence and presence of 20 µM tetradecanoyl-CoA (C14:0-CoA). The progress of β-oxidation was assayed as HClO$_4$ (5%, v/v)-soluble radioactivity.

the presence of NAD^+, if it is assumed that there exists a small rapidly cycling pool of NAD^+ and NADH which is tightly channelled between Complex 1 and the trifunctional protein [58,59]. This evidence is briefly reviewed below.

The CoA esters produced during β-oxidation of [U-^{14}C]hexadecanoate by isolated rat skeletal muscle mitochondrial fractions are shown in Fig. 7. Levels of hexadecanoyl-CoA reached approx. 9 nmol/mg of protein after 2 min of incubation; 3-hydroxyacyl-CoA and 2-enoyl-CoA esters were also detected (Fig. 7). The amounts of 3-hydroxyacyl-CoA and 2-enoyl-CoA esters for each chain length were comparable, due to the equilibrium of enoyl-CoA hydratase, and were approximately one-third of the amount of the corresponding saturated acyl-CoA esters. The concentrations of some CoA esters increased throughout the time course of the experiment rather than a steady state being reached (see, for example, tetradec-2-enoyl-CoA and 3-hydroxytetradecanoyl-CoA). There was a lag in the production of the shorter-chain CoA esters which was more pronounced in the absence of malate and which increased with decreasing chain length. A similar distribution of 3-hydroxy-, 2-enoyl- and saturated derivatives was observed in the acylcarnitine fraction. It should be pointed out that steady-state conditions were not obtained and therefore treatment of the results by formal control theory is not valid.

The production of 3-hydroxyacyl- and 2-enoyl-CoA esters by rat skeletal muscle and heart mitochondria oxidizing [U-^{14}C]hexadecanoylcarnitine or [U-^{14}C]hexadecanoate, in the absence of respiratory poisons, was unexpected. Previous studies of acyl groups formed from hexadecanoate (as CoA or carnitine esters, or free acids after alkaline hydrolysis) have shown generation of 3-hydroxyacyl- and 2-enoyl- groups only under conditions when the disposal of reducing equivalents via the respiratory chain is inhibited, e.g. state 4 conditions, ischaemia or impaired activity of Complex 1 due to rotenone inhibition or enzyme deficiency [64,66–68,70,75]. Most of these studies, however, were carried out on liver mitochondria. Previous studies of rat muscle mitochondria showed the production of tetradecanoate, dodecanoate and decanoate from hexadecanoate [76,77], and studies using rabbit heart mitochondria showed 3-hydroxyacid production from hexadecanoylcarnitine in the absence of rotenone and in the presence of 10 mM malate; this accumulation increased approx. 10-fold in the presence of 10 μM rotenone [78].

There are a number of possible mechanisms for the accumulation of 3-hydroxyacyl- and 2-enoyl-CoA esters. Inadequate oxygenation of the incubations can be excluded, since direct measurement of the NAD^+ and NADH concentrations in mitochondria showed that there were no gross changes in the NAD^+ redox state. The $NADH/NAD^+$ ratios obtained were comparable with those obtained by Moore et al. [75] in rabbit heart mitochondria and by Latipaa et al. [69] in perfused rabbit heart. The relationship between 3-hydroxyacyl-CoA dehydrogenases and Complex 1 [79,80]

Fig. 7   Acyl-CoA esters generated during β-oxidation of [U-^{14}C]hexadecanoate by isolated skeletal muscle mitochondria

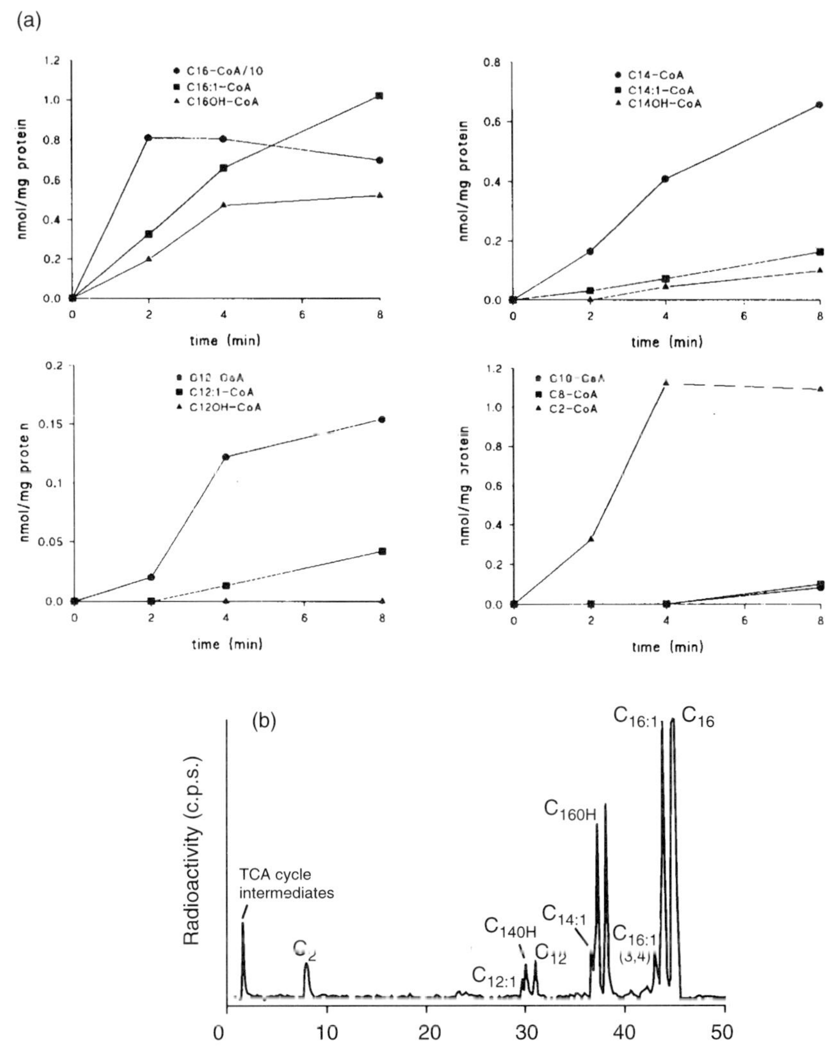

(a) *Time course of appearance of acyl-CoA esters generated by the β-oxidation of [U-^{14}C]hexadecanoate by intact rat skeletal muscle mitochondria. The conditions of incubation and analysis were as described in [58]. (b) Radiochromatogram of the acyl-CoA and 2-enoyl-CoA esters. The conditions of incubation and analysis were as described in [58]. The numbers indicate the carbon chain lengths of the acyl-groups; OH indicates 3-hydroxyderivatives; and :1 indicates Δ^2-enoyl esters. TCA cycle, tricarboxylic acid cycle.*

may be important for the control of β-oxidation flux. This interaction could result in a separate $NAD^+/NADH$ pool for 3-hydroxyacyl-CoA dehydrogenase, the postulated slower turnover rate of which, rather than the bulk-phase $NAD^+/NADH$ ratio, could determine the activity of 3-hydroxyacyl-CoA dehydrogenase. Alternatively, feedback inhibition of β-oxidation by an intermediate (e.g. succinyl-CoA) in the tricarboxylic cycle is a possible explanation. The function of this mechanism would be to maintain the generation of acetyl-CoA at a rate which corresponds to the demand for acetyl-CoA by the tricarboxylic acid cycle.

An additional explanation for the occurrence of 3-hydroxyacyl- and 2-enoyl-CoA esters could be the physiological activity ratios of the β-oxidation enzymes in muscle. Reichmann and De Vivo [81] compared the enzyme activities from a variety of tissues and found the acyl-CoA dehydrogenases to have the lowest activities, as also found by Jackson et al. [14] in human muscle. However, Reichmann and De Vivo measured 3-hydroxyacyl-CoA dehydrogenase activity in the non-physiological direction with a short-chain substrate. It is also difficult to interpret enzyme activity data in terms of intramitochondrial control, both because of differences in electron acceptors, assay conditions and mitochondrial preparations, and also because the measurement of enzyme activity in homogenates of disrupted mitochondria will not reflect any supramolecular organization which may be present within the intact mitochondrion.

Concluding remarks

Should the reader feel that the above discussion has led to few definite conclusions regarding the presence, or absence, of channelling during β-oxidation, our objective has been achieved. The evidence for channelling on the multifunctional enzymes of β-oxidation seems compelling. The same cannot be said for β-oxidation in general, although mitochondrial β-oxidation clearly does not operate as a sequence with free accumulation of intermediates. Peroxisomal β-oxidation, in contrast, exhibits extensive accumulation of intermediates, and yet shares some features thought to be typical of mitochondrial β-oxidation. It is appropriate at this point to direct the reader to the chapter in this book by Cornish-Bowden (Chapter 4), in which it is proposed that the low concentrations of intermediates found in mitochondrial β-oxidation do not necessitate the presence of channelling.

Studies of β-oxidation intermediates have revealed some striking differences. In the presence of an NAD^+ regenerator Δ^2-enoyl-CoA and 3-hydroxyacyl-CoA esters have never been detected from peroxisomal β-oxidation. However, in heart and skeletal muscle mitochondria metabolizing fatty acids these two intermediates are readily observed, even in the presence of appreciable concentrations of NAD^+. With liver mitochondria these two intermediates are primarily found when the respiratory chain has been blocked. This may represent operational differences between β-oxidation in non-ketogenic and ketogenic tissues.

Further work clearly is necessary if we are to gain insight into these basic aspects of a metabolic sequence that is fundamental to life.

The British Heart Foundation, Action Research, the Muscular Dystrophy Group of Great Britain, Nordisk Insulinfond and Fam. Blix's Fond are gratefully acknowledged for their support of some of the work described.

References

1. Lazarow, P.B. (1977) Science **197**, 580–581
2. Leighton, B., Tagliaferro, A.R. and Newsholme, E.A. (1987) J. Nutr. **117**, 1287–1290
3. Ganning, E.A., Brunk, U. and Dallner, G. (1984) Hepatology **4**, 541–547
4. Lock, E.A., Mitchell, A.M. and Elcombe, C.R. (1989) Annu. Rev. Pharmacol. **29**, 145–164
5. Osmundsen, H., Bremer, J. and Pedersen, J.I. (1991) Biochim. Biophys. Acta **1085**, 141–158
6. Reddy, J.K. and Mannaerts, G.P. (1994) Annu. Rev. Nutr. **14**, 343–370
7. Stern, J.R. and Del Campillo, A. (1956) J. Biol. Chem. **218**, 971–983
8. Hass, G.M and Hill, R.L. (1969) J. Biol. Chem. **244**, 6080–6086
9. Waterson, R.M. and Hill, R.L. (1972) J. Biol. Chem. **247**, 5258–5265
10. Stern, J.R., del Campillo, A. and Raw, I. (1956) J. Biol. Chem. **218**, 971–982
11. Wit-Peeters, E.M., Scholte, H.T., Van den Akker, F. and de Nie, I. (1971) Biochim. Biophys. Acta **231**, 23–31
12. Fong, J.C. and Schulz, H. (1981) Methods Enzymol. **71**, 390–398
13. Fong, J.C. and Schulz, H. (1977) J. Biol. Chem. **252**, 542–547
14. Jackson, S., Singh Kler, R., Bartlett, K., Briggs, H., Bindoff, L., Pourfarzam, M., Gardner-Medwin, D. and Turnbull, D.M. (1992) J. Clin. Invest. **90**, 1219–1225
14a. Jackson, S., Schaefer, J., Middleton, B. and Turnbull, D.M. (1995) Biochem. Biophys. Res. Commun. **214**, 247–253
15. Stern, J.R. (1957) Methods Enzymol. **1**, 559–567
16. Bradshaw, R.A. and Noyes, B.E. (1975) Methods Enzymol. **35**, 122–128
17. Osumi, T. and Hashimoto, T. (1980) Arch. Biochem. Biophys. **203**, 372–383
18. He, X.Y., Yang, S.Y. and Schulz, H. (1989) Anal. Biochem. **180**, 105–109
19. El-Fakhri, M. and Middleton, B. (1982) Biochim. Biophys. Acta **713**, 270–279
20. Middleton, B. (1972) Biochem. Biophys. Res. Commun. **46**, 508–515
21. Middleton, B. (1973) Biochem. J. **132**, 717–730
22. Middleton, B. and Bartlett, K. (1983) Clin. Chim. Acta **128**, 291–305
23. Seubert, W., Lamberts, I., Kramer, R. and Ohly, B. (1968) Biochim. Biophys. Acta **164**, 498–517
24. Staack, H., Binstock, J.F. and Schulz, H. (1978) J. Biol. Chem. **253**, 1827–1831
25. Uchida, Y., Izaik, K., Orii, T. and Hashimoto, T. (1992) J. Biol. Chem. **267**, 1034–1041
26. Carpenter, K., Pollit, R.J. and Middleton, B. (1992) Biochem. Biophys. Res. Commun. **183**, 443–448
27. Luo, M.J., He, X.Y., Sprecher, H. and Schulz, H. (1993) Arch. Biochem. Biophys. **304**, 266–271
28. Kerner, J. and Bieber, L. (1990) Biochemistry **29**, 4326–4334
29. Bock, R.M., Kramar, R. and Pavelka, M. (1980) in Peroxisomes and Related Particles in Animal Tissues, pp. 4–28, Springer-Verlag, Wien and New York
30. Huttinger, M., Pavelka, M., Goldenberg, H. and Kramar, R. (1981) Histochemistry **71**, 259–267

31. Appelkvist, E.L., Brunk, U. and Dallner, G. (1981) J. Biochem. Biophys. Methods **5**, 203–217
32. Wolvetang, E.J., Wanders, R.J., Schutgens, R.B., Berden, J.A. and Tager, J.M.(1990) Biochim. Biophys. Acta **1035**, 6–11
33. Krisans, S.K., Mortensen, R.M. and Lazarow, P.B. (1980) J. Biol. Chem. **255**, 9599–9607
34. Van Veldhoven, P.P., Just, W.W. and Mannaerts, G.P. (1987) J. Biol. Chem. **262**, 4210–4216
35. Schepers, L., Van Veldhoven, P.P., Casteels, M., Eyssen, H.J. and Mannaerts, G.P. (1990) J. Biol. Chem. **265**, 5242–5246
36. Palosaari, P.M., Vikinen, M. and Kiltunen, J.K. (1992) Prog. Clin. Biol. Res. **375**, 41–46
37. Miyazawa, S., Furuta, S., Osumi, T., Hashimoto, T. and Ui, N. (1981) J. Biochem. (Tokyo) **90**, 511–519
38. Bieber, L.L., Krahling, J.B., Clarke, P.R., Valkener, K.J. and Tolbert, N.E. (1981) Arch. Biochem. Biophys. **211**, 599–604
39. Novikov, V.D., Vanhove, G.F., Carchon, H., Asselberghs, S., Eyssen, H.J., Van Vedlhoven, P.P. and Mannaerts, G.P. (1994) J. Biol. Chem. **269**, 27125–27135
40. Hackenbrock, C.R. (1968) Proc. Natl. Acad. Sci. U.S.A. **61**, 598–605
41. Srere, P.A. (1987) Annu. Rev. Biochem. **56**, 89–124
42. Osmundsen, H. (1982) Int. J. Biochem. **14**, 905–914
43. Garland, P.B., Shepherd, D. and Yates, D.W. (1965) Biochem. J. **97**, 587–594
44. Sumegi, B. and Srere, P.A. (1984) J. Biol. Chem. **259**, 8748–8752
45. Izai, K., Uchida, Y., Orii, T., Yamamoto, S. and Hashimoto, T. (1992) J. Biol. Chem. **267**, 1027–1033
46. Alexson, S.E., Fujiki, Y., Shio, H. and Lazarow, P.B. (1985) J. Cell Biol. **101**, 294–304
47. Mannaerts, G.P., Van Veldhoven, P., Van Broekhoven, A., Vandebroek, G. and Debeer, L.J (1982) Biochem. J. **204**, 17–23
48. Yang, S.Y. and Schulz, H. (1983) J. Biol. Chem. **258**, 9780–9785
49. Furuta, S., Miyazawa, S., Osumi, T. and Hashimoto, T. (1980) J. Biochem. (Tokyo) **88**, 1059–1070
50. Nuttley, W.M., Aitchison, J.D. and Rachubinski, R.A. (1988) Gene **69**, 171–180
51. Yang, S.Y., Cuebas, D. and Schulz, H. (1986) J. Biol. Chem. **261**, 15390–15395
52. Yang, S.Y., Bittman, R. and Schulz, H. (1985) J. Biol. Chem. **260**, 2862–2868
53. Schulz, H. (1991) Biochim. Biophys. Acta **1081**, 109–120
54. Yu, S.Y., Cosly, S. and Schulz, H. (1989) J. Biol. Chem. **264**, 16489–16495
55. Lazarow, P.M. and de Duve, C. (1976) Proc. Natl. Acad. Sci. U.S.A. **73**, 2043–2046
56. Osmundsen, H., Neat, C.E. and Norum, K.R. (1979) FEBS Lett. **99**, 292–296
57. Christiansen, R.Z., Osmundsen, H., Borreback, B. and Bremer, J. (1978) Lipids **13**, 487–491
58. Eaton, S., Bhuiyan, A.K.M.J., Singh Kler, R., Turnbull, D.M. and Bartlett, K. (1993) Biochem. J. **289**, 161–168
59. Eaton, S., Turnbull, D.M. and Bartlett, K. (1994) Eur. J. Biochem. **220**, 671–681
60. Bartlett, K., Hovik, R., Eaton, S., Watmough, N.J. and Osmundsen, H. (1990) Biochem. J. **270**, 175–180
61. Sleboda, J., Pourfarzam, M., Bartlett, K. and Osmundsen, H. (1995) Biochim. Biophys. Acta **1258**, 309–318
62. Hovik, R., Brodal, B., Bartlett, K. and Osmundsen, H. (1991) J. Lipid Res. **32**, 993–999
63. Stewart, H.B., Tubbs, P.K. and Stanley, K.K. (1973) Biochem. J. **132**, 61–76
64. Stanley, K.K. and Tubbs, P.K.(1974) FEBS. Lett. **39**, 325–328
65. Osmundsen, H. and Bremer, J. (1977) Biochem. J. **164**, 621–633
66. Stanley, K.K. and Tubbs P.K. (1975) Biochem. J. **150**, 77–88
67. Bremer, J. and Wojtczak, B. (1972) Biochim. Biophys. Acta **280**, 515–530
68. Lopez-Cardozo, M., Klazinga, W. and Van Den Bergh, S.G. (1978) Eur. J. Biochem. **83**, 629–634
69. Latipaa, P.M., Karki, T.T., Hiltunen, J.K. and Hassinen, I.E. (1986) Biochim. Biophys. Acta **875**, 293–300
70. Watmough, N.J., Turnbull, D.M., Sherratt, H.S.A. and Bartlett, K. (1989) Biochem. J. **262**, 261–269

71. Davidson, B.V. and Schulz, H. (1982) Arch. Biochem. Biophys. **213**, 155–162
72. Powell, P.J., Lau, S.M., Killian, D. and Thorpe, C. (1987) Biochemistry **26**, 3704–3710
73. Singh Kler, R., Jackson, S., Bartlett, K., Bindoff, L.A., Eaton, S., Pourfarzam, M., Frerman, F.E., Watmough, M.J. and Turnbull, D.M. (1991) J. Biol. Chem. **266**, 22932–22938
74. Bartlett, K. and Eaton, S. (1994) Biochem. Soc. Trans. **22**, 432–436
75. Moore, K.H., Radloff, J.F. and Hull, F.E. (1980) Am. J. Physiol. **239**, H257–H265
76. Watmough, N.J., Bindoff, L.A., Birch-Machin, M.A., Jackson, S., Bartlett, K., Ragan, C.I., Poulton, J., Gardiner, R.M., Sherratt, H.S.A. and Turnbull, D.M. (1990) J. Clin. Invest. **85**, 177–184
77. Veerkamp, J.H., Van Moerkek, H.T.B., Glatz, J.F.C. and Van Hinsburgh, V.W.M. (1983) Biochim. Biophys. Acta **753**, 399–410
78. Moore, K.H., Radloff, J.F. and Hull, F.E. (1980) J. Mol. Cell. Cardiol. **14**, 451–459
79. Sumegi, B. and Srere, P.A. (1984) J. Biol. Chem. **259**, 15040–15045
80. Fukushima, T., Decker, R.V., Anderson, W.M. and Spivey, H.O. (1989) J. Biol. Chem. **264**, 16483–16488
81. Reichmann, H. and De Vivo, D.C (1991) Comp. Biochem. Physiol. **988**, 327–331
82. Ikeda, Y., Dabrowski, C. and Tanaka, K. (1985) J. Biol. Chem. **258**, 1066–1076
83. Finocchiario, G., Ito, K. and Tanaka, K. (1987) J. Biol. Chem. **262**, 7982–7989
84. Furuta, S., Miyazawa, S. and Hashimoto, T. (1981) J. Biochem. (Tokyo) **90**, 1739–1750
85. Gehring, U. and Repertinger, C. (1968) Eur. J. Biochem. **6**, 281–292
86. Frerman, F.E. and Goodman, S.I. (1985) Proc. Natl. Acad. Sci. U.S.A. **83**, 4517–4520
87. Dommes, V. and Kunau, W.H. (1984) J. Biol. Chem. **259**, 1789–1798
88. Palosaari, P.M. and Hiltunen, J.K. (1990) J. Biol. Chem. **265**, 2446–2449
89. Palossari, P.M., Kilponnen, J.M., Sormunen, R.T., Hassinen, I.E. and Hiltunen, J.K. (1990) J. Biol. Chem. **265**, 3347–3353
90. Luo, M.J., Smeland, T.E., Shoukry, K. and Shulz, H. (1994) J. Biol. Chem. **269**, 2384–2388
91. Miyazawa, S., Osumi, T. and Hashimoto, T. (1980) Eur. J. Biochem. **103**, 589–596

16

Nucleotide biosynthesis in mammals

Richard I. Christopherson and Eve Szabados

Department of Biochemistry, University of Sydney, Sydney,
NSW 2006, Australia

The current status of substrate channelling

Following the pioneering work of Gaertner and Davis and their co-workers
with *Neurospora crassa* on the channelling of intermediates of aromatic amino
acid biosynthesis [1] and of carbamoyl phosphate (CAP) as a precursor for
pyrimidines and arginine [2], the concept of substrate channelling by multi
functional enzymes and multienzyme complexes became well accepted [3]. A
number of possible selective advantages were proposed for such channelling
where enzymic activities, catalysing successive reactions in a metabolic
pathway, are found on a single particle in solution or interact in a dynamic
and transitory manner [4]. More recently, however, substrate channelling has
become very controversial [5]. For example, Cornish-Bowden [6,7] has
simulated a two-enzyme system where the intermediate may remain associated with the enzyme, or a controlled proportion may diffuse into the bulk
solvent, before binding as a substrate to the second enzyme. Variations in the
partitioning of the intermediate between the surface of the enzyme aggregate
and the bulk solvent produced only minor changes in its concentration [7].
This model used a 1:1 stoichiometric complex (E_2CE_3) between the
channelled intermediate (C) and the associated enzymes (E_2E_3).

$$A \overset{E_1}{\rightleftharpoons} B \overset{E_2}{\rightleftharpoons} C \overset{E_3}{\rightleftharpoons} D \tag{1}$$

Easterby has since developed a more general analysis of this system
(eqn. 1; [8]) and has shown that the analysis of Cornish-Bowden [7] holds
only under restricted conditions. Easterby [8] points out that changes to a
pre-existing channel should not be analysed to determine effects on pool
sizes; rather, the situation where no channel exists should be contrasted with
that where the channel is active. Easterby did not change the rate constants
along the channelled route, and the 'leakiness' of the channel or the distribu
tion of flux was accounted for by the channelling efficiency, α. The
'on-constant' for formation of the ES complex increased with channelling
because the channelled intermediate (C; eqn. 1) is encountered by the
enzyme, E_3, at a higher concentration. He defines the channelling advantage,

β, as the ratio of the effective on-constant in the channel to that in free solution, equivalent to the ratio of the total system volume to the volume occupied by the internalized pool of C. With this general analysis, Easterby demonstrated that the major kinetic advantage of channelling is reduction of pool sizes and a consequently reduced transition time.

An alternative approach to simulation of this system would be to assume that there is no physical channel but, because the catalytic sites for E_2 and E_3 are on the same particle in solution, the E_3 site is within a local concentration gradient of the product, C, radiating from the E_2 site (Fig. 1). At a given rate of production of C by E_2, the concentration of C will decrease with the inverse cube of the distance from E_2, rapidly approaching the concentration of C in the bulk solvent. This model would not require partitioning between the surface of the enzyme aggregate and the bulk solvent. The local concentration of C would be determined by the rate of its production, the distance between E_2 and E_3 and the temperature. With the current controversy about substrate channelling [5–8], this chapter on *de novo* nucleotide biosynthesis will emphasize associations of sequential enzymes *in vivo*, and a critical evaluation will be attempted where substrate channelling has been claimed.

The pathway for the *de novo* biosynthesis of pyrimidine nucleotides

The *de novo* biosynthesis of pyrimidine nucleotides is shown in Fig. 2. L-Glutamine is used as a substrate at reactions 1 and 9, catalysed by CAP synthetase and CTP synthetase respectively; a second amino acid, L-aspartate, is a substrate for reaction 2, catalysed by aspartate transcarbamylase. P-Rib-PP is an allosteric activator of CAP synthetase [9,10] and is a substrate for reaction 5, catalysed by orotate phosphoribosyltransferase. The end-product of the pathway, UTP, is a potent inhibitor of CAP synthetase [10,11], which shows apparent competitive kinetics with respect to ATP [9], a substrate showing positive homotropic co-operativity. The specific enzymic activity of CAP synthetase is low relative to that of subsequent enzymes in the pathway (Fig. 1; [12]) and, under normal conditions, flux through the *de novo* pathway may be regulated by cellular levels of P-Rib-PP, UTP and ATP. Lyons and Christopherson [9] have derived a velocity equation which describes such regulation of CAP synthetase. Under conditions of cellular growth where the availability of P-Rib-PP becomes limiting for pyrimidine biosynthesis, regulation of P-Rib-PP synthetase by ADP [13] may influence flux through the pathway, limiting the rates of reactions 1 and/or 5. Dihydro-orotase (reaction 3) and L-dihydro-orotate (DHO) dehydrogenase (reaction 4) may be inhibited by orotate [14,15], and orotate phosphoribosyl-transferase (reaction 5) may be inhibited by orotidine 5′-monophosphate (OMP), but these inhibitions are unlikely to have physiological significance.

There are two multifunctional proteins in the pathway for the *de novo* biosynthesis of pyrimidine nucleotides [16]. A trifunctional protein, called CAD or DHO synthetase, catalyses reactions 1, 2 and 3 of the pathway ($HCO_3^- \rightarrow CAP \rightarrow CA\text{-}asp \rightarrow DHO$; Fig. 2; [17]). The enzymic activities CAP synthetase, aspartate transcarbamylase and dihydro-orotase are contained in a single polypeptide chain of 243 kDa [18] which, in the native state, associates primarily as trimers and hexamers [17]. The three enzymic

---

Fig. 1   **Partial substrate channelling between associated enzymic activities E_2 and E_3**

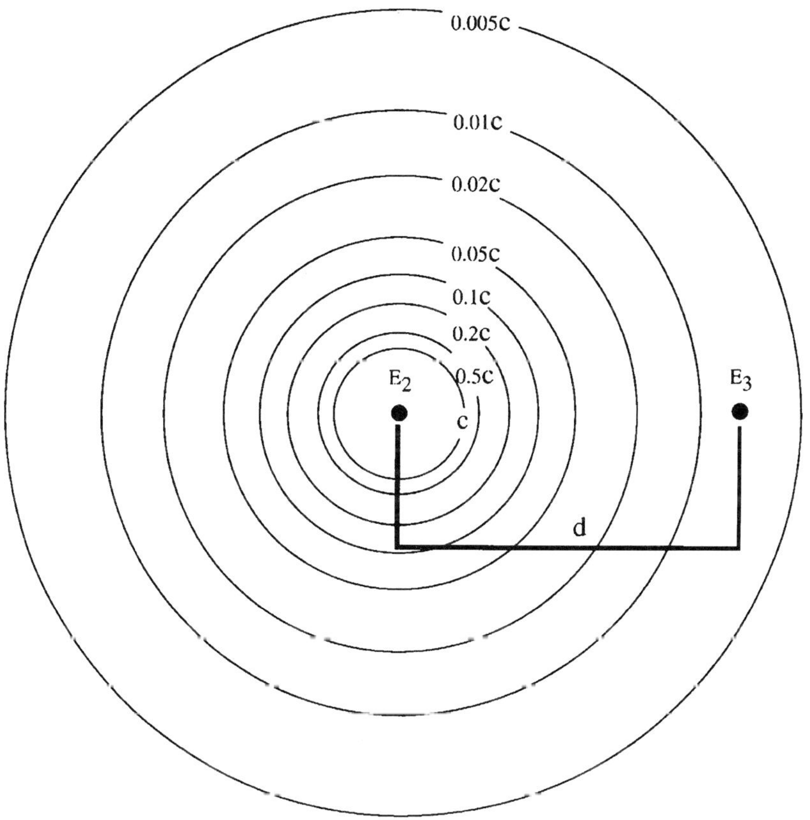

A concentration gradient of the product (C) of the enzymic activity E_2 is shown diffusing beyond E_3, for which C is a substrate. The concentration of C, denoted as c, decreases radially about E_2 as the inverse cube of the distance, as indicated by the contour lines starting at an arbitrary concentration, c, close to E_2. The catalytic sites for E_2 and E_3 are separated by a distance d. No allowance has been made in this figure for constraints on the radial diffusion of C by the enzyme complex or for the consumption of C by E_3.

activities are contained in discrete globular domains of the protein covalently connected by segments of polypeptide chain which are susceptible to digestion by proteases such as trypsin [19]. The aspartate transcarbamylase domain at the C-terminus is separated from the central dihydro-orotase domain by a large bridging region of 12.5 kDa consisting of multiple β-turns induced by proline residues [20]. The spatial arrangements of the catalytic

---

Fig. 2   The *de novo* pyrimidine biosynthetic pathway

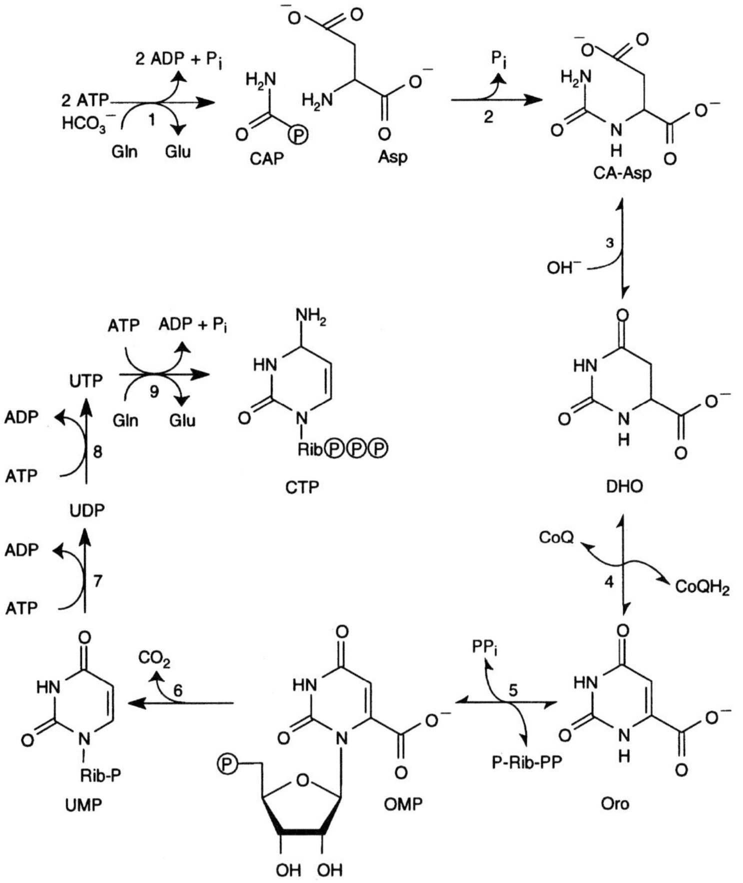

Abbreviations: CAP, carbamoyl phosphate; CA-asp, N-carbamoyl-L-aspartate; DHO, L-dihydro-orotate; Oro, orotate; OMP, orotidine 5'-monophosphate. Enzymes: 1, CAP synthetase II (EC 6.3.5.5); 2, aspartate transcarbamylase (EC 2.1.3.2); 3, dihydro-orotase (EC 3.5.2.3); 4, DHO dehydrogenase (EC 1.3.3.1); 5, orotate phosphoribosyltransferase (EC 2.4.2.10); 6, OMP decarboxylase (EC 4.1.1.23); 7, nucleoside monophosphate kinase (EC 2.7.4.4); 8, nucleoside diphosphate kinase (EC 2.7.4.6); 9, CTP synthetase (EC 6.3.4.2).

domains of CAD as the monomer (243 kDa) and the trimer have been proposed [21]. The trimer structure is based upon a trimer of aspartate transcarbamylase domains, which remains associated after proteolysis of CAD.

A bifunctional enzyme, UMP synthase, catalyses reactions 5 and 6 of the pyrimidine pathway (orotate → OMP → UMP; Fig. 2). The enzymic activities, orotate phosphoribosyltransferase and OMP decarboxylase, are contained in a protein of 51.5 kDa [22] which associates as a dimer in the presence of OMP or another ligand for the OMP decarboxylase active site [23]. Limited digestion of UMP synthase with trypsin or elastase produced a 28.5 kDa polypeptide with OMP decarboxylase activity, indicating that this activity is contained in a distinct globular domain [24]. The orotate phosphoribosyltransferase activity is rapidly lost during protease digestion.

DHO dehydrogenase, the enzyme catalysing reaction 4 of the pathway (DHO → orotate; Fig. 2), is located on the outer side of the mitochondrial inner membrane [15]. The immediate electron acceptor for this reaction is ubiquinone in mammals [25]. The *de novo* pyrimidine pathway is thus compartmentalized: DHO synthesized by trifunctional CAD in the cytosol must diffuse across the mitochondrial outer membrane to be oxidized to orotate, which in turn diffuses back into the cytosol to be a substrate for bifunctional UMP synthase. Thus, if a multienzyme complex catalysing the first six reactions of the pyrimidine pathway (HCO_3^- → CAP → CA-asp → DHO → orotate → OMP → UMP; Fig. 2) exists *in vivo*, CAD and UMP synthase would be associated with the mitochondrial outer membrane at contact points with the inner membrane. There is currently no evidence for such a complex. Mammalian cells contain two CAP synthases, the glutamine-dependent enzyme (CAP synthetase II) which is part of trifunctional CAD, and an ammonia-dependent enzyme (CAP synthetase I) which is found in the mitochondrial matrix. CAP synthetase I is found as 22–26% of the soluble protein in the matrix [26], and is normally used for urea and arginine biosynthesis. Under certain conditions (e.g. hyperammonaemia), CAP synthesized in the matrix by CAP synthetase I may be utilized for pyrimidine biosynthesis in the cytosol [27]

De novo biosynthesis of purine nucleotides

The pathway for the *de novo* biosynthesis of purine nucleotides is shown in Fig. 3. The amino acid L-glutamine is a substrate for reactions 1, 4 and 14, catalysed by amidophosphoribosyltransferase, FGAM synthetase and GMP synthetase respectively. Glycine is used as a substrate at reaction 2, and L-aspartate is used at reactions 7 and 11. P-Rib-PP shows positive homotropic co-operativity as a substrate for amidophosphoribosyltransferase [28], and this enzyme is subject to inhibition by AMP, IMP and GMP [29] and by polyglutamate derivatives of dihydrofolate [30]. The specific enzymic activity of amidophosphoribosyltransferase (P-Rib-PP → PRA) is low, and

Fig. 3   The *de novo* purine biosynthetic pathway

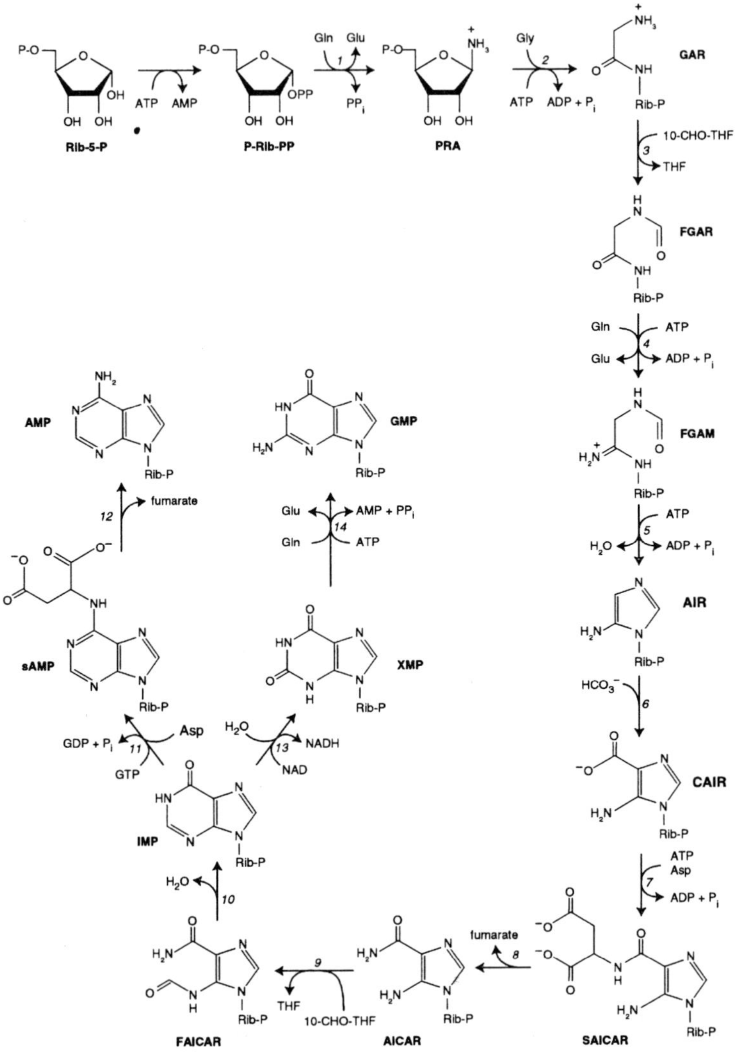

Abbreviations: Rib-5-P, ribose 5-phosphate; P-Rib-PP, 5-phosphoribosyl 1-pyrophosphate; PRA, 5-phosphoribosylamine; 10-CHO-THF, N^{10}-formyltetrahydrofolate; GAR, glycineamide ribotide; FGAR, N-formylglycineamide ribotide; FGAM, N-formylglycineamidine ribotide; AIR, 5-aminoimidazole ribotide; CAIR, 4-carboxy-5-aminoimidazole ribotide; SAICAR, N-succino-5-aminoimidazole-4-carboxamide ribotide; AICAR, 5-aminoimidazole-4-carboxamide ribotide; FAICAR, 5-formamidoimidazole-4-carboxamide ribotide; sAMP, N-succino-AMP. Enzymes: 1, amidophosphoribosyltransferase (EC 2.4.2.14); 2, GAR synthetase (EC 6.3.4.13); 3, GAR transformylase (EC 2.1.2.2); 4, FGAM synthetase (EC 6.3.5.3); 5, AIR synthetase (EC 6.3.3.1); 6, AIR carboxylase (EC 4.1.1.21); 7, SAICAR synthetase (EC 6.3.2.6); 8, adenylosuccinase (EC 4.3.2.2); 9, AICAR transformylase (EC 2.1.2.3); 10, IMP cyclohydrolase (EC 3.5.4.10); 11, sAMP synthetase (EC 6.3.4.4); 12, adenylosuccinase (EC 4.3.2.2); 13, IMP dehydrogenase (EC 1.2.1.14); 14, GMP synthetase (EC 6.3.4.1).

flux through the *de novo* pathway *in vivo* would be regulated by the end-products of the pathway, AMP, IMP and GMP. Inhibition of reaction 1 by dihydrofolate polyglutamates would signal the unavailability of N^{10}-formyltetrahydrofolate, required as a substrate at reactions 3 and 9 of the pathway [30]. The purine pathway is subject to further regulation at the branch point from IMP. XMP is a potent inhibitor of IMP cyclohydrolase (FAICAR $\rightarrow$ IMP; [31]), AMP inhibits adenylosuccinate synthetase (IMP $\rightarrow$ sAMP; [32]) and GMP inhibits IMP dehydrogenase (IMP $\rightarrow$ XMP; [33]).

There are four multifunctional proteins in the pathway for the *de novo* biosynthesis of purine nucleotides [34]. A trifunctional protein catalyses reactions 2, 3 and 5 catalysed by GAR synthetase, GAR transformylase and AIR synthetase, respectively (PRA $\rightarrow$ GAR $\rightarrow$ FGAR; FGAM $\rightarrow$ AIR; Fig. 3), and has a subunit molecular mass of 110 kDa [35]. The GAR synthetase and GAR transformylase domains may be separated by digestion of the trifunctional protein with chymotrypsin.

A bifunctional enzyme catalyses reactions 6 and 7 of the purine pathway (AIR $\rightarrow$ CAIR $\rightarrow$ SAICAR; Fig. 3) and contains the enzymic activities AIR carboxylase and SAICAR synthetase [36]. The chicken enzyme has a subunit molecular mass of 50 kDa and in the native state is found as hexamers or septamers. A second bifunctional enzyme, which we now call IMP synthase, containing AICAR transformylase and IMP cyclohydrolase activities, catalyses reactions 9 and 10 of the pathway (AICAR $\rightarrow$ FAICAR $\rightarrow$ IMP; Fig. 3; [31,37]). Human IMP synthase has a subunit molecular mass of 62.1 kDa and associates as a dimer [31]. A trifunctional enzyme, C_1-tetrahydrofolate (THF) synthase, containing 5,10-methylene-THF (5,10-CH_2-THF) dehydrogenase, 5,10-methenyl-THF (5,10-CH-THF) cyclohydrolase and 10-formyl-THF (10-CHO-THF) synthetase, catalyses the reactions 5,10-CH_2-THF $\rightarrow$ 5,10-CH-THF $\rightarrow$ 10-CHO-THF and THF $\rightarrow$ 10-CHO-THF [38]. The 10-formyl-THF produced is a substrate for GAR and AICAR transformylases catalysing reactions 3 and 9 of the pathway (Fig. 3). In higher eukaryotes the dehydrogenase and cyclohydrolase activities are found in one domain of the protein which is fused to a larger synthetase domain, forming a trifunctional enzyme [39]. The chicken enzyme has a subunit molecular mass of 95 kDa and is found in the native state as dimers [40].

There is a fifth enzyme which catalyses reactions 8 and 12 of the purine pathway (Fig. 3), but adenylosuccinate lyase has one active site with dual specificity, catalysing both reactions (SAICAR $\rightarrow$ AICAR; sAMP $\rightarrow$ AMP; Fig. 3). The rat enzyme has a subunit molecular mass of 52 kDa and associates as tetramers in the native state [41]. All 14 enzymic activities shown in Fig. 3 are cytosolic, and there is a variety of evidence for the association of sub-sets of these activities. The proposed existence of a 'pathway particle' or 'metabolon' for *de novo* purine biosynthesis will be discussed in a subsequent section.

Biosynthesis of deoxynucleotides

The pathways for the biosynthesis of the four deoxynucleoside triphosphates (dNTPs), dCTP, dTTP, dATP and dGTP, are shown in Fig. 4. The *de novo* pathways for the biosynthesis of pyrimidine (Fig. 2) and purine (Fig. 3) nucleotides provide the precursors for these interconversions, leading to the polymerization of RNA from NTPs and DNA from dNTPs. The enzymology of Fig. 4 will not be discussed, but the reactions shown are either cytosolic or nuclear. A variety of experiments in both prokaryotes and eukaryotes have shown that certain radiolabelled precursors of DNA may be preferentially incorporated into DNA without equilibration with subsequent cellular pools of intermediates [42]. The proposed existence of a multi-enzyme complex or 'replitase' able to convert some nucleosides, NMPs and NDPs to DNA will be discussed in a subsequent section.

Cellular levels of intermediates

As discussed in the first section, consideration of the cellular steady-state concentrations of intermediates (A, B, C, D...) in an unbranched metabolic pathway:

$$\xrightarrow{v} A \xrightarrow{E_1} B \xrightarrow{E_2} C \xrightarrow{E_3} D \xrightarrow{v} \tag{2}$$

with the kinetic parameters (K_m and V_{max}) for the enzymes (E_1, E_2, E_3...) and the flux (v) through the pathway can provide an indication of whether the intermediates are channelled between successive enzymes. As stated by Easterby [8], "the major kinetic advantage of channelling is a reduction of pool sizes". Traut [43] has compiled and analysed a valuable list of about 600 published concentrations for bases, nucleosides and nucleoside mono-, di- and tri-phosphates. However, intermediates from the *de novo* pyrimidine and purine pathways and catabolic pathways were generally omitted due to insufficient data. Cellular levels for some intermediates of the *de novo* pathways (Figs. 2 and 3) have been determined (e.g. [44,45]), but comprehensive lists of concentrations for the following intermediates:

$$HCO_3^- \xrightarrow{1} CAP \xrightarrow{2} CA\text{-}asp \xrightarrow{3} DHO \xrightarrow{4} orotate \xrightarrow{5} OMP \xrightarrow{6} UMP$$

$$\tag{3}$$

$$P\text{-}Rib\text{-}PP \xrightarrow{1} PRA \xrightarrow{2} GAR \xrightarrow{3} FGAR \xrightarrow{4} FGAM \xrightarrow{5} AIR \xrightarrow{6}$$

$$CAIR \xrightarrow{7} SAICAR \xrightarrow{8} AICAR \xrightarrow{9} FAICAR \xrightarrow{10} IMP \tag{4}$$

Fig. 4   **Conversion of nucleoside monophosphates into deoxynucleoside triphosphates and their polymerizations to form RNA and DNA**

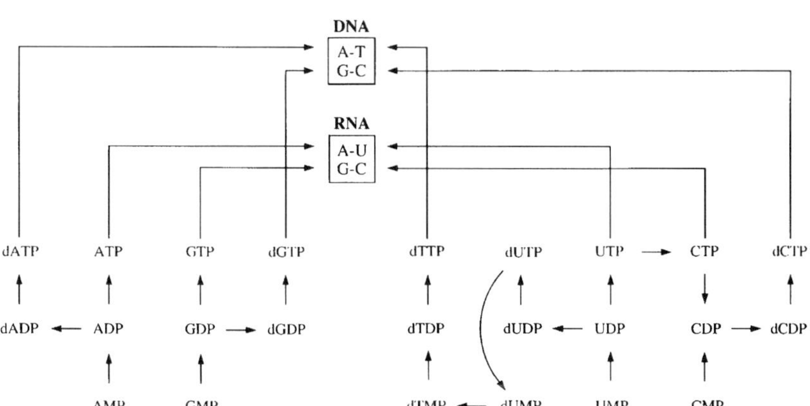

$$THF \xrightarrow{a} 5,10\text{-}CH_2\text{-}THF \xrightarrow{b} 5,10\text{-}CH\text{-}THF \xrightarrow{c} 10\text{-}CHO\text{-}THF$$

$$THF \xrightarrow{d} 10\text{-}CHO\text{-}THF \qquad (5)$$

determined concurrently from the same cell extract are not available. Low levels of some intermediates in cells, inconsistent with the kinetic parameters of enzymes and the observed metabolic flux, would provide some evidence for channelling in growing cells.

Substrate channelling in *de novo* pyrimidine biosynthesis

The first report of experimental data supporting substrate channelling in these pathways was from Lue and Kaplan in 1970 [46] with bifunctional CAP synthetase/aspartate transcarbamylase from yeast. Using [^{14}C]bicarbonate as a substrate for the bifunctional enzyme ($HCO_3^- \rightarrow CAP \rightarrow CA\text{-}asp$; Fig. 2), they found that exogenous unlabelled CAP could not dilute the label recovered in CA-asp. In addition, ornithine transcarbamylase in the reaction mixture could not compete on even terms with aspartate transcarbamylase for CAP produced by the bifunctional enzyme. More recent research with this yeast enzyme [47] shows that the channelling of CAP is not absolute and may result from a privileged diffusion between the two catalytic sites (cf. Fig. 1).

The subject of this chapter is, however, substrate channelling in mammalian systems where the first three reactions of the *de novo* pyrimidine pathway ($HCO_3^- \rightarrow CAP \rightarrow CA\text{-}asp \rightarrow DHO$; Fig. 2) are catalysed by a trifunctional protein called CAD or DHO synthetase. Evans and his co-workers [48] demonstrated catalytic synergy for the overall reaction with no apparent lag time for the formation of $[^{14}C]$DHO from $[^{14}C]$bicarbonate, and suggested that the equivalent system of unlinked enzymes would take 1 h to attain a comparable rate of synthesis of DHO. Christopherson and Jones [49] found that when the overall reaction, $HCO_3^- \rightarrow CAP \rightarrow CA\text{-}asp \rightarrow DHO$, catalysed by CAD was coupled to the enzymic sequence $DHO \rightarrow orotate \rightarrow OMP$ by addition of appropriate enzymes and substrates, CAP and CA-asp reached steady-state levels of approx. 0.20 μM and 7.1 μM, respectively. Consideration of the K_m and V_{max} values of aspartate trans-carbamylase and dihydro-orotase, determined under the same conditions as the overall rate of synthesis of DHO by CAD, indicated that the local concentrations of CAP at the active site of aspartate transcarbamylase and of CA-asp at the dihydro-orotase site must be 2.2- and 3.1-fold higher, respectively than their average concentrations in the bulk solvent. Similar concentrations were predicted by calculation of steady-state concentrations from ratios of the rate constants for the three activities. A high local concentration of CA-asp at the third site was also indicated by a 3.6-fold reduction in the transient time for dihydro-orotase activity from that predicted. Competition experiments performed with exogenous CAP and CA-asp indicated only partial channelling of the two intermediates. Considerably more DHO was actually synthesized from endogenous CA-asp, which consequently accumulated to a lesser degree than expected. The partial channelling of CAP and CA-asp by CAD was supported by two procedures of kinetic analysis: by a $^{14}C/^{3}H$ competition experiment and by a reduction in the predicted transient time from 4.7 min to 1.3 min [49]. The low steady-state concentrations of CAP (0.2 μM) and CA-asp (7.1 μM) prevailing during the overall reaction:

$$HCO_3^- \xrightarrow{k_1} CAP \xrightarrow{k_2} CA\text{-}asp \xrightarrow{k_3} DHO \tag{6}$$

are primarily due to the favourable ratios of the rate constants:

$$[CAP]_{ss} = k_1/k_2 \tag{7}$$

$$[CA\text{-}asp]_{ss} = k_1/k_3 \tag{8}$$

where the subscript ss denotes the steady-state concentration [49]. Maintenance of these low concentrations would prevent futile cycling of CAP and possible toxic side-effects of CA-asp [50].

Recently, a cDNA encoding the entire trifunctional CAD protein of 243 kDa has been cloned and expressed in *Escherichia coli* [21]. The purified recombinant protein had kinetic parameters similar to those obtained for native CAD and was subject to regulation by P-Rib-PP and UTP. Recombinant CAD also exhibited partial channelling, like the native trifunctional protein, but a mutant CAD, lacking the 12 kDa bridging region between the aspartate transcarbamylase and dihydro-orotase domains, did not channel CAP [21]. These results suggest that partial channelling of CAP is due to the close proximity of the active sites for CAP synthetase and aspartate transcarbamylase. CAP is inherently unstable under physiological conditions, with a half-time for decomposition of 42 min [51]. Maintenance of a low steady-state concentration of CAP (0.2 μM) would therefore provide a selective advantage, but can be attributed more to the high V_{max}/K_m ratio for aspartate transcarbamylase than to substrate channelling [49].

The bifunctional enzyme UMP synthase catalyses the conversion orotate $\rightarrow$ OMP $\rightarrow$ UMP (Fig. 2). Steady-state concentrations of OMP are very low (50–100 nM [52]), indicating that UMP synthase is very efficient at decarboxylating the OMP synthesized by the phosphoribosyltransferase. Channelling of OMP by UMP synthase has been proposed from experiments where endogenous OMP synthesized from orotate was competed with exogenous OMP with different radiolabelling [53]. A subsequent re-evaluation of these data by numerical simulation suggested that preferential utilization by the decarboxylase of OMP synthesized by the phosphoribosyltransferase was not required to account for the results [54]. However, this re-evaluation by McClard was flawed. He stated that "such channelling could only be operative if the number of active sites of the second enzyme either approximates or exceeds the number of molecules of the transient species, in this case [6-^{14}C]OMP". This requirement applies only to complete or stoichiometric channelling where a single molecule of the channelled species is sequestered; the partial channelling of CAP by CAD described above only requires that the subsequent enzyme (aspartate transcarbamylase) operates at a higher local concentration of the channelled substrate (CAP) than that prevailing in the bulk solvent ([49]; Fig. 1). Thus UMP synthase does not need "to sequester greater that 200 OMP molecules" for OMP channelling, as stated by McClard [54]. More recent data suggest that the complex steady-state kinetics of UMP synthase in the presence of OMP and cycling of orotate $\rightarrow$ OMP $\rightarrow$ orotidine $\rightarrow$ orotate may explain the original data interpreted as channelling of OMP [55]. Further support for the channelling of OMP by UMP synthase might be obtained from short-term competition experiments with pure UMP synthase where only small proportions of exogenous OMP were consumed by the decarboxylase, and the kinetic parameters of the phosphoribosyltransferase and decarboxylase used for simulations were evaluated under the same conditions used for channelling in the presence of the substrates(s) (or analogues) for the other enzymic activity.

A metabolon for *de novo* purine biosynthesis?

Substrate channelling has not been reported for the trifunctional enzyme catalysing reactions 2, 3 and 5 of the *de novo* purine pathway or for the bifunctional enzyme catalysing reactions 6 and 7 (see Fig. 3). We have purified the bifunctional enzyme, IMP synthase, catalysing reactions 9 and 10 from human CCRF-CEM leukaemia cells [31]. Four types of experiments, first used to analyse substrate channelling for CAD by Christopherson and Jones [49], have been performed to characterize possible channelling of FAICAR by IMP synthase (E. Szabados and R.I. Christopherson, unpublished work).

$$\text{AICAR} + 10\text{-CHO-THF} \xrightarrow{k_1} \text{FAICAR} \xrightarrow{k_2} \text{IMP} + \text{H}_2\text{O} \tag{9}$$

The kinetic parameters (K_m and V_{max}) were determined for AICAR transformylase and IMP cyclohydrolase under the conditions used for the overall reaction (eqn. 9). Progress curves for the conversion $[^3\text{H}]\text{AICAR} \rightarrow [^3\text{H}]\text{-}$ $\text{FAICAR} \rightarrow [^3\text{H}]\text{IMP}$ were determined and the intermediate, FAICAR, was found to reach a steady-state concentration of $0.118\ \mu\text{M}$. Four types of experiment to test for channelling of FAICAR were performed, with the following results.

(i) The observed rate of synthesis of IMP was found to be 13.4-fold higher than that calculated by substitution of the observed steady-state concentration of FAICAR ($0.118\ \mu\text{M}$) into the appropriate form of the Michaelis–Menten equation. The local concentration of FAICAR giving rise to this higher rate of IMP synthesis may be calculated from a rearranged form of the Michaelis–Menten equation:

$$[\text{FAICAR}] = vK_m/(V_{max} - v) \tag{10}$$

The local FAICAR concentration obtained was $1.57\ \mu\text{M}$, 13.3-fold higher than that prevailing in the bulk solvent.

(ii) At saturating concentrations of 10-CHO-THF and AICAR, the AICAR transformylase reaction has a zero-order rate constant, k_1, determined from the V_{max}; the first-order rate constant, k_2, for the IMP cyclohydrolase reaction can be determined from the ratio V_{max}/K_m. Under these conditions, the steady-state concentration of FAICAR can be calculated [49,56]:

$$[\text{FAICAR}]_{ss} = k_1/k_2 \tag{11}$$

The local concentration of FAICAR at the IMP cyclohydrolase site was calculated as $1.60\ \mu\text{M}$, in close agreement with the value calculated in (i) of $1.57\ \mu\text{M}$ FAICAR required to sustain the observed rate of the cyclohydrolase reaction.

(iii) Because the maximal rate of the cyclohydrolase reaction is well in excess of the operating rate of the first activity (the V_{max} is 35.6-fold higher), and the steady-state concentration of FAICAR ($0.118\ \mu\text{M}$) is well below the K_m for FAICAR under the conditions for the overall reaction ($64\ \mu\text{M}$), the equation formulated by Easterby [57] can be used to calculate the predicted transient time (τ).

$$\tau = 1/k_2 \tag{12}$$

However, the value obtained for IMP synthase was 0.43 s, below the limit of detection using the stopped-time chromatographic assay of Szabados and Christopherson [58]. No detectable lag was seen in the synthesis of IMP from AICAR and thus the observed and predicted transient times could not be compared as a test for the channelling of FAICAR by IMP synthase.

(iv) The fourth test used to characterize substrate channelling for CAD by Christopherson and Jones [49] was a competition experiment between endogenous and exogenous substrate with different radiolabels. For IMP synthase, only ^{3}H-labelled AICAR and FAICAR were available and competition experiments have been run in duplicate using:

$$[^3\mathrm{H}]\mathrm{AICAR} \rightarrow \quad [^3\mathrm{H}]\mathrm{FAICAR}\ (\text{endogenous}) \quad \rightarrow [^3\mathrm{H}]\mathrm{IMP} \qquad (13)$$
$$+\ \text{unlabelled FAICAR (exogenous)}$$

and the opposite radiolabelling with unlabelled AICAR and [^{3}H]FAICAR. A series of incubations was performed concurrently with increasing concentrations of added exogenous FAICAR. The amount of IMP synthesized from AICAR decreased as the concentration of exogenous FAICAR increased, but not as rapidly as might have been predicted if the endogenous and exogenous FAICAR (eqn. 13) had mixed completely. However, the analysis of these data has been complicated by the fact that the added exogenous FAICAR progressively inhibits AICAR transformylase, and the presence of AICAR and 10-CHO-THF at saturating concentrations increases the apparent K_m of FAICAR for the cyclohydrolase from 6.2 μM to 64 μM. Thus for IMP synthase, experiments (i) and (ii) provided evidence for an increase (13.3-fold) in FAICAR concentration at the cyclohydrolase site relative to that prevailing in the bulk solvent. Such a higher local concentration could be attributed to the close proximity of the transformylase and cyclohydrolase sites on a single enzyme molecule in solution (cf. Fig. 1).

The only other report of substrate channelling in *de novo* purine biosynthesis relates to trifunctional C_1-THF synthase, which provides 10-CHO-THF for the two transformylase reactions of the pathway [39]. This enzyme contains 5,10-CH-THF dehydrogenase, 5,10-CH-THF cyclohydrolase and 10-CHO-THF synthetase, catalysing the reactions shown in Scheme 1. MacKenzie and his co-workers have shown that the dehydrogenase and cyclohydrolase activities of human C_1-THF synthase are simultaneously inactivated upon chemical modification, and affinity labelling has shown that they share a common folate binding site [39]. Consistent with the spatial overlap of these two catalytic sites, the 5,10-CH-THF is channelled from the dehydrogenase to the cyclohydrolase [59]. The synthesis of 10-CHO-THF from 5,10-CH$_2$-THF proceeds without a lag, and approx. 60% of the 5,10-CH-THF is converted preferentially into 10-CHO-THF [60].

Rowe and his co-workers have partially purified the enzymes of the *de novo* purine pathway from pigeon liver and identified a particular inter-relationship between them which was preserved during the purification procedure [61]. There was some differential partitioning of individual enzyme

Scheme I

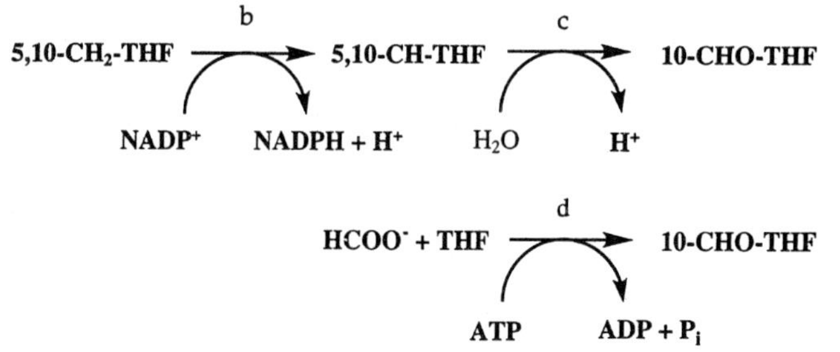

$$5,10\text{-CH}_2\text{-THF} \xrightarrow{\ b\ } 5,10\text{-CH-THF} \xrightarrow{\ c\ } 10\text{-CHO-THF} \qquad (14)$$

$$\text{NADP}^+ \quad \text{NADPH} + \text{H}^+ \qquad \text{H}_2\text{O} \qquad \text{H}^+$$

$$\text{HCOO}^- + \text{THF} \xrightarrow{\ d\ } 10\text{-CHO-THF}$$

$$\text{ATP} \qquad \text{ADP} + \text{P}_i$$

activities during chromatography on controlled pore glass in the presence of 2% (w/v) poly(ethylene glycol), but the enzymic activities catalysing reactions 1, 2 and 4 (P-Rib-PP → PRA → GAR; FGAR → FGAM; Fig. 3) co-chromatographed. However, in subsequent work with human lymphocytes, no evidence was obtained for the existence of a multienzyme complex for purine biosynthesis [62]. Trifunctional C_1-THF synthase has been co-purified 325-fold from chicken liver with serine hydroxymethyltransferase (reaction a, eqn. 5; Ser + THF → 5,10-CH_2-THF + Gly), GAR transformylase (reaction 3, Fig. 3; GAR → FGAR) and AICAR transformylase (reaction 9, Fig. 3; AICAR → FAICAR) after chromatography on hydroxyapatite and GAR–Sepharose [40]. As described above, multifunctional enzymes catalyse reactions 2, 3 and 5, reactions 6 and 7, reactions 9 and 10 and three reactions leading to the synthesis of 10-CHO-THF. If it is assumed that all of the reports listed above are correct, then the overlap between the multienzyme complexes described by Rowe and co-workers [61] and Caperelli and co-workers [40] with the known multifunctional enzymes provides direct evidence for a large multienzyme aggregate consisting of the enzymic activities catalysing the first 10 reactions of the *de novo* purine pathway and four enzymic activities leading to the synthesis of 10-CHO-THF. There is currently no evidence to implicate the enzymes catalysing reactions 6, 7 and 8 of the purine pathway in this putative complex. Fig. 5 shows a cartoon of this proposed 'pathway particle' or 'metabolon' supported by genetic evidence in yeast for a structural role for the trifunctional enzyme which produces 10-CHO-THF [63]. In the presence of adequate cytoplasmic levels of 10-CHO-THF, genetic deletions of C_1-THF synthase result in inactivation of the *de novo* purine pathway. Point mutations giving expression of full-length but inactive C_1-THF synthase (reactions b, c and d; Scheme 1), however, result in purine synthesis, suggesting that the trifunctional enzyme is required for an active metabolon (Fig. 5).

The association of enzymes of the *de novo* pathway with folate enzymes forming a multienzyme complex or metabolon could result in channelling of 10-CHO-THF, as shown in Fig. 5. The substrates P-Rib-PP, serine and THF could feed into the metabolon at amidophosphoribosyl-transferase (reaction 1) and serine hydroxymethyltransferase (reaction a) respectively. Other substrates would feed into the metabolon at reactions indicated in Fig. 3, and the final product, IMP, would emerge from IMP cyclohydrolase (reaction 10; Fig. 5). The glycine produced by serine hydroxymethyltransferase could even be transferred as a substrate to GAR synthetase (reaction 2). PRA, the product of amidophosphoribosyltransferase (reaction 1) and the substrate for GAR synthetase (reaction 2), is very unstable, with a half-life of 38 s at 37 °C [64], and is therefore probably channelled. Associations between some of the enzymes of such a metabolon would be fragile and may be disrupted when cell extracts are prepared. Currently, the only experimental evidence *in vitro* for substrate channelling

---

Fig. 5   **Proposed metabolon for the *de novo* biosynthesis of purine nucleotides**

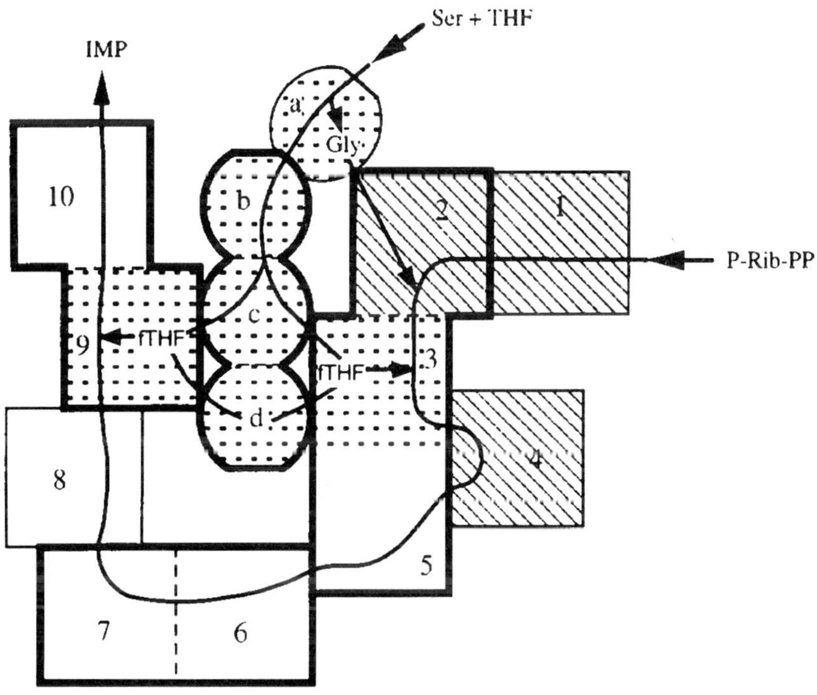

Enzymes of the purine pathway are numbered 1–10 as for Fig. 3 and eqn. (4); folate-metabolizing enzymes are lettered a–d as for eqn. (5). Enzymic activities covalently linked as multifunctional proteins are surrounded by heavy lines. Enzymic activities which co-purified are indicated by diagonal stripes [61] and stipling [40]. Abbreviation: fTHF, 10-CHO-THF.

between enzymes of this putative metabolon are between reactions 9 and 10 (E. Szabados and R.I. Christopherson, unpublished work) and reactions b and c [39]. The proposal of a metabolon for *de novo* purine biosynthesis remains speculative. Further evidence for interactions between mammalian purine enzymes and for channelling of intermediates *in vitro* or in growing cells is required before this concept will be accepted.

DNA synthesis by a replitase?

Evidence for the existence of a large multienzyme complex in mammals which provides dNTPs in the vicinity of DNA replication and catalyses their polymerization has been reviewed recently by Reddy and Fager [65]. The most significant data consistent with the existence of a replitase in mammalian cells will be briefly discussed here. Reddy and Pardee [66] reported that in Chinese hamster embryo fibroblast cells (CHEF/18) in S phase of the cell cycle, a multienzyme complex (including DNA polymerase, thymidine kinase, dihydrofolate reductase and nucleoside diphosphate kinase) was formed which rapidly sedimented in sucrose gradients. This complex was only found in cells synthesizing DNA and was associated with the nuclear fraction. They found that NDPs were incorporated into DNA by permeabilized cells more efficiently than dNTPs. Incubation mixtures required the presence of dithiothreitol for activation of ribonucleotide reductase, and formaldehyde and THF for thymidylate synthase activity. Reddy and Pardee proposed that a multienzyme complex or replitase channels NDPs directly to the site of their incorporation into DNA and that free dNTPs have limited access to DNA polymerase of this replitase (Fig. 6). They suggested that the replitase could be associated with the nuclear membrane matrix in intact cells.

Reddy and Pardee [67] subsequently showed that there was rapid and specific channelling of NDPs into DNA through reactions beginning with ribonucleotide reductase and terminating with DNA polymerase in permeabilized CHEF/18 cells. [^{3}H]CDP was incorporated into DNA without dilution by added exogenous unlabelled dCTP, showing that the endogenous [^{3}H]dCTP formed did not equilibrate with a cellular dCTP pool (Fig. 6). The rate of incorporation of CDP into DNA was limited by the initial step, catalysed by ribonucleotide reductase (reaction 1, Fig. 6). They proposed that free dNTPs, which are not effectively incorporated into DNA, may function as allosteric regulators of ribonucleotide reductase or as substrates for DNA repair [67]. In a third paper from these workers [68] the replitase was found to contain DNA polymerase, thymidine kinase, dihydrofolate reductase, NDP kinase and, in addition, ribonucleotide reductase and thymidylate synthase. The concentrations of free dNTPs formed from NDPs were far too low to sustain the observed rates of incorporation of NDPs into DNA. Such a result could be attributed to high local concentrations of dNTPs within the replitase. Radiolabelled thymidine microinjected into the cytoplasm of mammalian cells is efficiently incorporated into DNA [69], and thymidine kinase has been found associated with the replitase fraction (Fig. 6).

Fig. 6 shows the proposed assembly of the replitase on the nuclear membrane with the dNTP synthesizing complex in the cytoplasm and the replication apparatus in the nucleus [65]. Incorporation of four different precursors through dNTPs into DNA is shown. ^{3}H-labelled CDP is incorporated into DNA with minimal accumulation of intermediates [66]. ^{3}H-labelled thymidine, dUMP and deoxyuridine are channelled directly into DNA without significant accumulation of [^{3}H]dTTP [70,71]. There is evidence for enzymes 1, 2, 6, 7, 8, 9 and 10 in the dNTP synthesizing complex and for DNA polymerase, 3'5' exodeoxyribonuclease and DNA topoisomerase II activities (enzymes 3, 4 and 5; Fig. 6) in the replication apparatus in the nucleus [65]. However, the existence of the replitase remains controversial [72]; some radiochemical labelling studies suggest that the free dNTP pool is readily used for replication [73]. The physical properties of the replitase should be further characterized and more rigorous tests for substrate channelling could be applied, for example experiments (i)–(iv) described above for IMP synthase.

Fig. 6   **Proposed replitase for the synthesis of dNTPs and their polymerizations to form DNA**

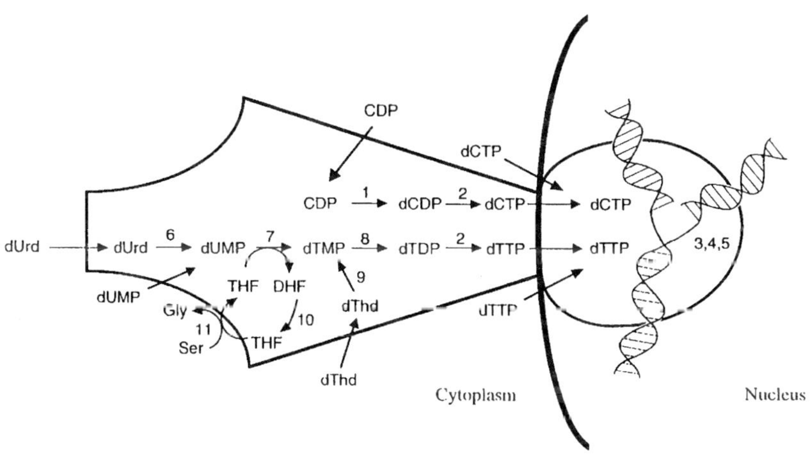

The numbers denote the following enzymes: 1, ribonucleotide reductase; 2, nucleoside diphosphate kinase; 3, DNA polymerase; 4, 3'5' exodeoxyribonuclease; 5, DNA topoisomerase II; 6, uridine kinase; 7, thymidylate synthase; 8, thymidylate kinase; 9, thymidine kinase; 10, dihydrofolate reductase. Abbreviations: dThd, deoxythymidine; dUrd, deoxyuridine. The dNTP synthesizing complex and replication apparatus are shown assembled on opposite sides of the nuclear membrane (heavy line). Modified from Reddy and Fager [65].

Multienzyme complexes and substrate channelling: from controversy to fact

A variety of selective advantages have been proposed for the existence of multifunctional enzymes and multienzyme complexes [74]. However, they may dissociate or be subject to proteolysis when cells are broken. Cell extracts should therefore be prepared in solvents that resemble 'synthetic cytoplasm', containing, for example, glycerol (30%, v/v), poly(ethylene glycol), dimethyl sulphoxide, sucrose, dextran or polyvinylpyrrolidone, where the ordered array of hydrogen bonds in water has been disrupted and the additive occupies space between water molecules, excluding protein molecules and promoting their association. Such cell extracts should be prepared in the presence of protease inhibitors, kept cold and processed rapidly to minimize proteolysis and denaturation. Interactions between protein subunits of a putative multienzyme complex can be established by protein affinity chromatography [75]. A purified enzyme available in relatively large quantities (perhaps recombinant) is covalently attached as a ligand to Sepharose. A crude cell-free extract is then passed through the affinity column and enzymes which are candidates for the complex are assayed in the eluate. The retardation or binding of such an enzyme provides some evidence for such an interaction within a multienzyme complex *in vivo*.

The concept of substrate channelling has become controversial [7], and rigorous testing by several independent procedures is required to be sure that the next enzyme in the metabolic sequence is operating at a local concentration of substrate which is higher than that prevailing in the bulk solvent (Fig. 1). Experimental tests (i)–(iv) listed for the description of channelling of FAICAR by IMP synthase can be generally applied to most enzyme systems. Such experiments must be performed with care. The kinetic parameters for each enzyme of the reaction sequence may be different in the presence of substrates for the other enzymes, either because they act as competitive inhibitors, or because they change the K_m and/or V_{max} via induced conformational changes (non-competitive inhibition). An increase in the K_m for the 'channelled' intermediate may affect the results of experiment (iv), where increasing concentrations of exogenous substrate are competed with endogenous substrate with a different radiolabel. If the apparent K_m for the proposed channelled intermediate is high enough, addition of the exogenous substrate will simply make the enzyme work at a faster rate. The result would be no apparent decrease in formation of the product from the endogenous substrate. However, endogenous and exogenous substrate may have mixed completely, and the conclusion that substrate channelling had occurred would be incorrect.

A fifth approach for the detection of substrate channelling is to add a different enzyme activity that is also able to use the proposed channelled intermediate. For example, ornithine transcarbamylase has been added to assays for CAD to determine whether CAP is channelled to aspartate transcarbamylase [76]. A sixth and quite elegant test is to use multifunctional proteins which lack the first or second enzymic activities due to point mutations, e.g. the bifunctional CAP synthetase/aspartate transcarbamylase from yeast [47]. The two mutant enzymes are mixed to determine whether the reaction sequence $HCO_3^- \rightarrow CAP \rightarrow CA\text{-asp}$ is slower with a higher steady-state concentration of the intermediate. For multienzyme complexes which are too unstable to extract, pulse-labelling of a metabolic pathway can be done with intact cells growing in culture. The progress curves obtained for radiolabelling of intermediates can be compared with computer simulations based upon the kinetic parameters of the constituent enzymes determined *in vitro*. If correct simulations of the time courses for radiolabelling of intermediates require a high local concentration of a particular intermediate, then substrate channelling could be proposed. However, there are difficulties in transposing kinetic parameters determined *in vitro* to intact cells growing in culture. Identification of multienzyme complexes and their ability to channel intermediates will remain a challenge, and a multifaceted experimental approach must be used before controversy becomes fact.

This work was supported by Project Grant 950124 from the National Health and Medical Research Council of Australia.

References

1. Gaertner, F.H., Ericson, M.C. and DeMoss, J.A. (1970) J. Biol. Chem. **245**, 595–600
2. Williams, L.G., Bernhardt, S.A. and Davis, R.H. (1971) J. Biol. Chem. **246**, 973–978
3. Gaertner, F.H. (1978) Trends Biochem. Sci. **3**, 63–65
4. Spivey, H.O. and Merz, J.M. (1989) BioEssays **10**, 127–130
5. Ovádi, J. (1991) J. Theor. Biol. **152**, 135–141
6. Cornish-Bowden, A. (1991) Eur. J. Biochem. **195**, 103–108
7. Cornish-Bowden, A. (1993) Eur. J. Biochem. **213**, 87–92
8. Easterby, J.S. (1993) J. Mol. Recognit. **6**, 179–185
9. Lyons, S.D. and Christopherson, R.I. (1985) Eur. J. Biochem. **147**, 587–592
10. Tatibana, M. and Shigesada, K. (1972) J. Biochem. (Tokyo) **72**, 549–560
11. Levine, R.L., Hoogenraad, N.J. and Kretchmer, N. (1971) Biochemistry **10**, 3694–3699
12. Jones, M.E. (1980) Annu. Rev. Biochem. **49**, 253–279
13. Becker, M.A., Raivio, K.O. and Seegmiller, J.E. (1979) Adv. Enzymol. **49**, 281–306
14. Christopherson, R.I. and Jones, M.E. (1980) J. Biol. Chem. **255**, 3358–3370
15. Chen, J.J. and Jones, M.E. (1976) Arch. Biochem. Biophys. **176**, 82–90
16. Shoaf, W.T. and Jones, M.E. (1973) Biochemistry **12**, 4039–4051
17. Coleman, P.F., Suttle, D.P. and Stark, G.R. (1977) J. Biol. Chem. **252**, 6379–6385
18. Kim, H., Kelly, R.E. and Evans, D.R. (1992) J. Biol. Chem. **267**, 7177–7184
19. Davidson, J.N., Rumsby, P.C. and Tamaren, J. (1981) J. Biol. Chem. **256**, 5220–5225
20. Williams, N.K., Simpson, R.J., Moritz, R.L., Peide, Y., Crofts, L., Minasian, E., Leach, S.J., Wake, R.G. and Christopherson, R.I. (1990) Gene **94**, 283–288
21. Guy, H.I. and Evans, D.R. (1994) J. Biol. Chem. **269**, 23808–23816
22. McClard, R.W., Black, M.J., Livingstone, L.R. and Jones, M.E. (1980) Biochemistry **19**, 4699–4706
23. Traut, T.W. (1982) Trends Biochem. Sci. **7**, 255–257
24. Floyd, E.E. and Jones, M.E. (1985) J. Biol. Chem. **260**, 9443–9451
25. Forman, H.J. and Kennedy, J. (1975) J. Biol. Chem. **250**, 4322–4326

26. Raijman, L. and Jones, M.E. (1976) Arch. Biochem. Biophys. **175**, 270–278
27. Wendler, P.A., Blanding, J.H. and Tremblay, G.C. (1983) Arch. Biochem. Biophys. **224**, 36–48
28. Schoettle, S.L. and Christopherson, R.I. (1994) Proc. Aust. Soc. Biochem. Mol. Biol. POS-1-44
29. Holmes, E.W. (1980) Adv. Enzyme Regul. **19**, 215–231
30. Sant, M.E., Lyons, S.D., Phillips, L. and Christopherson, R.I. (1992) J. Biol. Chem. **267**, 11038–11045
31. Szabados, E., Hindmarsh, E.J., Phillips, L., Duggleby, R.G. and Christopherson, R.I. (1994) Biochemistry **33**, 14237–14245
32. Van den Berghe, G., Bontemps, F. and Vincent, M.F. (1991) in Purine and Pyrimidine Metabolism in Man VII (Harkness, R.A., Elion, G.B. and Zollner, N., eds.), pp. 281–286, Plenum Press, New York and London
33. Okada, M., Shimura, K., Shiraki, H. and Nakagawa, H. (1983) J. Biochem. (Tokyo) **94**, 1605–1613
34. Henikoff, S. (1987) BioEssays **6**, 8–13
35. Daubner, S.C., Schrimsher, J.L., Schendel, F.J., Young, M., Henikoff, S., Patterson, D., Stubbe, J. and Benkovic, S.J. (1985) Biochemistry **24**, 7059–7062
36. Patey, C.A.H. and Shaw, G. (1973) Biochem. J. **135**, 543–545
37. Benkovic, S.J. (1984) Trends Biochem. Sci **9**, 320–322
38. MacKenzie, R.E. (1973) Biochem. Biophys. Res. Commun. **53**, 1088–1095
39. Pelletier, J.N. and MacKenzie, R.E. (1994) Biochemistry **33**, 1900–1906
40. Caperelli, C.A., Benkovic, P.A., Chettur, G. and Benkovic, S.J. (1980) J. Biol. Chem. **255**, 1885–1890
41. Casey, P.J. and Lowenstein, J.M. (1987) Biochem. J. **246**, 263–269
42. Moyer, J.D. and Herderson, J.F. (1985) CRC Crit. Rev. Biochem. **19**, 45–61
43. Traut, T.W. (1994) Mol. Cell. Biochem. **140**, 1–22
44. Kemp, A.J., Lyons, S.D. and Christopherson, R.I. (1986) J. Biol. Chem. **261**, 14891–14895
45. Sant, M.E., Poiner, A., Harsanyi, M.C., Lyons, S.D. and Christopherson, R.I. (1989) Anal. Biochem. **182**, 121–128
46. Lue, P.F. and Kaplan, J.G. (1970) Biochim. Biophys. Acta **220**, 365–372
47. Penverne, B., Belkaid, M. and Herve, G. (1994) Arch. Biochem. Biophys. **309**, 85–93
48. Mally, M.I., Grayson, D.R. and Evans, D.R. (1980) J. Biol. Chem. **255**, 11372–11380
49. Christopherson, R.I. and Jones, M.E. (1980) J. Biol. Chem. **255**, 11381–11395
50. Christopherson, R.I., Traut, T.W. and Jones, M.E. (1981) Curr. Top. Cell Regul. **18**, 59–77
51. Allen, C.M. and Jones, M.E. (1964) Biochemistry **3**, 1238–1247
52. Traut, T.W. and Jones. M.E. (1977) Biochem. Pharmacol. **26**, 2291–2296
53. Traut, T.W. and Jones, M.E. (1977) J. Biol. Chem. **252**, 8374–8381
54. McClard, R.W. and Shokat, K.M. (1987) Biochemistry **26**, 3378–3384
55. Traut, T.W. (1989) Arch. Biochem. Biophys. **268**, 108–115
56. McClure, W.R. (1969) Biochemistry **8**, 2782–2786
57. Easterby, J.S. (1973) Biochim. Biophys. Acta **293**, 552–558
58. Szabados, E. and Christopherson, R.I. (1994) Anal. Biochem. **221**, 401–404
59. Hum, D.W. and MacKenzie, R.E. (1991) Protein Eng. **4**, 493–500
60. Cohen, L. and MacKenzie, R.E. (1978) Biochim. Biophys. Acta **522**, 311–317
61. Rowe, P.B., McCairns, E., Madsen, G., Sauer, D. and Elliott, H. (1978) J. Biol. Chem. **253**, 7711–7721
62. McCairns, E., Fahey, D., Sauer, D. and Rowe, P.B. (1983) J. Biol. Chem. **258**, 1851–1856
63. Barlowe, C.K. and Appling, D.R. (1990) Mol. Cell. Biol. **10**, 5679–5687
64. Schendel, F.J., Cheng, Y.S., Otvos, J.D., Wehrli, S. and Stubbe, J. (1988) Biochemistry **27**, 2614–2623
65. Reddy, G.P.V. and Fager, R.S. (1993) Crit. Rev. Eukaryotic Gene Expression **3**, 255–277
66. Reddy, G.P.V. and Pardee, A.B. (1980) Proc. Natl. Acad. Sci. U.S.A. **77**, 3312–3316
67. Reddy, G.P.V. and Pardee, A.B. (1982) J. Biol. Chem. **257**, 12526–12531
68. Noguchi, H., Reddy, G.P.V. and Pardee, A.B. (1983) Cell **32**, 443–451
69. Wawra, E. (1988) J. Biol. Chem. **263**, 9908–9912

70. Wickremasinghe, R.G., Yaxley, J.C. and Hoffbrand, A.V. (1982) Eur. J. Biochem. **126**, 589–596
71. Reddy, G.P.V. (1989) J. Mol. Recognit. **2**, 75–83
72. Muller, E.G.D. (1994) J. Biol. Chem. **269**, 24466–24471
73. Matthews, C.K. and Slabaugh, M.B. (1986) Exp. Cell Res. **162**, 285–295
74. Bisswanger, H. and Schmincke-Ott, E. (1980) Multifunctional Proteins, John Wiley & Sons, New York
75. Formosa, T., Barry, J., Alberts, B.M. and Greenblatt, J. (1991) Methods Enzymol. **208**, 24–45
76. Otsuki, T., Mori, M. and Tatibana, M. (1982) J. Biochem. (Tokyo) **92**, 1421–1437

Subject index